Atlas of Orthopedic Oncology Volume 1

Ajay Puri
Wan Faisham Nu'man Bin Wan Ismail
Editors

Atlas of Orthopedic Oncology Volume 1

An Anatomical Guide to Resections of Soft Tissue Sarcomas, Pelvic Resection and Major Amputations

Springer

Editors
Ajay Puri
Department of Surgical Oncology
Tata Memorial Centre
Mumbai, Maharashtra, India

Wan Faisham Nu'man Bin Wan Ismail
Prince Court Medical Centre
Universiti Sains Malaysia
Kuala Lumpur, Kuala Lumpur, Malaysia

ISBN 978-981-95-8957-9 ISBN 978-981-95-8958-6 (eBook)
https://doi.org/10.1007/978-981-95-8958-6

This Springer imprint is published by the registered company Springer Nature Singapore Pte Ltd.
The registered company address is: 152 Beach Road, #21-01/04 Gateway East, Singapore 189721, Singapore

Foreword

Having had the opportunity to witness the factors over the past five decades that were important in achieving our current levels of success in musculoskeletal oncology, one clinical factor that is clear is one that was emphasized by Bill Enneking: while surgeons have little control over the development of metastatic disease, it is the responsibility of surgeons to achieve adequate clear margins, to minimize the chance of local recurrence with the subsequent adverse consequences. This two-volume book is a great asset for surgeons of all levels of training and experience to achieve the resection goals, promoting precision surgery and confidence in resections. Following this anatomical approach advocated by the authors allows the surgeon to avoid important adjacent structures, and maximize functional recovery!

The Case Atlas format highlights the tremendous volume of experience and expertise of Professor Faisham and colleagues, providing comprehensive step-by-step surgical planning and resection tips; the high definition photographs with clear anatomical structures enhance further understanding of the resection principles! The volume on bone tumours likewise provides well-illustrated, clear steps to the resection, and offers a variety of reconstructions ranging from simple effective techniques to more sophisticated techniques, depending on the circumstances!

All of our tumour patients will benefit from the knowledge imparted in this two-volume case formatted book!

Emeritus Professor Orthopaedic Surgery
Mayo Clinic, Rochester, MN, USA

Franklin H. Sim

Introduction

In cancer treatment, surgical procedures play a crucial role in removing tumours, preventing their spread and restoring function and aesthetics. Collaborative approach for sarcoma entails close cooperation between surgical, medical and radiation oncologists, pathologists and radiologists, with surgical oncologists playing a crucial role. This collaboration ensures comprehensive and tailored care for each patient. Understanding sarcoma behaviour, the surgical anatomy, compartmentalization concept and margin are important to achieve oncological margin and improve local control and the survival of patients with sarcoma. Preoperative planning with advance radiology, including CT scan, MRI and PET scan, is important for surgical execution for good margin as well as minimized contamination.

The purpose of this atlas is to illustrate radiological evaluations and detailed surgical techniques with anatomical correlation for each procedure. Each anatomical procedure of bone and soft tissue sarcoma are written in detail from simple resection to complex procedures, such as limb salvage with advance microsurgical and flap technique.

Each chapter starts with a simple and important introduction, anatomical description of the surgical structures of limb salvage surgery, anatomical compartmentalization concept for sarcoma growth and relevant structures to achieve surgical oncological margin. Important vital structures related to specific area of sarcoma have been highlighted to achieve optimum functional outcome and, most importantly, to avoid surgical complication to the vital structures. This atlas will facilitate readers in understanding the anatomic correlation of important structures in specific regions for surgical planning for sarcoma resection. Potential sarcoma infiltration, compartmentalization concept and anatomical barrier of sarcoma have been described in a concise manner for better understanding. Potential areas of infiltration and contamination by sarcoma for evaluation and surgical planning have also been highlighted.

Preoperative radiological assessment and the importance of sarcoma extension and surgical margin, which plays a crucial role in achieving local control, have been explained. This atlas also provides concise critical points used during most limb salvage surgeries combined with labelled preoperative MRI as well as step-by-step live surgery photographs. Each topic will highlight the radiological evaluation, including an MRI, as part of the assessment prior surgery. Relevant structures related to sarcoma involvement, specific areas of involvement and important neurovascular structures, which are critical for major decision, are also discussed. The assessment includes a series of important labelled combine images of MRIs for a better understanding of this crucial part of sarcoma management. The assessment includes combine axial, sagittal, or coronal with labelling for better understanding of each level evaluation of sarcoma. Serial MRI images for evaluation of vital structures are also included.

The main part of this atlas is the step-by-step surgical procedures with high-quality labelled surgical photos for all the anatomical region of sarcoma management. The procedures start with general surgical access and each anatomical layer of surgical procedures for sarcoma resection. Vital structures, including the major vessels and nerves, and other relevant important structures have been labelled for a better understanding of its correlation with the main sarcoma prior resection. This atlas has been designed to describe simple to complicated procedures, including different surgical approaches, and modifications for sarcoma resection. Options of bone and joint reconstruction have been described in detail and advanced techniques of microsurgeries and flaps are also included. Surgical procedures have been presented in a clear and easily comprehensible manner using both important anatomical and surgical landmarks. Attractive labels and arrows are inserted alongside the figures. The cases illustrated comprise the main surgical approach of each anatomical site with a view to share the surgical principles to achieve oncological margin and optimum function in complex heterogenicity of sarcoma in general.

This book aims to share armamentarium of surgical procedures to all orthopaedic oncology surgeons who dedicate their lifelong journey to salvage limb for patients with sarcoma. It will also be a valuable reference and excellent guidebook for junior surgeons and trainees' in orthopaedic surgical oncology specialty.

Contents

Editors and Contributors

About the Editors

Ajay Puri currently serves as the Chief of Orthopaedic Oncology and Professor and Head of Surgical Oncology at the Tata Memorial Centre. He has held esteemed positions including founder President of the Indian Musculoskeletal Oncology Society, Past President of the Asia Pacific Musculoskeletal Tumor Society, and past Chairman of the Indian Orthopaedic Association (Oncology). He is a member of the Global Steering Committee of the International Sarcoma Kindred Study (ISKS), the largest multi-institutional international trial aimed at understanding the genetic background of sarcomas. He has pioneered the development of a low-cost indigenous megaprosthesis, extensively used in India and other Asian and African nations. Additionally, he has popularized novel methods of biological reconstruction after oncologic resection. He serves on the editorial board of the *Journal of Bone & Joint Surgery* (formerly JBJS [Br]), *Bone & Joint-360*, *Bone & Joint Open*, and *Sarcoma.* He has published numerous papers and book chapters, establishing himself as a leading authority in Orthopaedic Oncology.

Wan Faisham is an orthopaedic oncology surgeon at Prince Court Medical Center, a prestigious oncology centre in Malaysia. He previously served as a professor and consultant surgeon at Universiti Sains Malaysia and is renowned as one of the pioneers of limb salvage surgery for orthopaedic cancer. Throughout his career, he has been involved in numerous clinical research endeavours and multidisciplinary collaborations in oncology. For his significant contributions to the field, he has been honoured with five distinguished awards and appointed as the International Advisor to the Asian Pacific Musculoskeletal Oncology Society. He has authored over 100 research papers in medical journals and 4 textbooks related to his expertise. Currently, he is a leading figure in oncology applicable to sarcomas in Malaysia and is recognized as an orthopaedic oncology expert within ASEAN and the Asia Pacific region. He is actively involved in training both national and international orthopaedic oncology fellows. His research interests primarily focus on survival and functional outcomes following surgery for orthopaedic cancer. Internationally, his surgical method utilizing allograft and vascularized tissue has been recognized as a trademark in the field.

Contributors

Nawaz Hussain Mohamed Amir KPJ Ipoh Specialist Hospital, Ipoh, Perak, Malaysia

Domenico Andrea Campanacci Orthopaedic Oncology Unit, Careggi University Hospital, Florence, Italy

Wei Guo Musculoskeletal Tumor Center, Peking University People's Hospital, Beijing, China

Ahmad Sukari Halim Reconstructive Sciences Department, School of Medical Sciences, Universiti Sains Malaysia, Kubang Kerian, Kelantan, Malaysia

Syurahbil Abdul Halim Orthopaedic Oncology Reconstructive Unit, Universiti Sains Malaysia, Kubang Kerian, Kelantan, Malaysia

Katsuhiro Hayashi Department of Orthopedic Surgery, Graduate School of Medical Sciences, Kanazawa University, Kanazawa, Japan

Wan Faisham Nu'man Bin Wan Ismail Prince Court Medical Center, Kuala Lumpur, Malaysia

Orthopaedic Oncology Reconstructive Unit, Universiti Sains Malaysia, Kubang Kerian, Kelantan, Malaysia

Lee Jeys Royal Orthopaedic Hospital NHS Trust, Birmingham, UK

Vineet Kurisunkal Royal Orthopaedic Hospital NHS Trust, Birmingham, UK

Haijie Liang Musculoskeletal Tumor Center, Peking University People's Hospital, Beijing, China

Danielle Maes Queen Elizabeth Hospital NHS Trust, Birmingham, UK

Shinji Miwa Department of Orthopedic Surgery, Graduate School of Medical Sciences, Kanazawa University, Kanazawa, Japan

Francesco Muratori Orthopaedic Oncology Unit, Careggi University Hospital, Florence, Italy

Mohammad Bin Paiman Hand and Microsurgery - Orthopaedic Department, Universiti Sains Malaysia, Kubang Kerian, Kelantan, Malaysia

Ashwin Prajapati Department of Surgical Oncology, Tata Memorial Centre, Mumbai, Maharashtra, India

Ajay Puri Department of Surgical Oncology, Tata Memorial Centre, Mumbai, Maharashtra, India

Kumaran Rasappan National University Hospital, Singapore, Singapore

Arman Zaharil Mat Saad Plastic Reconstructive & Microsurgery, MSU Medical Centre, Management and Science University of Malaysia, Shah Alam, Selangor, Malaysia

Roberto Scanferla Orthopaedic Oncology Unit, Careggi University Hospital, Florence, Italy

Guido Scoccianti Orthopaedic Oncology Unit, Careggi University Hospital, Florence, Italy

Maurizio Scorianz Orthopaedic Oncology Unit, Careggi University Hospital, Florence, Italy

Rudra Pratap Singh Department of Surgical Oncology, Tata Memorial Centre, Mumbai, Maharashtra, India

Wan Azman Wan Sulaiman Reconstructive Sciences Department, School of Medical Sciences, Universiti Sains Malaysia, Kubang Kerian, Kelantan, Malaysia

Yuta Taniguchi Department of Orthopedic Surgery, Graduate School of Medical Sciences, Kanazawa University, Kanazawa, Japan

Hiroyuki Tsuchiya Department of Orthopedic Surgery, Graduate School of Medical Sciences, Kanazawa University, Kanazawa, Japan

Zulmi Wan Prince Court Medical Center, Kuala Lumpur, Malaysia

Kwok Chuen Wong Orthopaedic Oncology, Department of Orthopaedics and Traumatology, Prince of Wales Hospital, The Chinese University of Hong Kong, Hong Kong SAR, China

Sahran Yahaya Orthopaedic Oncology Reconstructive Unit, Universiti Sains Malaysia, Kubang Kerian, Kelantan, Malaysia

Norazman Mat Zin Orthopaedic Oncology Reconstructive Unit, Universiti Sains Malaysia, Kubang Kerian, Kelantan, Malaysia

Resection Soft Tissue Sarcoma: Lower Limb

Buttockectomy 'Glutectomy'

Wan Faisham Nu'man Bin Wan Ismail

Introduction

Tumour of the gluteus maximus is usually confined to its muscle compartment. Resection is tolerated with minimal functional disability. Patients with resection are able to ambulate well and climb stairs without difficulty.

Surgical Anatomy

The gluteus maximus originates from the alar of the iliac crest and sacral lamina and is distally inserted at the iliotibial band and proximal femur 3–4 cm below the greater trochanter.

- The area below the gluteus muscle 'the retro gluteal space' consists of all short rotator muscles of the femur.
- The sciatic nerve passes below the piriformis with the inferior gluteal artery through the retro gluteal space. However, it is rarely involved and can be isolated for oncological margins.
- The retro gluteal space where the sciatic nerve lies is rarely involved. However, in large tumours, the sciatic nerve and other nearby muscles, gluteus medius and minimi should be evaluated for infiltration. The origin and attachment of the gluteus maximus in the upper femur and sacrum are important landmarks for a buttockectomy.

W. F. N. B. W. Ismail (✉)
Prince Court Medical Center, Kuala Lumpur, Malaysia

Orthopaedic Oncology Reconstructive Unit, Universiti Sains Malaysia, Kubang Kerian, Kelantan, Malaysia

A. Puri, W. F. N. B. W. Ismail (eds.), *Atlas of Orthopedic Oncology Volume 1*,
https://doi.org/10.1007/978-981-95-8958-6_1

Assessment

An MRI assessment of the surrounding bony attachment infiltration and retro gluteal space includes:

- Sacrum and ilium origin of the gluteus maximus
- Ischiorectal fossae space
- Sciatic nerve infiltration
- Sacrotuberus ligament and lamina of sacrum
- Short rotator muscles of the hip joint and intra pelvic extension to the sciatic notch

Surgical Steps

Resection involves complete removal of the gluteus maximus muscle and ligation of the inferior gluteal vessels.

- A large skin flap exposing the entire gluteus is required.
- Distal tendinous and muscular part of the attachment to the proximal femur shaft are elevated for exploration of the sciatic nerve and assessment of the retro gluteal space.
- The origin of the gluteus maximus at the sacrum, pelvic brim, and ligament is assessed and detached for completion of resection.

Total Gluteus Maximus Resection 'Buttokectomy'

1. Sciatic nerve
2. Inferior gluteal vessels
3. Iliac wing shows no activity on bone scan (Fig. 1f)

MRI image of large sarcoma involving the entire gluteus maximus. The sciatic nerve and retro gluteal space and all the attachments are free with good oncological margin (Fig. 1a–e).

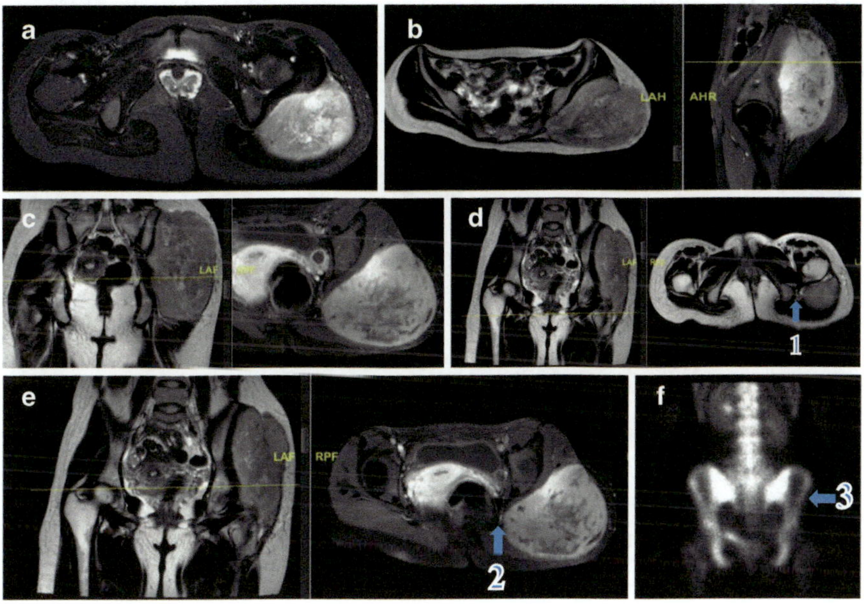

A large flap exposing the entire gluteus is required for a buttockectomy. A large curvilinear incision centred at the gluteus muscle and straight longitudinal incision over the greater trochanter to the gluteus insertion (Fig. 1g, h).

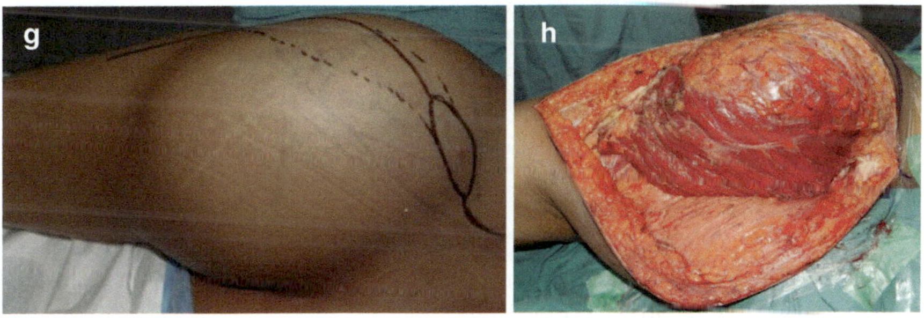

1. Gluteal insertion
2. Sciatic nerve
3. Gluteus medius
4. Piriformis muscle
5. Iliac wing

The origin of the gluteus maximus at the sacrotuberous, sacrospinous ligament, and lamina of the sacrum is identified. The insertion over the lateral femur is detached and the entire gluteus maximus is mobilised from the deeper structures and brought medially. The inferior gluteal artery is identified below the piriformis muscle and ligated for haemostasis (Fig. 1i, j). Total buttockectomy radical margin in high-grade sarcoma can be achieved by detaching both the origin and attachment (Fig. 1k).

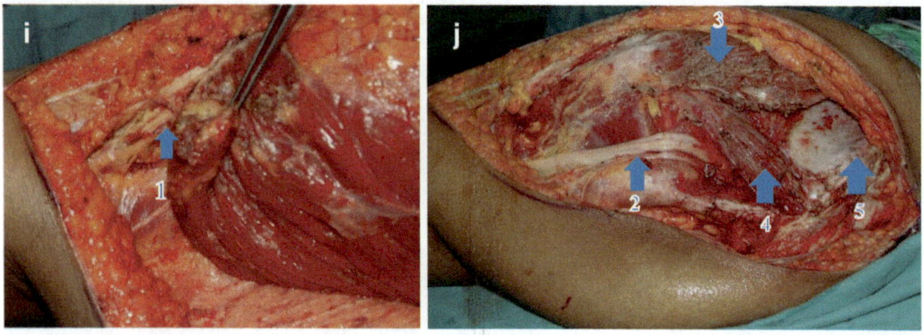

1. Sacrotuberous ligament
2. Sacral lamina

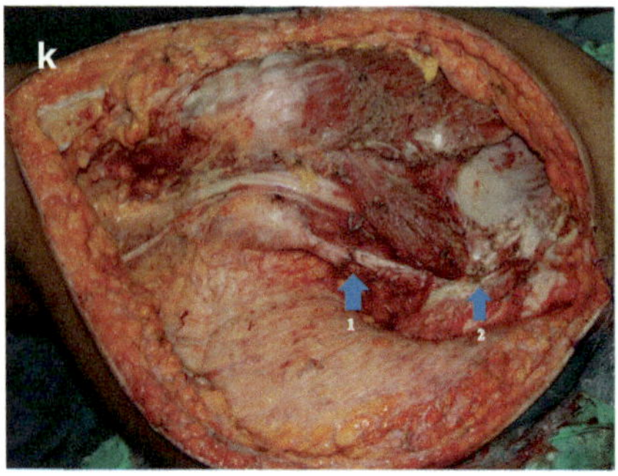

2 years after surgery—Radiograph and MRI image showed post-radiation osteopenia with no local recurrence (Fig. 1l–n).

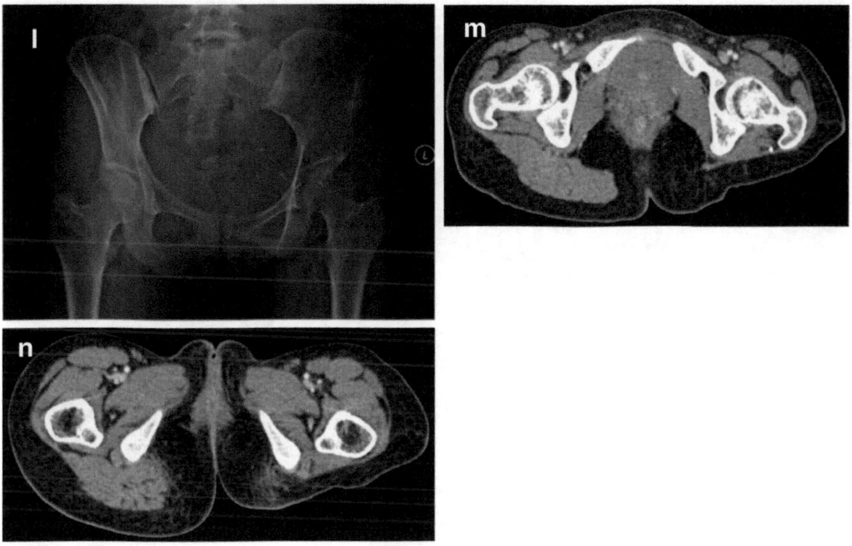

Buttock Sarcoma with Skin Infiltration

Heterogeneous high-grade sarcoma with central necrosis and surrounding oedema over the skin requiring compartment resection of the gluteus maximus for good oncological margins (Fig. 2a–e).

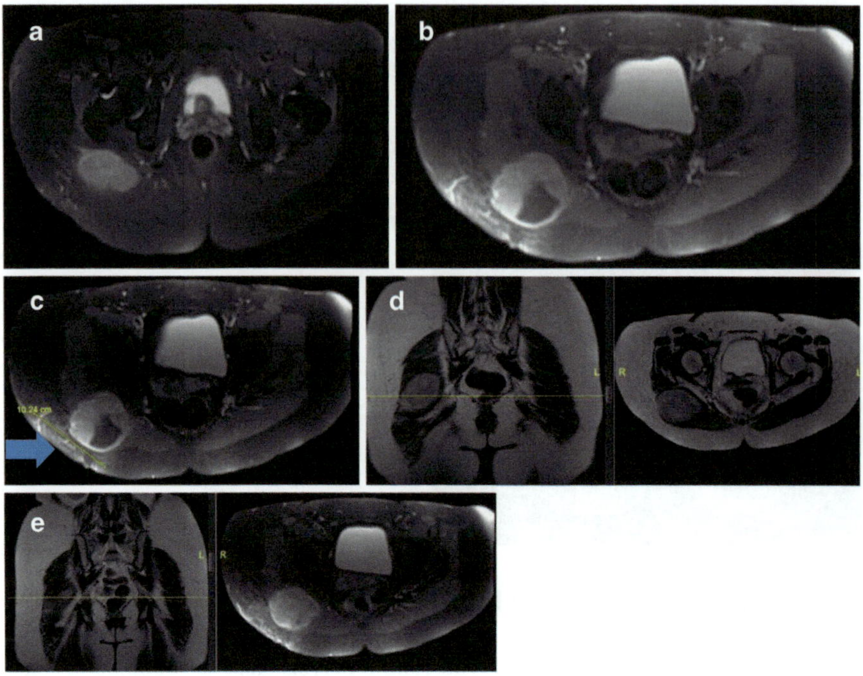

Resection of entire gluteus maximus with wide margin of skin infiltration over biopsied scars. Mobilisation of entire gluteus maximus from the femur insertion above the sciatic nerve, final resection at the medial border of sacrum and iliac wing(Fig. 2f–i).

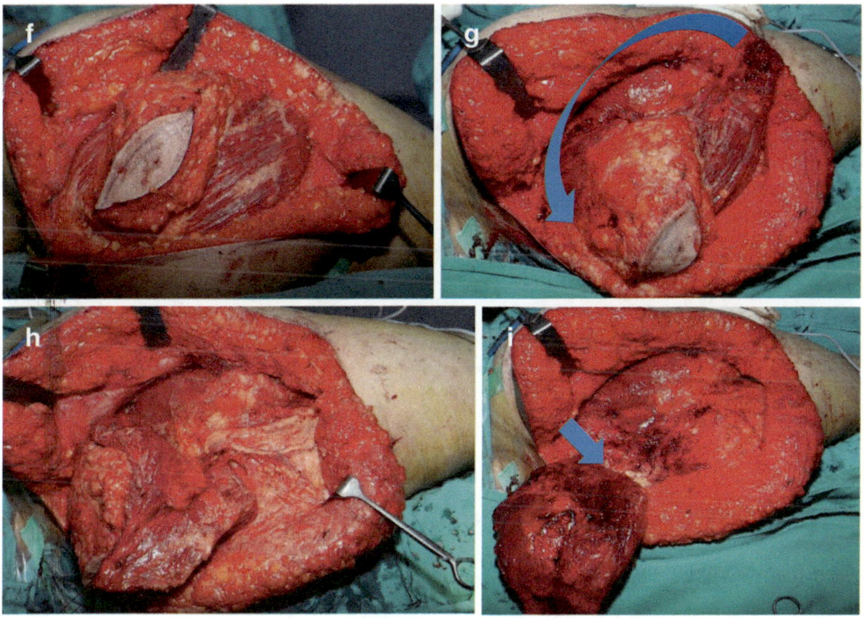

Gluteal Sarcoma with Sciatic Nerve Involvement

MRI image sarcoma arising from the gluteus maximus in close proximity to the sciatic nerve up to the level of the greater sciatic notch (Fig. 3a–e). Resection of the sciatic nerve will significantly cause functional disability. Resection of the gluteus maximus muscle and exploration of the sciatic nerve inferiorly after detaching the insertion at the proximal femur. Epineural resection and partial sciatic nerve resection are performed for complete margins (Fig. 3f–j).

1. Sarcoma proximity to sciatic nerve and no clear plane to the gluteus maximus
2. Greater sciatic notch
3. Multiple nodular lesions within sciatic nerve

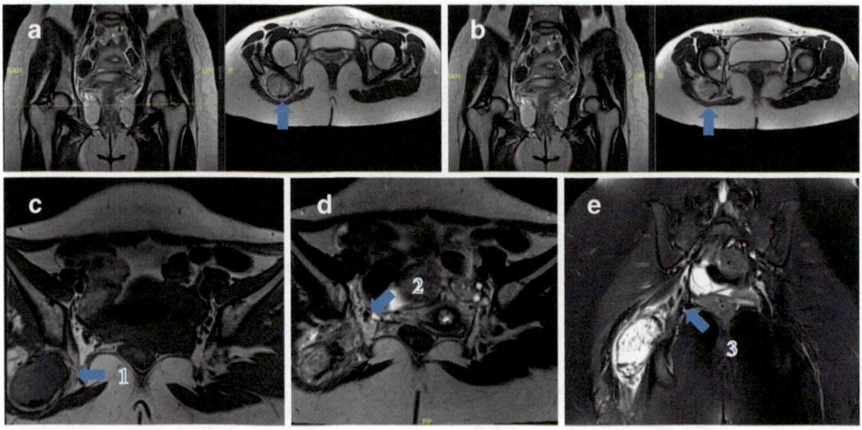

• Epineural clearance from tumour abutting the sciatic nerve

The hip and knee joint are maintained in extension and flexion respectively to minimise traction injury to the nerve during procedures.

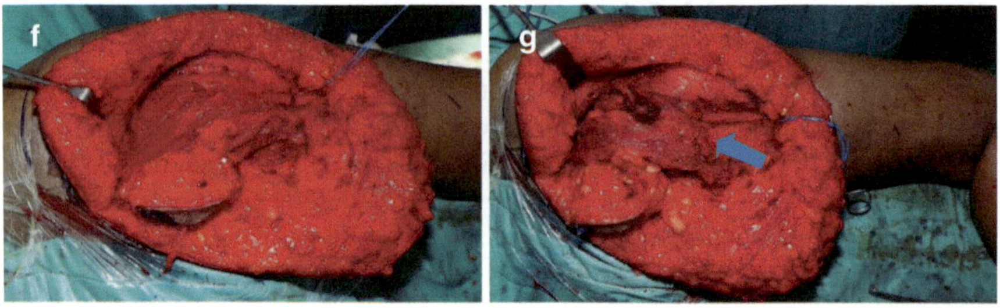

Brachytherapy tubes are inserted for delivering local high-dose radiation to control the disease locally (Fig. 3k, l). Early-focus high-dose radiation minimises the risk of local recurrence in cases with narrow surgical margins. Follow-up CT scan showed no local recurrence at 1 year (Fig. 3m, n).

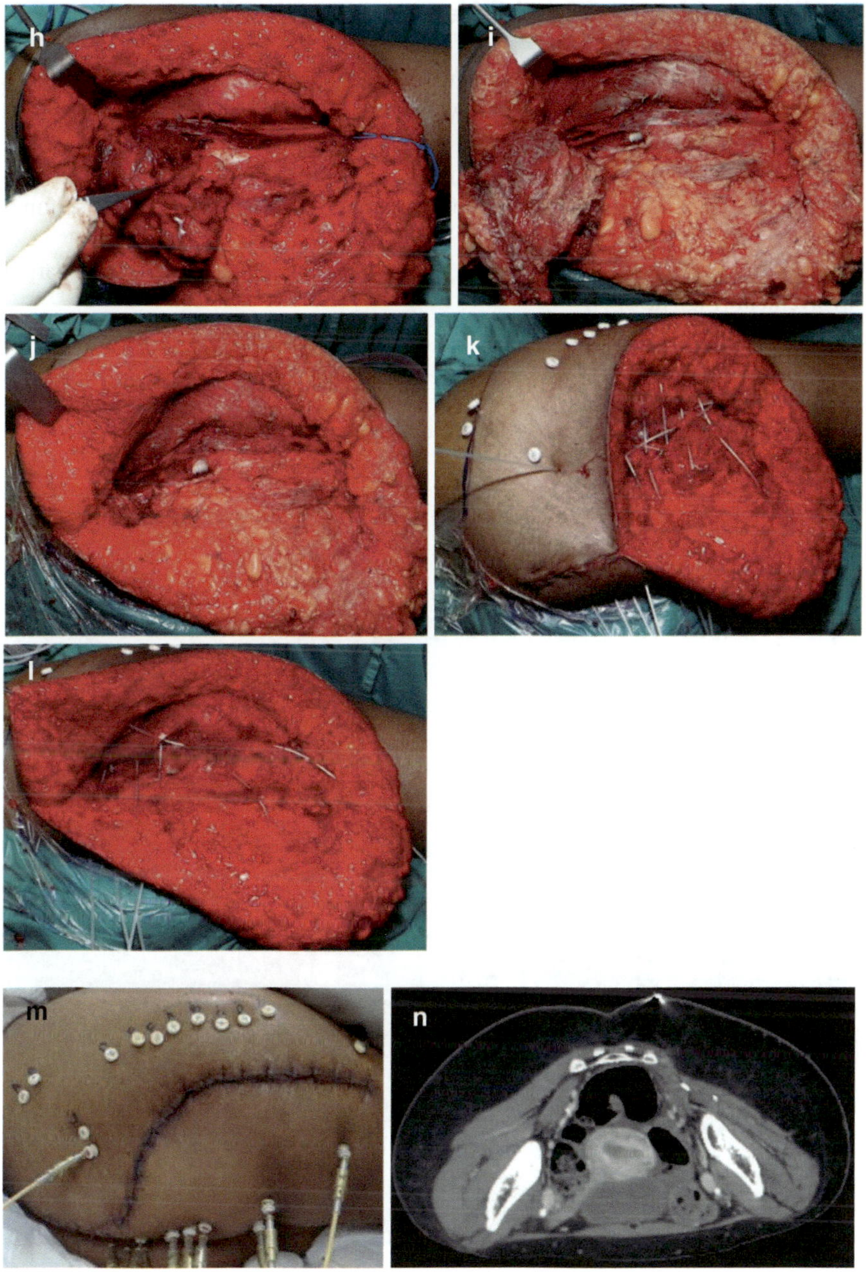
h
i
j
k
l
m
n

Benign Lipoblastoma in Children

Tumour arising from the gluteus medius muscle is rare. Resection of the muscle causes loss of abduction and limping with Trendelenburg gait. A case of lipoblastoma below the gluteus medius, which stretched the entire muscle in a 4-year-old child. The anterior part of the gluteus medius is mobilised with the superior gluteal nerve and vessels. Marginal resection of the tumour is an option to minimise functional deficit (Fig. 4g–j).

MRI image of lipoblastoma arising below gluteus medius muscle with partial involvement (Fig. 4a–f)

1. Gluteus medius
2. Stretch gluteus maximus
3. Superior gluteal vessels exit from sciatic foreman

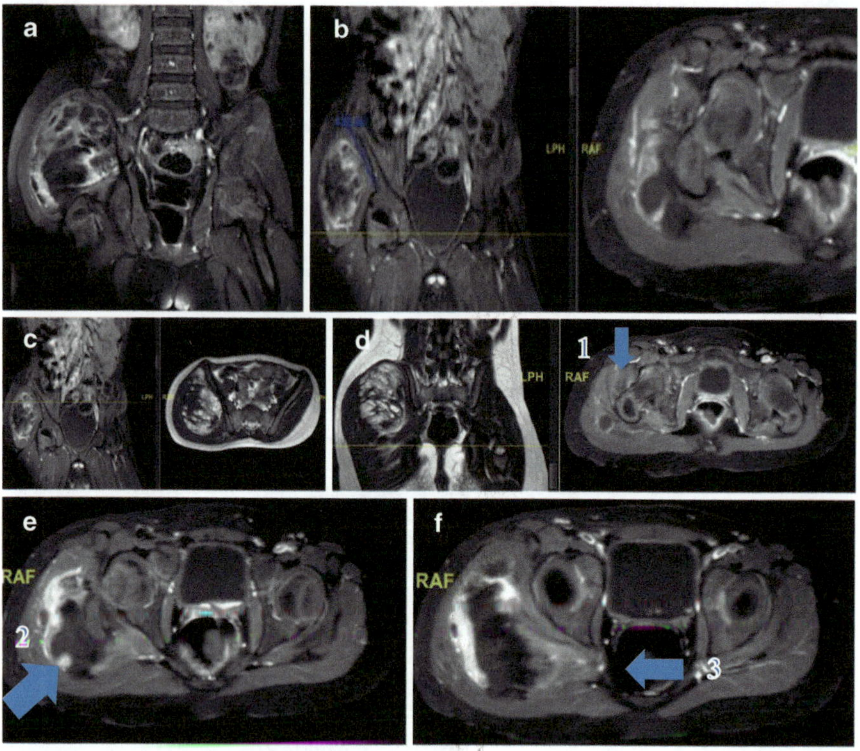

Exploration of the superior gluteal neurovascular structures and elevation of the anterior gluteus medius from the tumour.

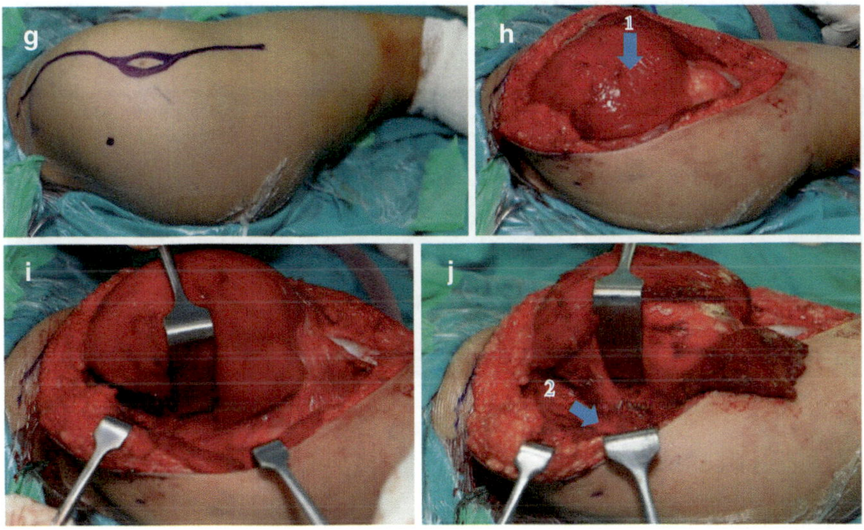

1. Gluteus medius
2. Gluteus maximus
3. Superior gluteal nerve

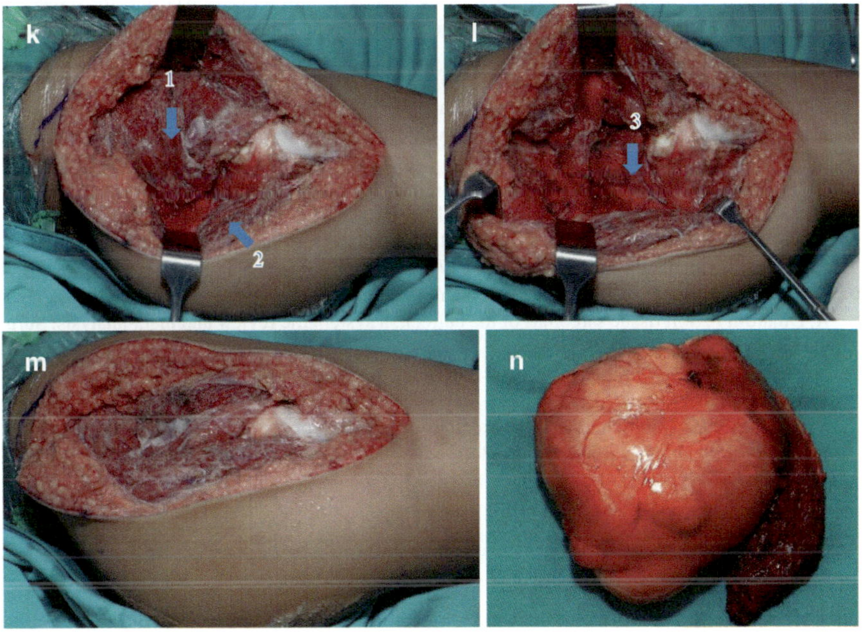

Marginal resection of lipoblastoma with preservation of the gluteus medius for abduction strength (Fig. 4k–n).

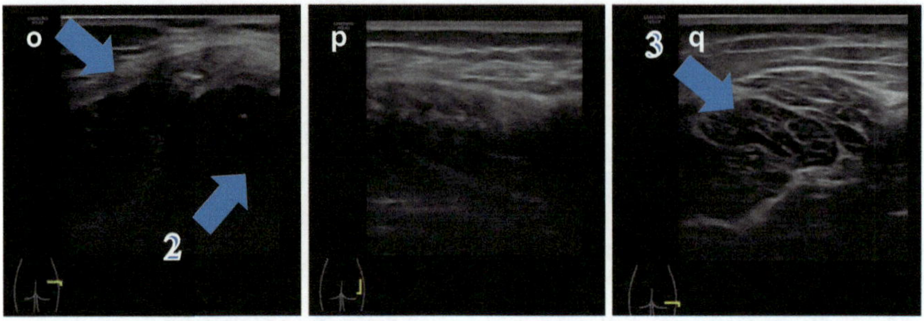

1. Gluteus medius
2. Femoral head
3. Gluteus maximus

Follow-up local ultrasound showed no evidence of local recurrence (Fig. 4o–q).

Suggested Reading

1. Bonaddio Jr VA, Payne R, Harbaugh K, Rizk E, Fox E. Infragluteal exposure for resection of subgluteal tumors: a surgical technique for accessing the sciatic nerve and notch. Cureus. 2021;13(11).
2. Ham SJ, Pras E, Hoekstra HJ. Buttockectomy as a limb saving procedure for locally advanced soft tissue sarcoma of the buttock region. Eur J Surg Oncol. 1998;24(3):184–7.
3. Karakousis CP. Tumor in the buttock area. Atlas of operative procedures in surgical oncology. Springer; 2015. p. 305–9.
4. Kubo T, Sugita T, Shimose S, et al. Nerve tolerance to high-dose-rate brachytherapy in patients with soft tissue sarcoma: a retrospective study. BMC Cancer. 2005;5:79.
5. Malawer MM, Wittig JC, Bickels J. Operative techniques in orthopaedic surgical oncology. Lippincott Williams & Wilkins; 2015. p. 217–22.
6. Sacco R, Lalevee M, Pellegrino P, Ferro A, Yasmine B, Andre G, Matthieu G, Hamza A, Piana R, Dujardin F. Soft tissue sarcomas of the buttock: a systematic review and meta-analysis. Surg Oncol. 2022;45:101883.
7. Sugarbaker PH, Chretien PA. A surgical technique for buttockectomy. Surgery. 1982;91(1):104–7.
8. Sugarbaker PH, Chretien PA. Buttockectomy. In: Atlas of extremity sarcoma surgery. JB Lippincott Philadelphia; 1984. p. 125–34.

Adductor Thigh Resection

Wan Faisham Nu'man Bin Wan Ismail

Introduction

The adductor muscle group is a common site for soft tissue sarcoma of the thigh. It consists of the adductor magnus, brevis, longus, and gracilis muscles. A wide resection margin is possible in most cases and functional deficits following surgical procedures are minimal.

Surgical Anatomy

The adductor muscle compartment consists of the adductor magnus, brevis and longus, and gracilis muscles and is supplied by the obturator nerve and artery.

- All originate from the symphysis pubis, inferior pubic ramus, ischium, and obturator fascia—proximal tumour extension will infiltrate and involve this structure.
- The superficial femoral artery and vein that lie anterior and lateral to the compartment must be explored prior to resection.
- The profunda femoris artery passes through the adductor brevis and travels along the linear aspera—proximal ligation of this artery will minimise bleeding during resection. It should be included together with the margin, especially in a large tumour extending to the linear aspera.

W. F. N. B. W. Ismail (✉)
Prince Court Medical Center, Kuala Lumpur, Malaysia

Orthopaedic Oncology Reconstructive Unit, Universiti Sains Malaysia, Kubang Kerian, Kelantan, Malaysia

A. Puri, W. F. N. B. W. Ismail (eds.), *Atlas of Orthopedic Oncology Volume 1*,
https://doi.org/10.1007/978-981-95-8958-6_2

- The medial hamstring shares a similar origin from the ischium and there is no intermuscular septum separating it from the adductor. Large tumour of the adductor can involve this compartment and requires combined resection. Sciatic nerve will be displaced laterally and must be explored prior to the resection.

Assessment

Detailed preoperative surgical evaluation of the superficial femoral artery and other proximal anatomic structures, including the pelvic floor, sciatic nerve and hip joint, is important. Surgical planning can be either for a partial adductor or complete adductor compartment resection. A good oncology margin is key for controlling the disease locally.

An MRI is used to determine whether a portion of the adductor or the entire compartment is to be resected.

- Careful evaluation of the entire course of the superficial femoral artery and its relationship with the tumour
- Careful evaluation of the adductor origin from the symphysis pubis, inferior pubic rami, ischium, and obturator membrane for tumour extension
- Closed proximity with the psoas attachment and hip capsule
- Extension to the femoral bone near the linear aspera in large tumour
- Correlation with the adductor opening of the adductor magnus muscle in distal tumour

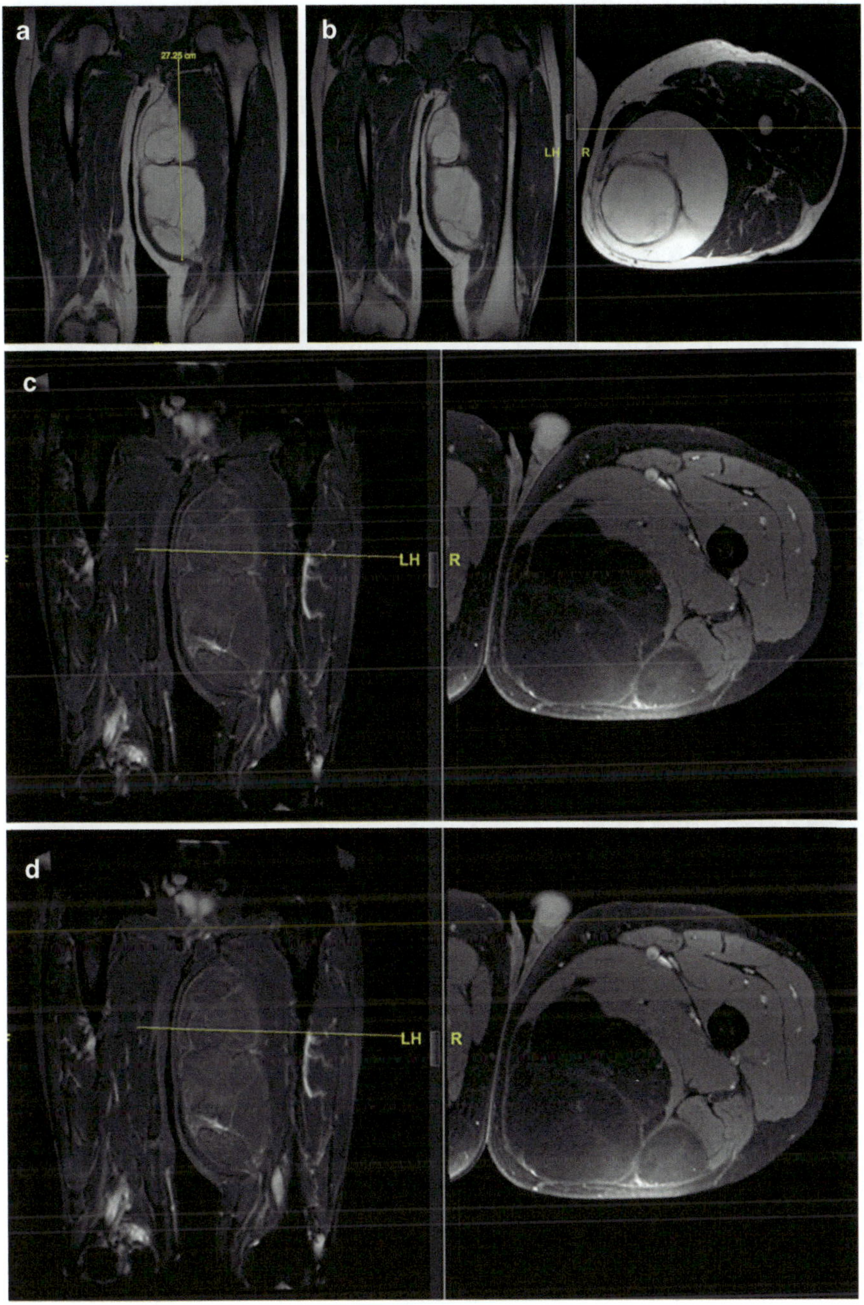
a
27.25 cm
b
LH
R
c
LH
R
d
LH
R

- Superficial femoral artery

The adductor is a common site for liposarcoma. Evaluation of resection length with its margin can accurately be determined by an MRI. Assessment showed that the proximal part of the tumour involves the medial hamstring that must be resected in total with the adductor compartment (Fig. 1a–d).

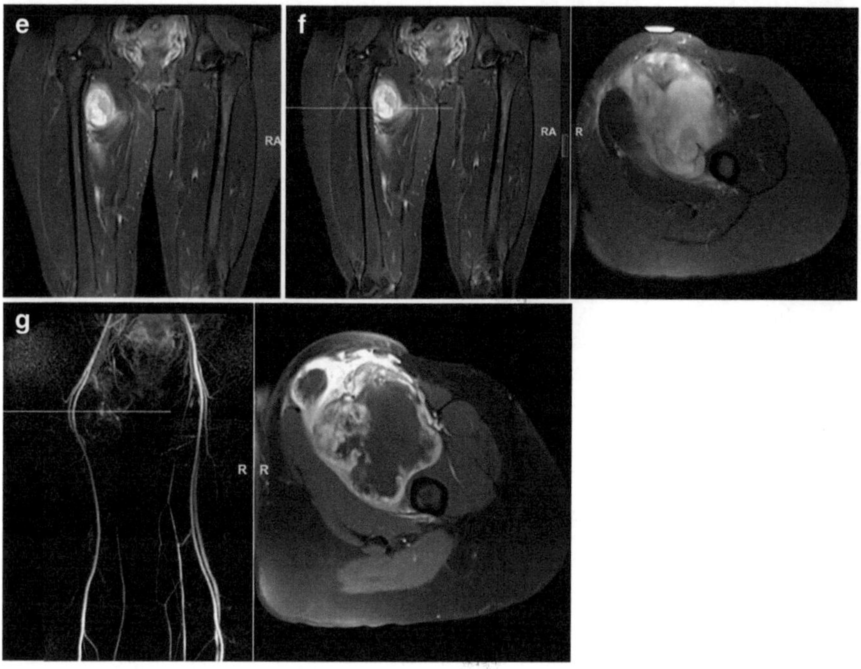

1. Superficial femoral vessels
2. Profunda femoral artery

Pleomorphic sarcoma of the adductor with closed proximity with the superficial femoral vessels should be evaluated with an MRI angiography for patency and involvement of the vessels. The capsule of hip joint and psoas tendon attachment is free from tumour infiltration (Fig. 1e–g).

The superficial femoral artery and vein that lie anterior and lateral to the compartment must be explored prior resection. The profunda femoris vessels lie medial to the compartment and supplies it. They must be ligated in proximity of the tumour for better margin and to minimise bleeding. Exploration and preservation of the superficial femoral vessels, nerve, and muscle are crucial for surgical success.

Surgical Steps (Fig. 2a–d)

Three important steps:

- The profunda femoral vessels must be identified and ligated
- The obturator artery must be identified and ligated during adductor origin detachment
- The tendinous part of the adductor origin must be detached prior to distal resection to prevent muscle retraction

Reconstruction involves closure of the sartorial muscle over the main vessels of the deep fascia and prolonged vacuum drainage to allow tissue adhesion and prevent seroma.

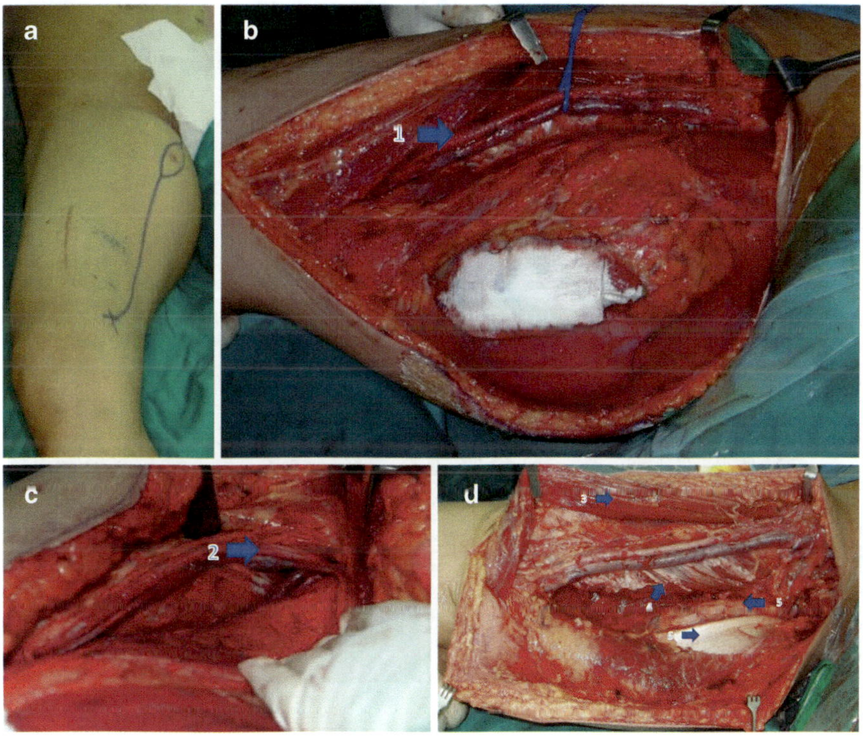

1. Superficial femoral vessels
2. Profunda femoral vessels
3. Sartorius muscle
4. Vastus medialis
5. Sciatic nerve
6. Ischial part of adductor magnus

Resection of Adductor and Posterior Compartment

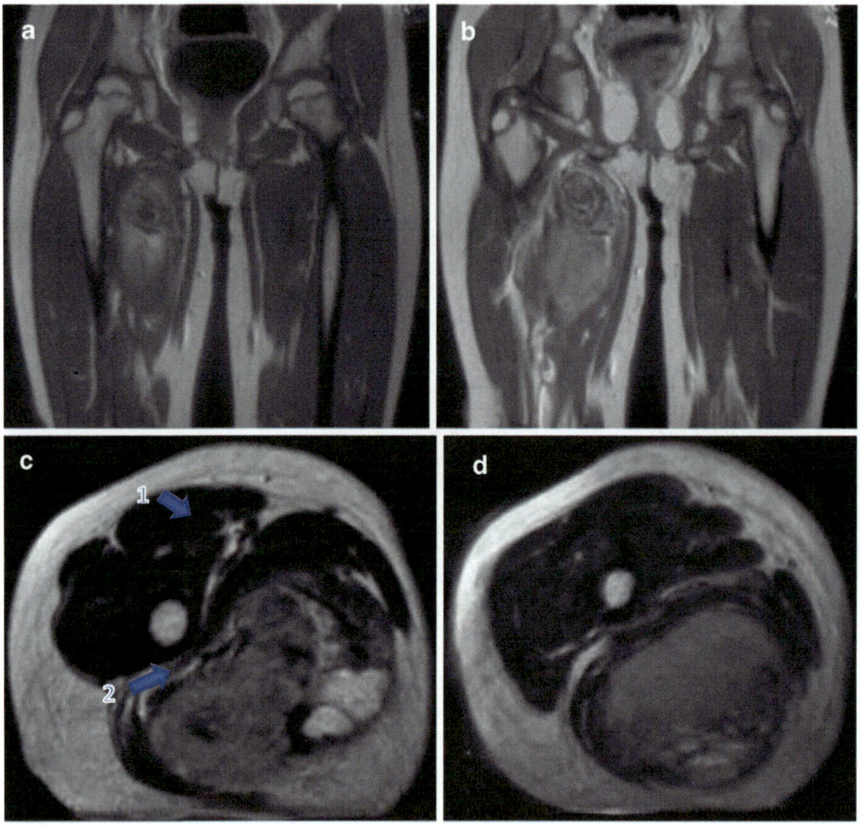

Large adductor magnus tumour with posterior extension involves medial hamstring as it shares a similar origin from the ischium and there is no intermuscular septum separating it (Fig. 3a d). Resection of both compartment requires mobilisation of adductor compartment from femoral vessels and mobilisation of sciatic nerve.

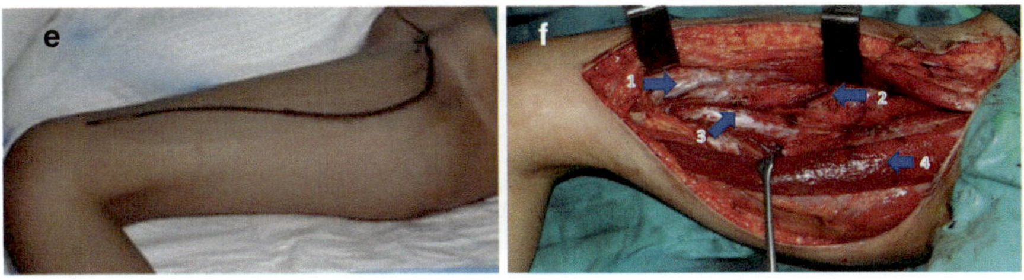

Mobilisations of these entire adductor and posterior compartment leaving biceps femoris muscle which is not involved on MRI evaluation. The profunda femoral vessels which is not involve by the tumor is preserved (Fig. 3e–g).

1. Femoral vessels
2. Profunda femoral vessels
3. Biceps femoris muscle tendon
4. Gracilis
5. Sciatic nerve

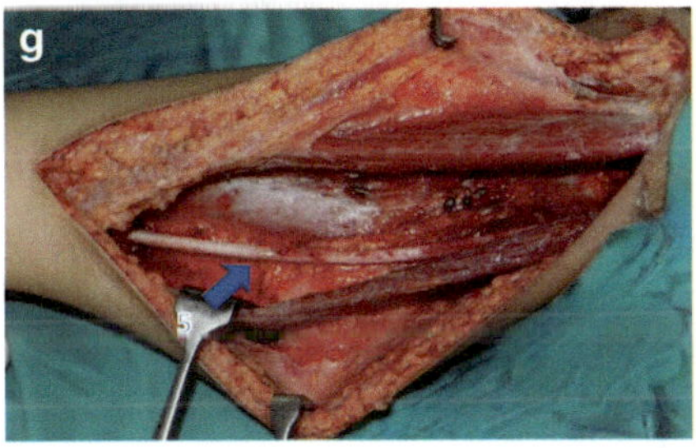

Adductor Sarcoma with Posterior Compartment Closely Attach to Linear Aspera

Adductor tumour with posterolateral extension closely attached to the periosteum and linea aspera. Detailed MRI assessment of the profunda femoris vessels and bone involvement is important to achieve good oncological margin (Fig. 4a–c).

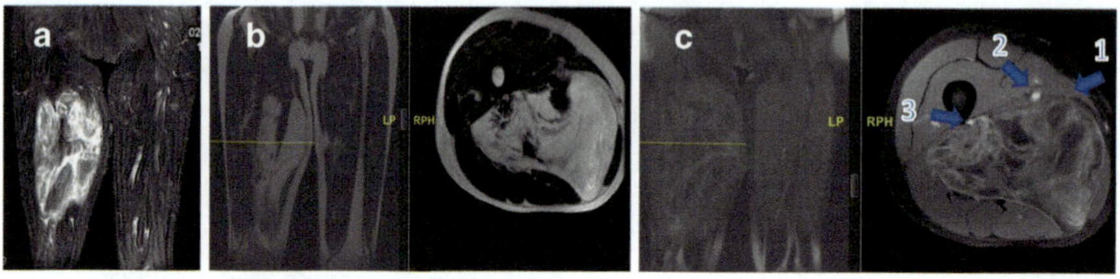

1. Sartorius loosely attached to the tumour
2. Superficial femoral vessels
3. Profunda femoral vessels and tumour closely attached to linea aspera

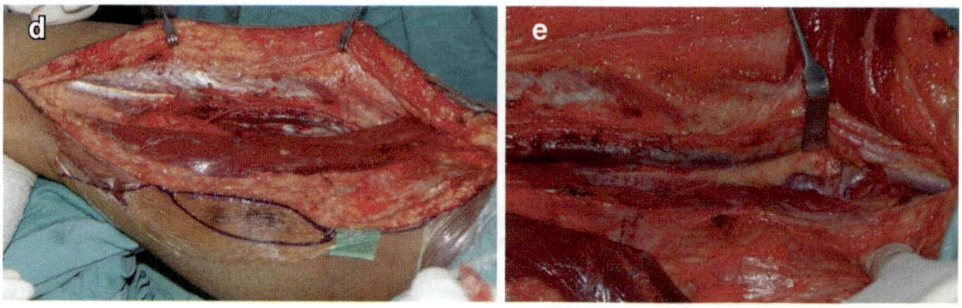

Exploration of the femoral vessels is the primary step for evaluating tumour extension. The femoral neurovascular sheath can be included within the resection for better oncological margin. There is no intermuscular septum separating the adductor from the medial hamstring of the posterior compartment. Extension of tumour to the medial hamstring is possible (Fig. 4d–f).

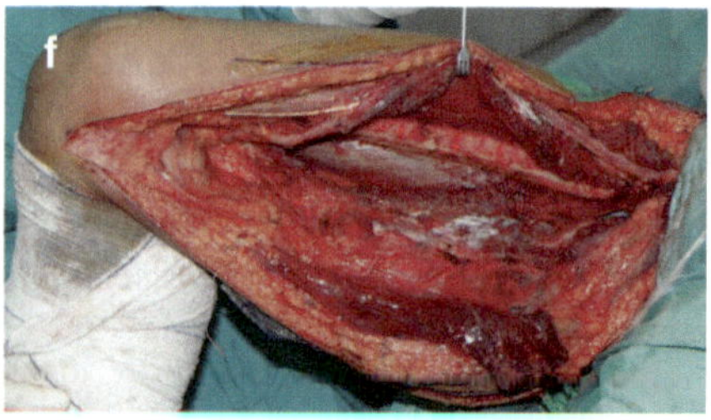

Evaluation of the margin for extra-compartment resection is important for tumour clearance. Part of vastus medialis is included in the margin and the periosteum is cleared to the linea aspera for oncological margin. Care must be taken to ensure good haemostasis of the profunda femoral artery and its branch during this procedure.

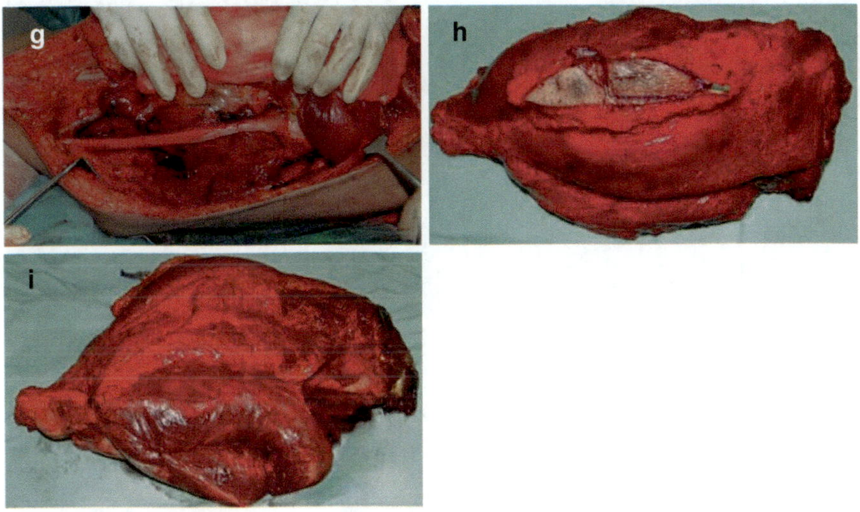

The sciatic nerve that lies between the medial and lateral hamstring must be protected prior final resection of the hamstring origin at the ischial tuberosity. The adductor muscle attachment is detached from its origin and the linea aspera attachment is free to create a plane between the medial and lateral hamstring. The sciatic nerve is protected and mobilised prior to final mobilisation of tumour and resection (Fig. 4g–j).

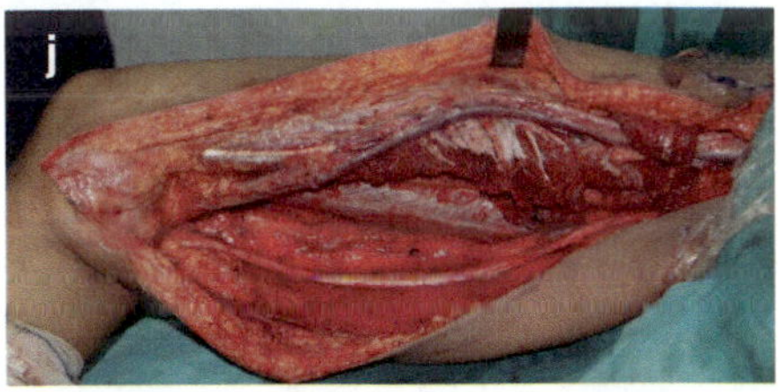

Adductor Sarcoma with Pubic Rami Involvement

The superior and inferior pubic rami are the closest margins and occasionally involved in large sarcomas. Resection of the pelvic bone (type III) is done by elevating the inguinal ligament to expose the space of Retzius. The pubic bone is resected at the level of the symphysis pubis and medial wall of the acetabulum to achieve oncological margin.

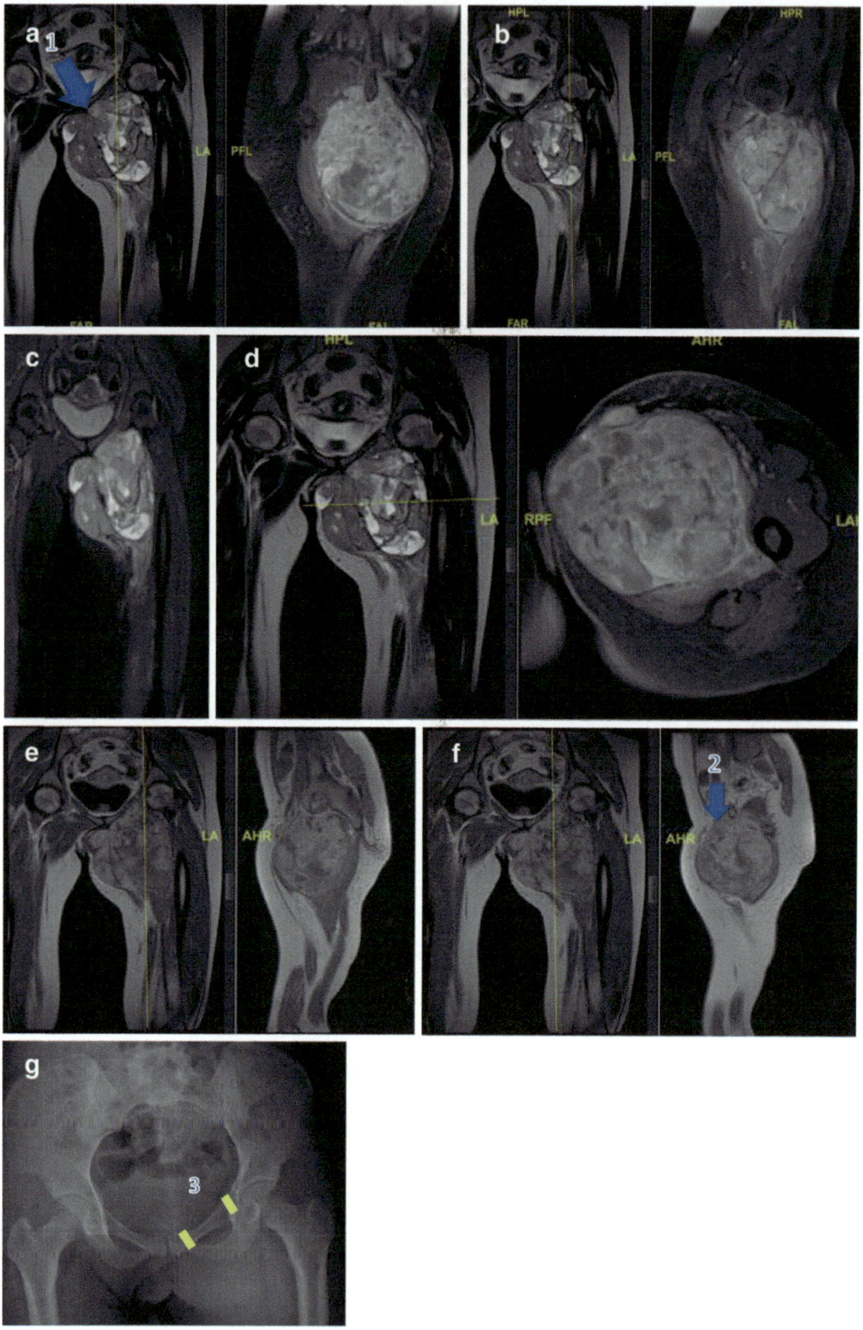
a
1
LA
PFL
FAR
b
HPL
HPR
LA
PFL
FAR
FAL
c
d
HPL
AHR
LA
RPF
e
LA
AHR
f
2
LA
AHR
g
3

Pleomorphic sarcoma proximal adductor attached to superior pubic rami and obturator membrane. The superficial femoral vessels closely attached to the tumour border displaced laterally (Fig. 5a–f).

1. Obturator membrane
2. Superior pubic rami involved
3. Plan osteotomy (Fig. 5g)

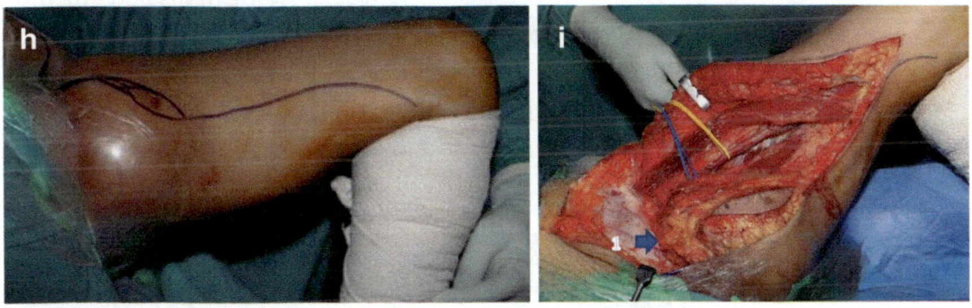

Resection of proximal adductor compartment with muscle origin to the superior pubic rami (Fig. 5h–k).

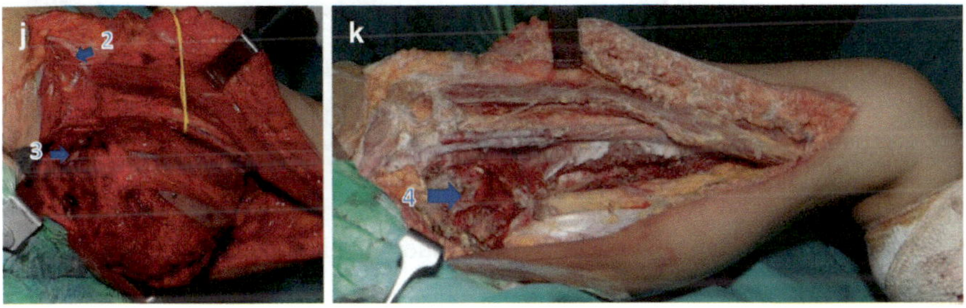

1. Inguinal ligament
2. Anterior superior iliac spine—lateral cutaneous nerve
3. Medial wall acetabulum
4. Obturator defect
5. Prolene mesh

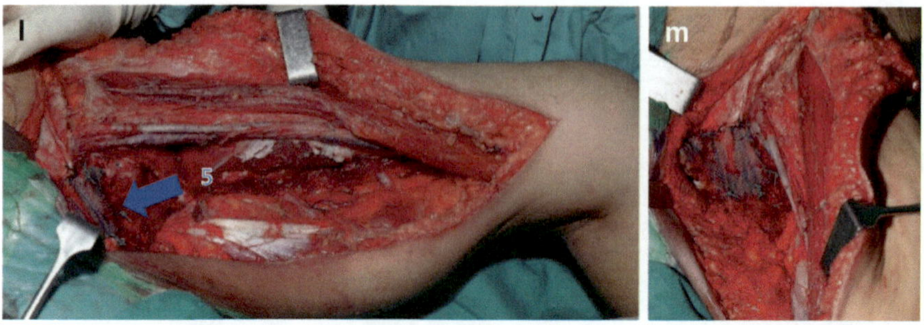

Resection of the pubic bone will create a defect over the pelvic floor. Reconstruction is done with prolene mesh to close the defect and prevent hernia (Fig. 5l, m).

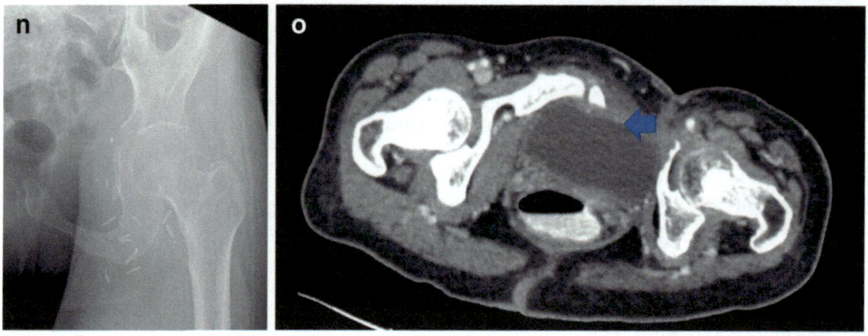

- Prolene mesh reconstruction prevent bladder herniation, CT scan evaluation 2 years after surgery (Fig. 5n, o).

Suggested Reading

1. Pradhan A, Cheung YC, Grimer RJ, Abudu A, Peake D, Ferguson PC, Griffin AM, Wunder JS, O'Sullivan B, Hugate R, Sim FH. Does the method of treatment affect the outcome in soft-tissue sarcomas of the adductor compartment? J Bone Joint Surg. 2006;88-B:1480–6.
2. Karakousis CP. Tumor in the medial thigh atlas of operative procedures in surgical oncology. Springer Science; 2015. p. 323–9.
3. Karakousis CP. Refinements of surgical technique in soft tissue sarcomas. J Surg Oncol. 2010;101:730–8.
4. Grainger MF, Grimer RJ, Carter SR, Tillman RM. Wound complications following resection of adductor compartment tumours. Sarcoma. 2001;5(4):203–7.
5. Malawer M, Sugarbaker P. Adductor muscle group excision. Operative technique. In: Orthopaedic surgical oncology. Lippincott Williams & Wilkins; 2012. A Wolters Kluwer.
6. Rudiger HA, Ngan SY, Choong PF. Surgical outcome of soft tissue sarcomas of the adductor compartment. J Orthop Surg. 2009;17(3):284–7.
7. Tanaka A, Okamoto M, Kito M, Yoshimura Y, Aoki K, Suzuki S, Takazawa A, Komatsu Y, Ishida T, Takahashi J. Influence of the adductor compartment resection on muscle strength and postoperative function in soft-tissue sarcoma of the thigh. Jpn J Clin Oncol. 2022;52(4):370–4.

Quadriceps Compartment Resection

Wan Faisham Nu'man Bin Wan Ismail,
Arman Zaharil Mat Saad, Wan Azman Wan Sulaiman,
Zulmi Wan, and Ahmad Sukari Halim

Introduction

The quadriceps of the thigh is important for knee extensor and anti-gravity function for ambulation. Resection of this compartment will interfere with proper ambulation. Preservation of part of the quadriceps with intact innervation and good margin of tumour clearance are keys for surgical success.

Surgical Anatomy

The quadriceps consists of the rectus femoris, vastus lateralis, medialis and intermedius muscle. Each compartment muscle group has its own perimysium for oncological margin, especially for localised tumour. Exploration of the femoral nerve and its motor branch with preservation of the remaining muscle motor unit prior to resection of the muscle group compartment is important.

W. F. N. B. W. Ismail (✉)
Prince Court Medical Center, Kuala Lumpur, Malaysia

Orthopaedic Oncology Reconstructive Unit, Universiti Sains Malaysia,
Kubang Kerian, Kelantan, Malaysia

A. Z. M. Saad
Plastic Reconstructive & Microsurgery, MSU Medical Centre, Management and Science University of Malaysia, Shah Alam, Selangor, Malaysia

W. A. W. Sulaiman · A. S. Halim
Reconstructive Sciences Department, School of Medical Sciences, Universiti Sains Malaysia,
Kubang Kerian, Kelantan, Malaysia

Z. Wan
Prince Court Medical Center, Kuala Lumpur, Malaysia

A. Puri, W. F. N. B. W. Ismail (eds.), *Atlas of Orthopedic Oncology Volume 1*,
https://doi.org/10.1007/978-981-95-8958-6_3

- The superficial femoral artery and vein lay medial to the anterior compartment and must be explored when tumour is adjacent to them.
- The femoral triangle is a key structure for exploring the femoral vessels and identification of branches of femoral nerve for specific compartment muscle resection. The branch of femoral nerve starts dividing below the inguinal ligament and supplies the main muscle groups.
- The branch of the lateral circumflex vessels (profunda femoral artery) transverse behind the sartorius and rectus femoris muscle and supplies the muscle compartment.
- The nerve to the vastus medialis traversing within the subsatorial canal can be preserved for adequate strength for walking if another muscle compartment is resected.
- The vastus medialis, lateralis and intermedius muscles originate from the femur and inter muscular septum and only the rectus femoris origin lies superficially from the anterior inferior iliac spine pelvis. They all blend to form the quadriceps tendon attached to the patella.
- The medial septum that separates the vastus medialis from the adductors is thin in the upper thigh and becomes well defined in the lower thigh.
- The lateral septum, which is thicker and separates the vastus laterals from the posterior compartment, is a good anatomical barrier.

Assessment

Detailed evaluation of tumour extension to examine whether it involves single or multiple muscle compartments is important for oncological margin and planning for reconstruction of quadriceps function.

- The superficial femoral artery and vein, which pass through the medial wall of the sub-sartorial canal and are separated from the vastus medialis by the thick fascia, permit a safe resection margin.
- Large tumour on the medial compartment extending to the adductor has a high possibility of involving the femoral vessels and may require a bypass graft.
- Tumour in the vastus intermedius has a poor plane with the periosteum. A resection margin must include the periosteum for better margin. Evaluation of the anterior cortex of the femur for tumour infiltration is important for a definitive oncological margin.

Surgical Steps (Fig. 1)

- Exploration of the femoral vessels in the subsartorial canal is crucial in medially located tumour in the vastus medals and intermedius.
- The sartorius muscle is preserved with proximal septum innervation for quadriceps reconstruction.

- Exploration of the femoral triangle for branches of the femoral nerve and descending circumflex vessels is important for definitive muscle or group resection. It is important in a proximally situated tumour.

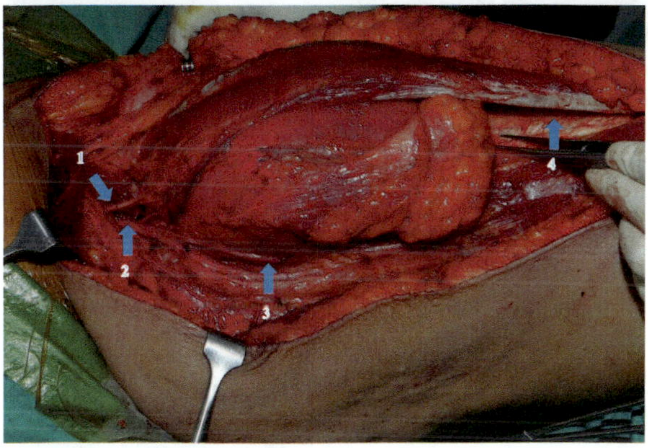

The rectus femoris has good tendinous parts separated from the vastus intermedius and can be retained with good margin provided the branch of the femoral nerve and circumflex vessels are preserved.

1. Femoral nerve—branch to rectus and vastus lateralis
2. Femoral nerve—branch to saphenous and motor to vastus medialis
3. Motor branch to vastus medialis
4. Intertendinous plane—vastus intermedius and rectus femoris

In large tumours, when the entire quadriceps is involved and needs to be resected, options for reconstruction as anti-gravity motor include:

- A gracilis muscle transpositional flap
- Combination of a gracilis and short head transpositional flap
- Free motorised muscle flap (latissimus dorsi)

Limited Resection of the Quadriceps Muscle

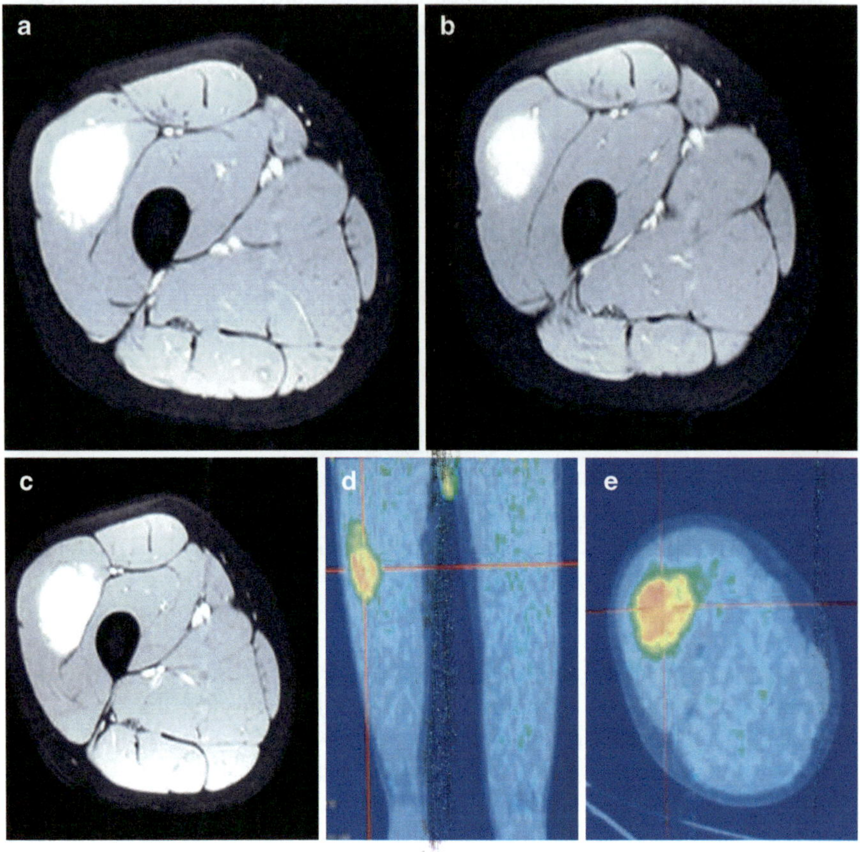

Sarcoma confined to the vastus lateralis with clear border to the intermedius group. Superior and inferior margin of 5 cm and cuff of soft tissue are adequate for oncological margin. MRI image and PET scan evaluation prior resection (Fig. 2a–e).

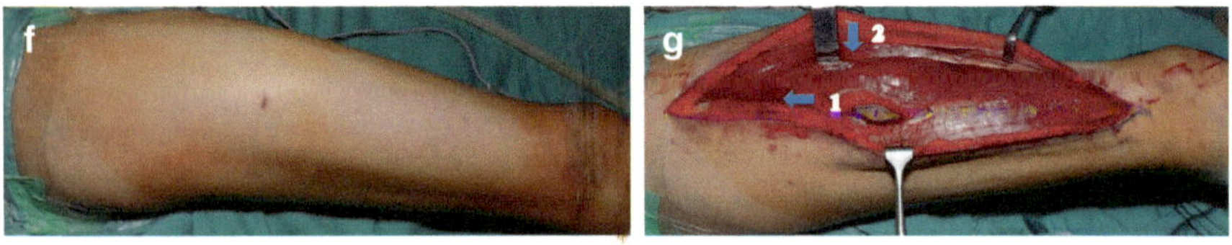

Biopsy was done directly to the tumour through the vastus lateralis compartment. A medial and lateral flap was created to visualise the vastus lateralis covering the tumour. The rectus femoris was elevated for exploration of the medial septum of the vastus lateralis (Fig. 2f and g).

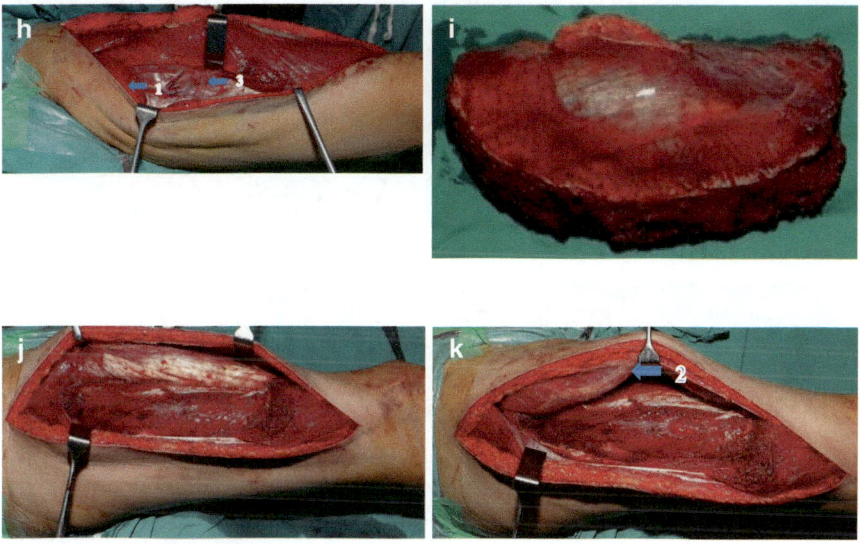

1. Tensor fascia latae muscle
2. Rectus femoris
3. Vastus intermedius

Tumour within the vastus lateralis was elevated medially through the septum above the intermedius group. The entire mid portion was removed till the lateral septum with 5 cm superior and inferior cuff of normal tissue (Fig. 2h–k).

Lateral Compartment Thigh Resection

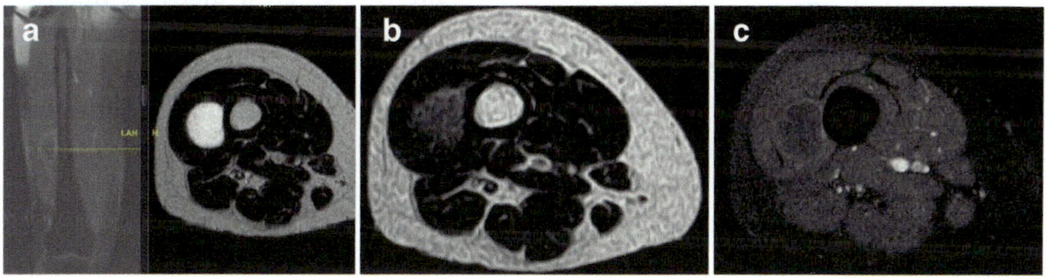

Sarcoma involving the vastus lateralis and intermedius and closely attached to the periosteum (Fig. 3a–c) is resected with good quality margin without major vessels and nerve exploration. The oncological margin of tumour extension is guided by proper evaluation via an MRI. The periosteum is included for better quality resection margin (Fig. 3d–h).

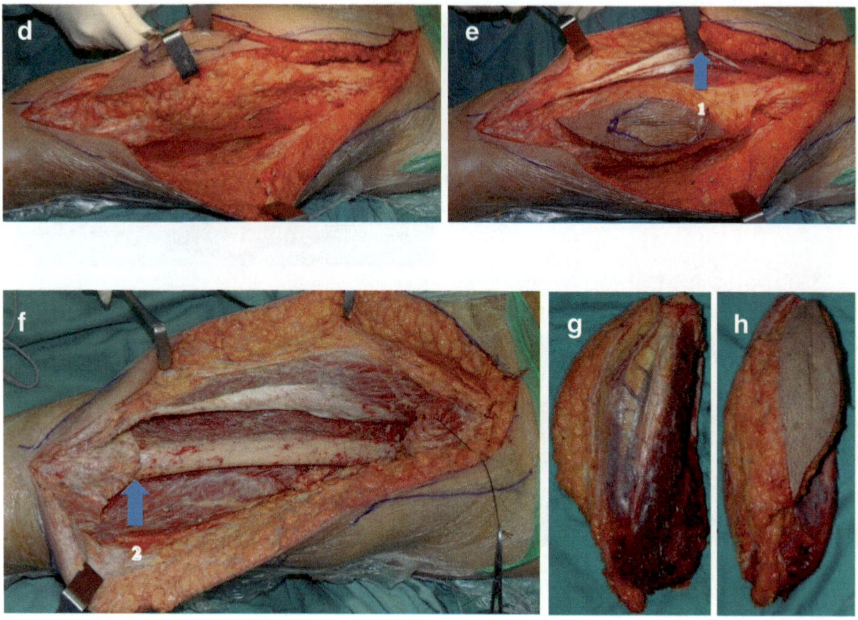

1. Rectus femoris
2. Remnant of vastus lateralis tendon—parapatellar tissue

Rectus Femoris Resection

Isolated rectus femoris sarcoma is rare. Resection of the entire rectus weakens the quadriceps. However, the remaining quadriceps is adequate to maintain anti-gravity muscle for standing and walking. The rectus femoris has clear plane boundaries with the peripheral muscle of the vastus medialis and lateralis at proximal part; however, it is blended distally. It is separated from the vastus intermedius by a strong layer of tendon. However, it becomes blended with the tendinous part of quadriceps muscle and attached to the patella.

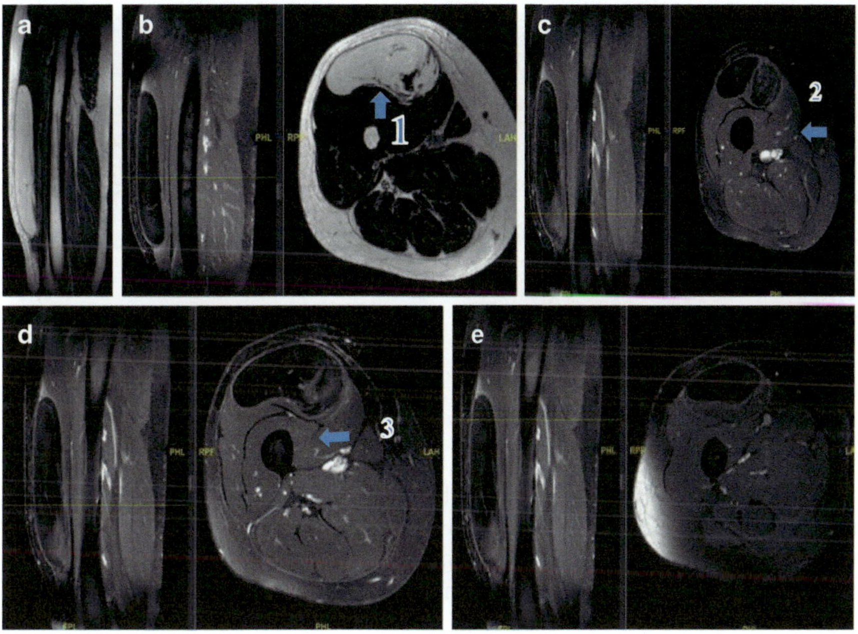

- 1. Rectus femoris
- 2. Vastus medialis
- 3. Vastus intermedius

MRI image of liposarcoma rectus femoris muscle (Fig. 4a–e).
Good-quality margin is possible for complete rectus femoris resection.

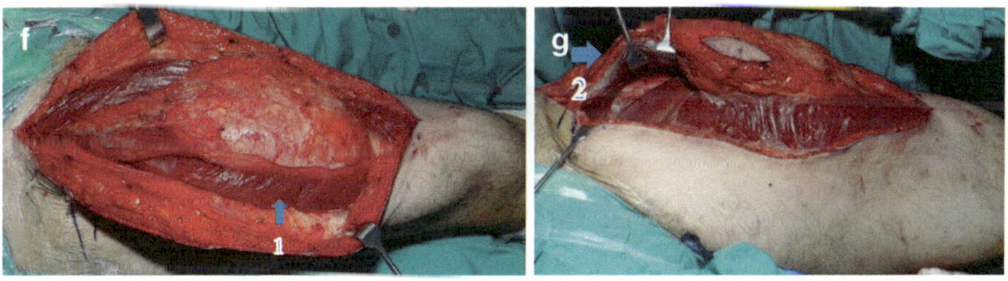

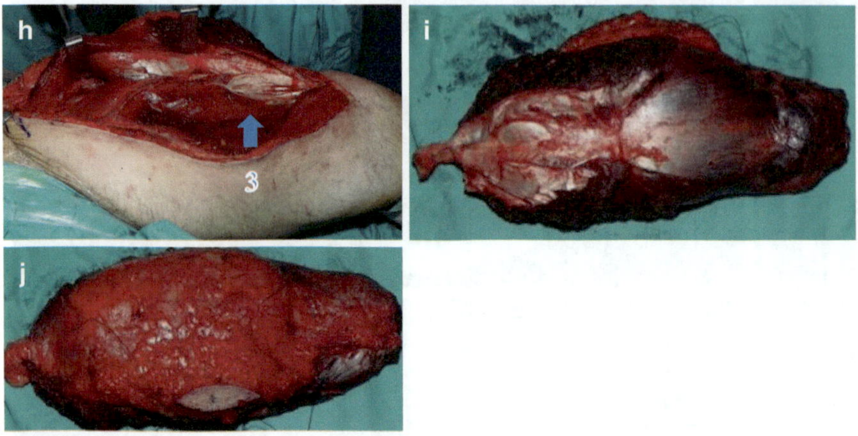

The distal and peripheral margins of the tumour to the vastus medals and lateralis are achieved with cuff 1–2 cm of normal tissue. The distal part of the rectus femoris tendon is elevated from the vastus intermedius. Both the vastus medialis and lateralis are mobilised and apposed with running suture for final reconstruction (Fig. 4f–k).

1. Vastus medialis
2. Rectus femoris elevate from vastus intermedius
3. Vastus lateralis

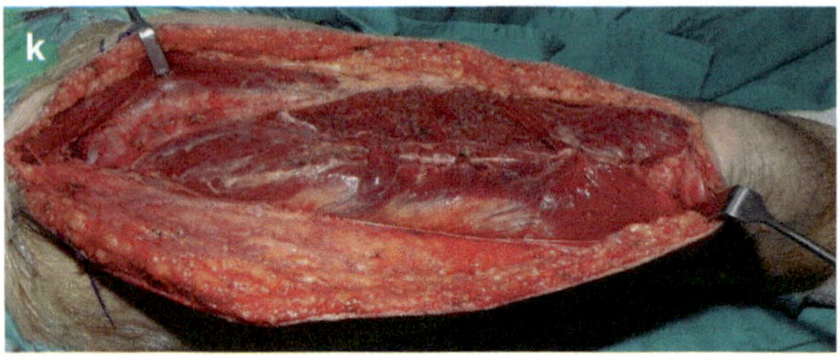

Proximal Medial Quadricep Resection

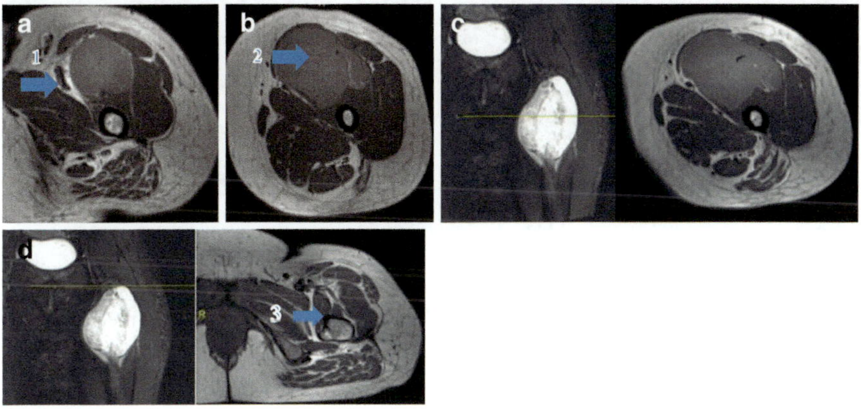

MRI image of soft tissue sarcoma proximal quadriceps compartment (Fig. 5a–d)

1. Superficial femoral artery
2. Vastus medialis and intermedius
3. Superior border of vastus medialis

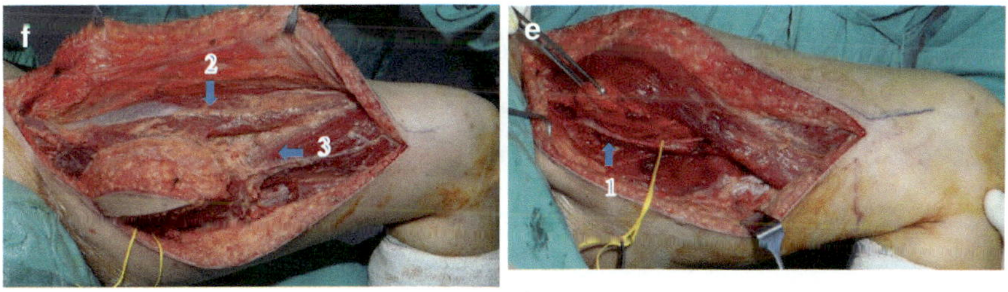

Tumour situated in the vastus medialis and intermedius muscle compartment is usually in close proximity with the femoral vessels. The rectus femoris muscle compartment has good boundaries to the vastus medialis and intermedius and should be preserved with proximal motor and vascular supply (Fig. 5e–g).

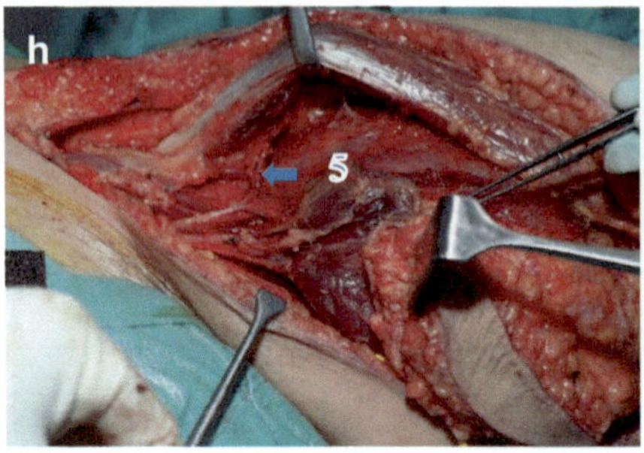

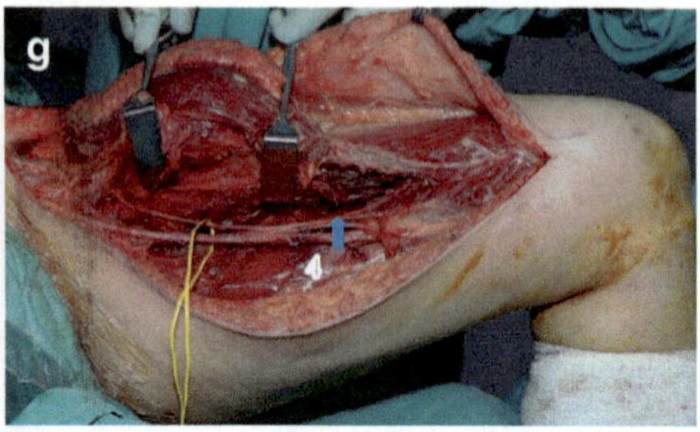

The lateral fasciocutaneous flap is created for mobilisation of the proximal rectus femoris with nerve and vascular supply. The entire proximal vastus medialis and intermedius muscle are resected above the periosteum unilateral to inter muscular septum (Fig. 5h)

1. Superficial femoral artery
2. Rectus femoris
3. Vastus medialis
4. Saphenous nerve and nerve to distal vastus medialis
5. Femoral branch to rectus femoris and vastus lateralis

Exploration is required through the entire course within the vessels sheath fascia for good-quality margin. Branches of the nerve to the vastus medialis distally should be preserved for additional quadriceps strength (Fig. 5i).

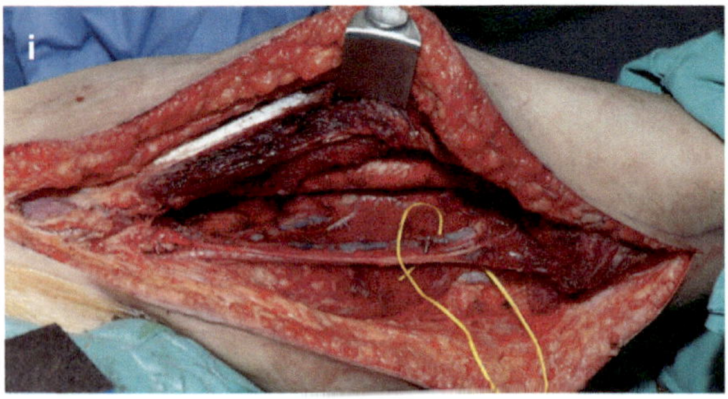

Large Proximal Quadricep Resection

In large proximal quadriceps tumour, exploration of the femoral vessels and mobilisation is required as it is in close proximity to the tumour. The proximal femoral nerve branches were evaluated for compartment resection of the involved specific quadricep muscle group.

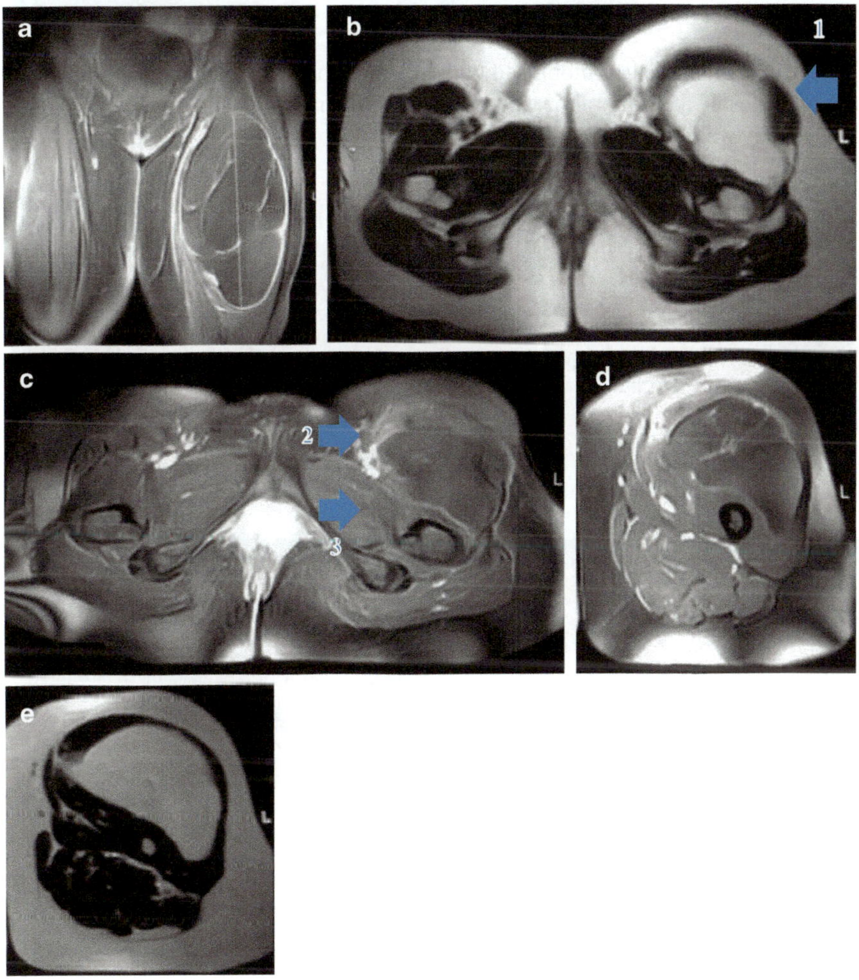

MRI of low-grade liposarcoma quadricep compartment proximal thigh (Fig. 6a–e)

1. Rectus femoris
2. Superficial femoral artery
3. Vastus medialis

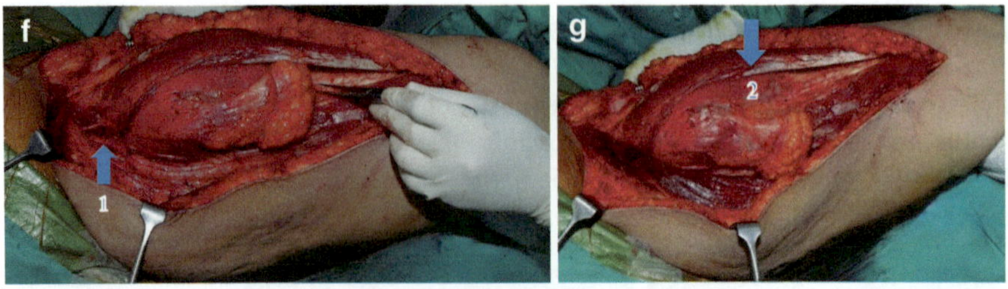

The rectus femoris was mobilised with intact motor branch for extensor function, and branches of the femoral nerve to rectus, vastus medialis and cutaneous saphenous nerves were maintained (Fig. 6f–k).

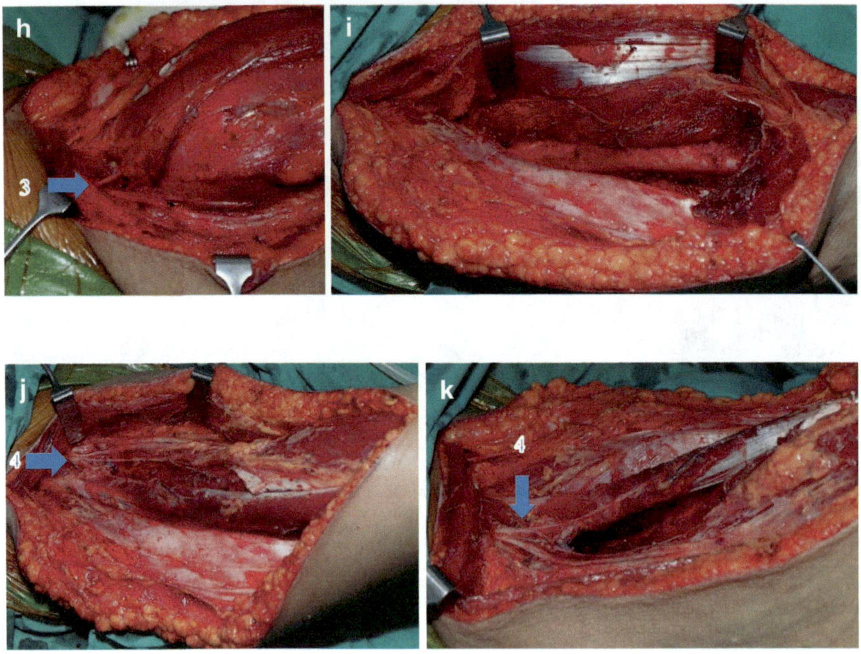

1. Superficial femoral artery and branch of femoral nerve
2. Rectus femoris
3. Proximal femoral nerve and branch
4. Branches femoral nerve
   - Vastus lateralis
   - Rectus femoris
   - Saphenous nerve and motor to vastus medialis

Large Sarcoma—Complete Quadriceps Resection

A large sarcoma situated at the proximal part and anterior of the thigh usually involves the entire quadriceps sparing the vastus medialis muscle. Exploring the subsartorial canal and preserving the motor branch of the femoral nerve to the vastus medialis are adequate for knee extension and ambulation.

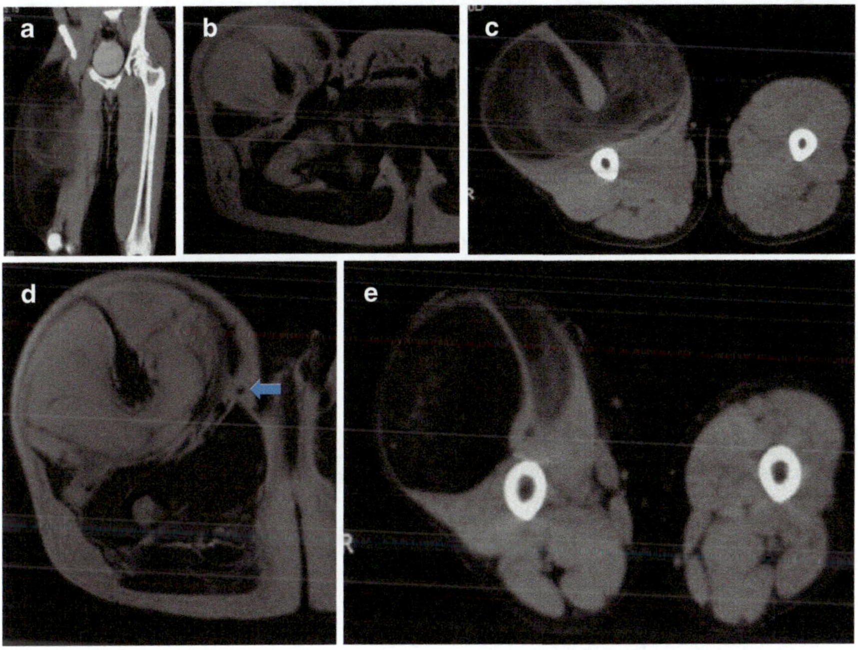

The MRI showed that the entire quadricep is involved, except for the vastus medialis muscle group. The superficial femoral vessels were explored, and the saphenous branch and nerve to the vastus medialis were maintained for motor and sensory function (Fig. 7a–e).

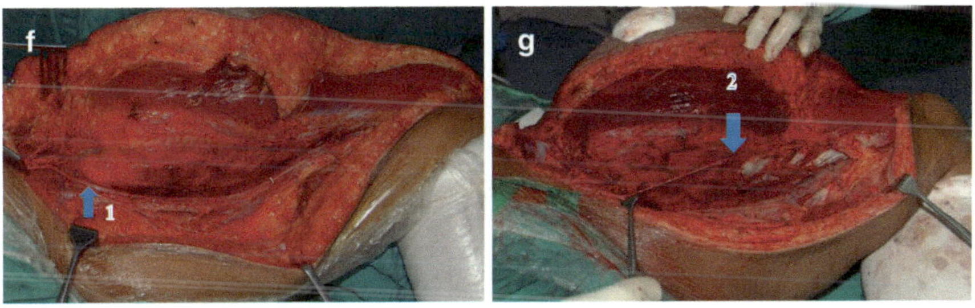

The entire quadriceps was elevated from the lateral intermuscular septum and periosteum of the femur. The vastus medialis with branch of the nerve and saphenous branch were preserved (Fig. 7f–j). A rotational gracilis muscle transfer is an option to improve quadriceps strength as anti-gravity while walking.

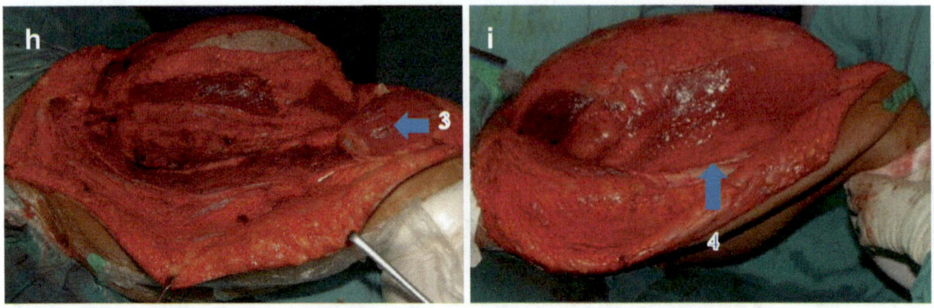

1. Superficial femoral vessels and saphenous nerve
2. Nerve to vastus medialis
3. Distal part vastus medialis
4. Vastus lateralis—lateral intermuscular septum

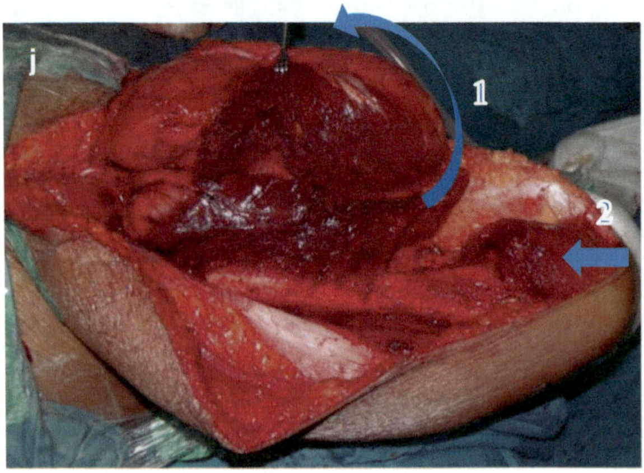

1. Entire quadriceps elevated from lateral intermuscular septum and femur after detach rectus femoris tendon from quadricep tendon and distal vastus medialis (Fig. 7j).
2. The medial and lateral parapatellar soft tissues are maintained for stability.

The tendinous part of the gracilis insertion is attached to the remnant quadriceps tendon. The motor nerve of the gracilis from the obturator branch is maintained to provide extensor function (Fig. 7k–m).

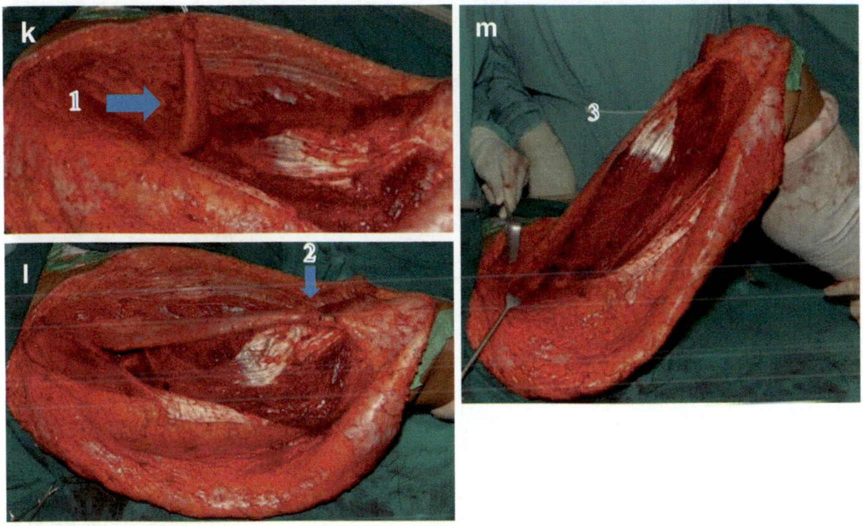

1. Mobilisation of gracilis flap with intact nerve and vessels
2. Repair to the remnant of quadriceps tendon
3. Assessment of tension in knee flexion

Distal Quadriceps Resection with Motorised Latissimus Dorsi Flap

Sarcoma over the quadriceps with distal thigh extension sometimes involves the medial and lateral soft tissue stabiliser of the patella. The tendinous part of the rectus femoris and patella can be preserved in low- to intermediate-grade malignancy to maintain extensor mechanism. However, to maintain patella stability and tracking, soft tissue knee reconstruction with flap is required, especially in massive tissue loss. The flap can also be motorised to improve quadriceps function.

MRI and CT scan image of distal thigh quadriceps sarcoma (Fig. 8a–g).

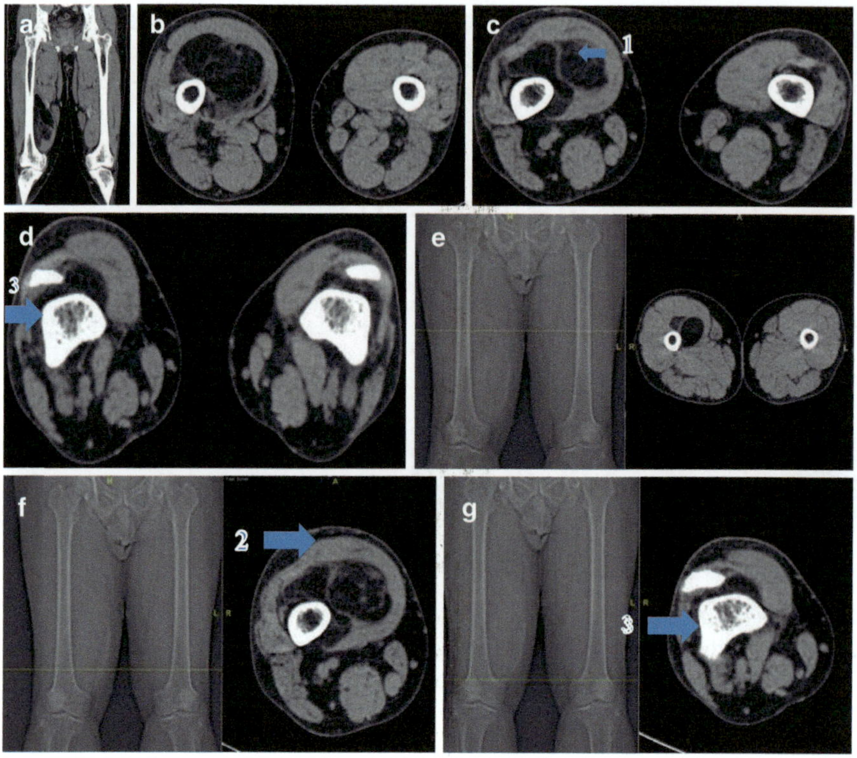

1. Vastus intermedius and vastus medialis infiltration
2. Rectus femoris muscle and tendon with good plane
3. Suprapatellar pouch infiltration

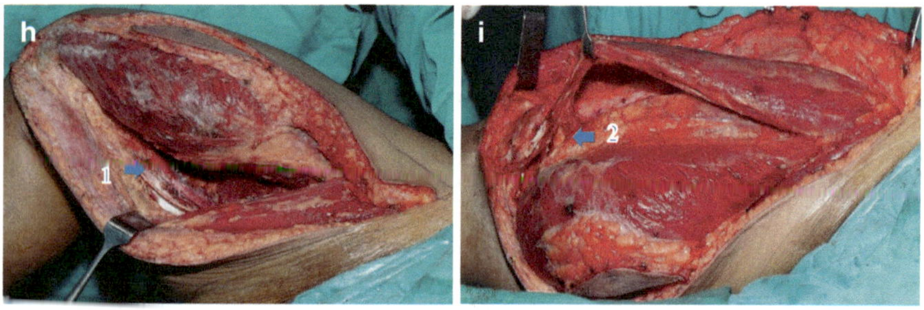

Elevation of the rectus femoris from the vastus intermedius. The entire vastus medialis, lateralis, suprapatellar pouch fat and both the patella retinaculum were removed to achieve oncological margin. The patella is stabilised with a latissimus dorsi flap. The quadricep function is augmented by motorising this flap (Fig. 8h–n).

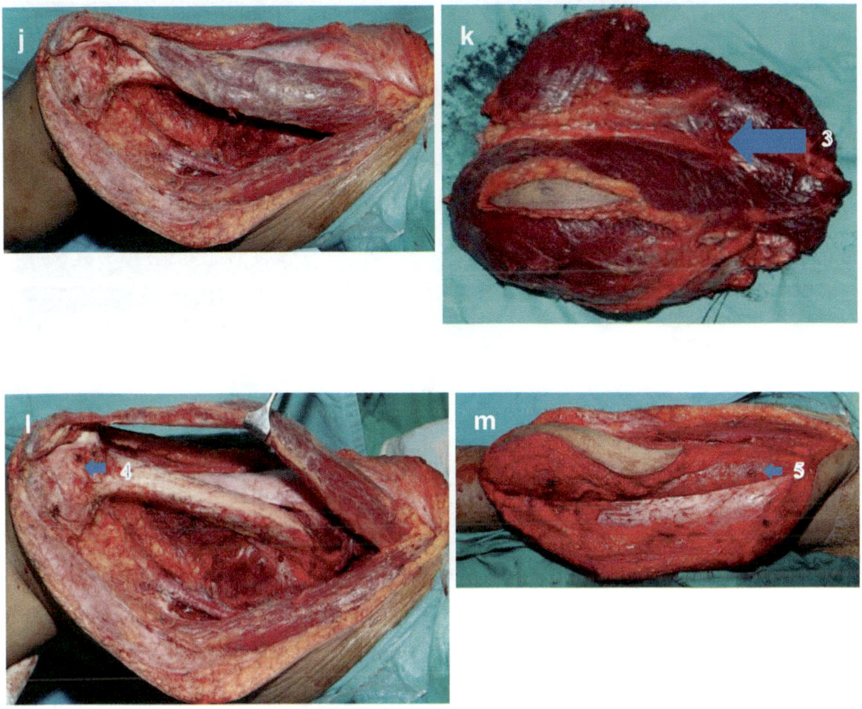

1. Superficial femoral vessels
2. Suprapatellar fat and synovium
3. Plane between rectus femoris and vastus intermedius
4. Parapatellar fascia remove with vastus medialis, lateralis and intermedius for oncological margin
5. Latissimus dorsi flap

Resection of Entire Quadriceps and Motorised Latissimus Dorsi Flap

When the entire compartment is removed and total extensor mechanism loss for anti gravity ambulation function, knee fusion is an option. A motorised latissimus dorsi flap, whereby the thoracodorsal nerve is connected to the proximal femoral nerves, is used as an anti-gravity function. Good tissue tension with early faradic stimulation is required to achieve good extension power and minimise extension lag.

MRI image of sarcoma with extension to the entire quadriceps (Fig. 9a–d).

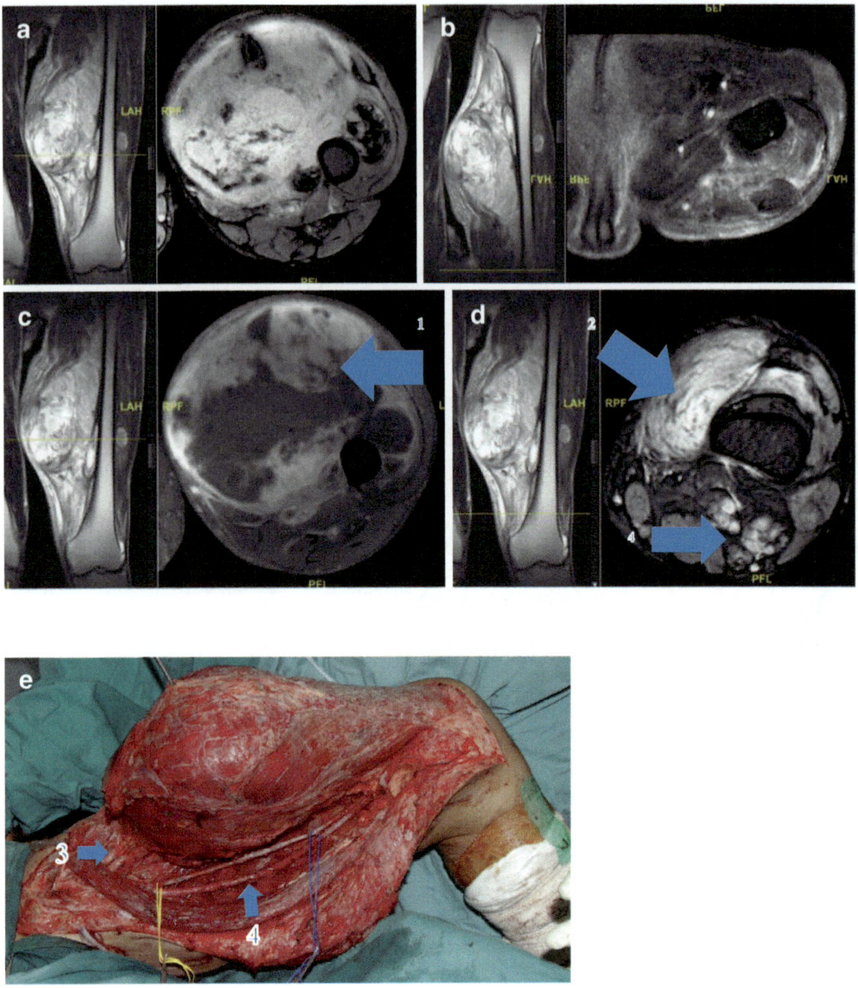

1. Heterogeneous lesion involves entire quadriceps
2. Distal thigh involvement of vastus medialis and intermedius muscle
3. Thickened femoral nerve branch
4. Femoral artery

A case of neurofibromatosis with neurofibrosarcoma over the anterior thigh. The tumour involved the middle to distal femur with poor plane to the rectus and was closely attached to the medial patella. Multiple neurofibromatous lesions over the subcutaneous and along the sciatic nerve were noted (Fig. 9e).

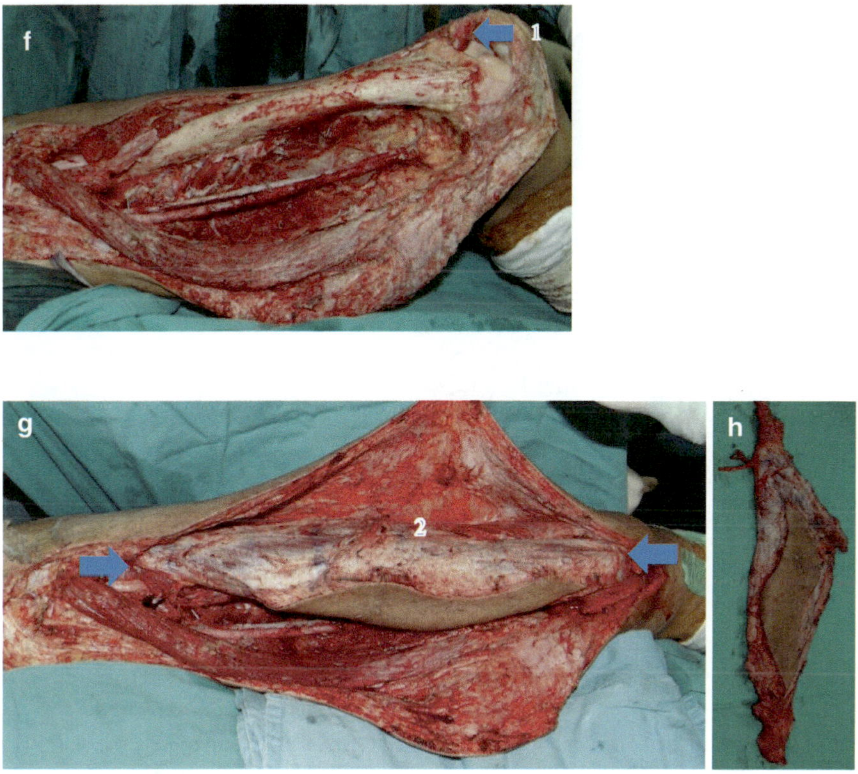

1. Remnant quadriceps tendon (Fig. 9f)
2. A motorised latissimus dorsi flap inserted over superior border of patella and remnant of quadriceps origin (Fig. 9g and h)

Expected functional outcome: Normal ambulation with good range of knee motion; however, extension weakness remained with significant extensor lag (Fig. 9i–k).

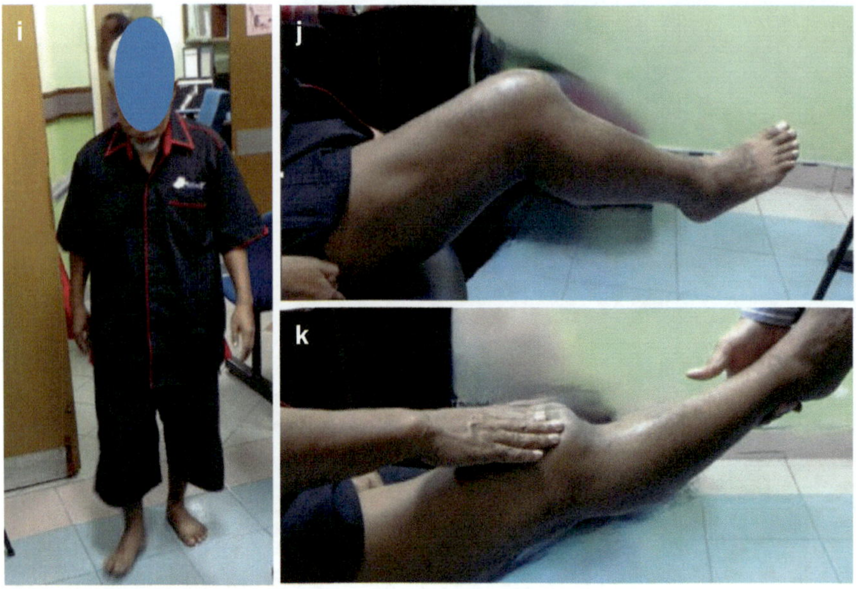

Total Quadriceps Sarcoma with Anterior Femur Infiltration

Resection of entire quadriceps results in knee extensor mechanism loss for walking. Sarcoma infiltrating to the bone or circumferentially surrounding the bone is at risk of positive margin and local recurrence. Furthermore, direct extension of tumour to involve bone or neurovascular structures is associated with high local recurrence and decreased survival due to its early aggressiveness.

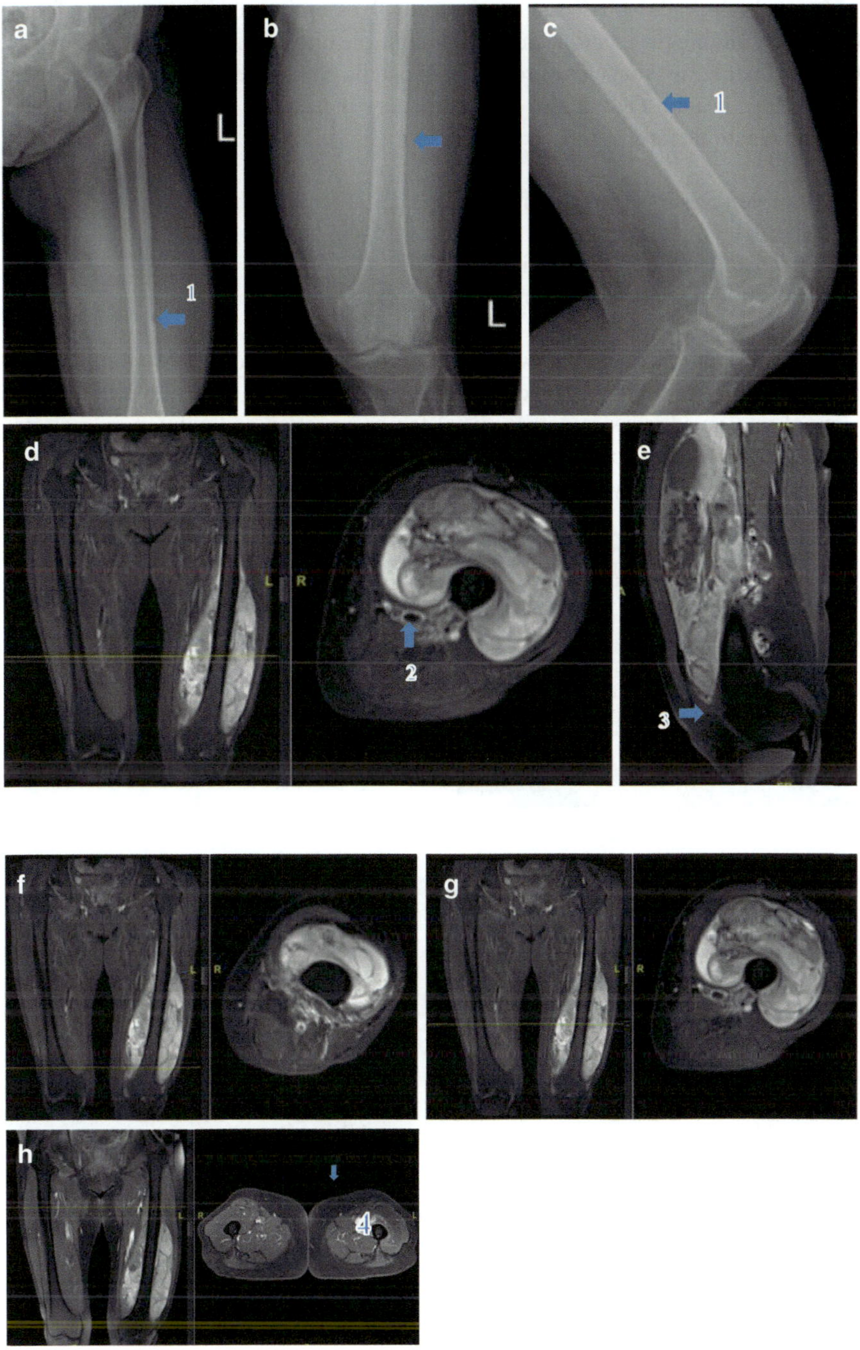
a
L
1
b
L
c
1
d
L
R
2
e
3
f
g
h
4

Large high-grade soft tissue sarcoma involves entire quadriceps circumferentially surrounding the anterior femur with multiple direct infiltration to anterior cortex. The distal extension close proximity to patella and entire suprapatellar synovial pouch (Fig. 10a–h). Patient also had pulmonary metastases and had poor response to early chemotherapy.

1. Multiple invasions over the anterolateral distal femur
2. Superficial femoral artery
3. Suprapatellar pouch extension
4. Vastus intermedius—superior margin

The decision to resect bone was based on radiologic evidence of multiple bone invasion and circumferential involvement of the quadriceps to the femoral bone. In view of total quadriceps resection, distal femur resection and pulmonary metastases, we performed resection with knee arthrodesis and early radiotherapy and subsequent targeted therapy to improve her quality of life.

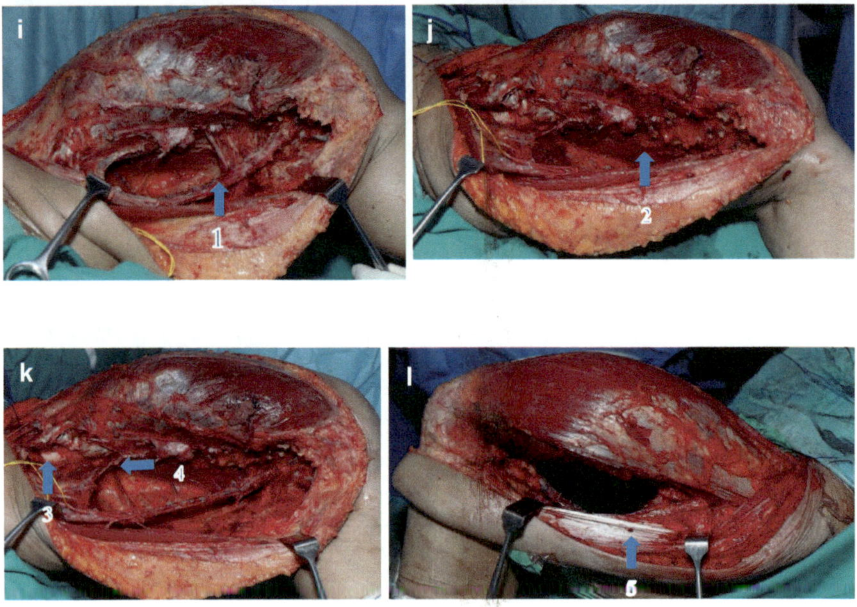

Exploration of femoral vessels from subsatorial canal, mobilisation of posterior compartment leaving short head biceps origin as oncological margin (Fig. 10i and j). A skin flap was raised laterally to the lateral intermuscular septum to expose the entire quadriceps (Fig. 10k–m).

1. Superficial femoral artery
2. Short head biceps origin
3. Superior margin—femoral bone

4. Profunda femoral artery
5. Iliotibial band

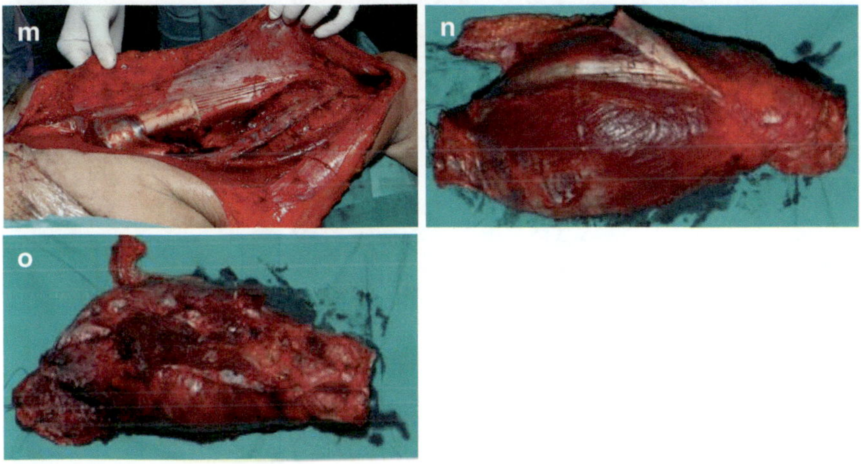

Resection of entire quadriceps with distal femur and entire knee joint including patella with good oncological margin. Reconstruction using intercalary cemented prosthesis (Fig. 10m–q).

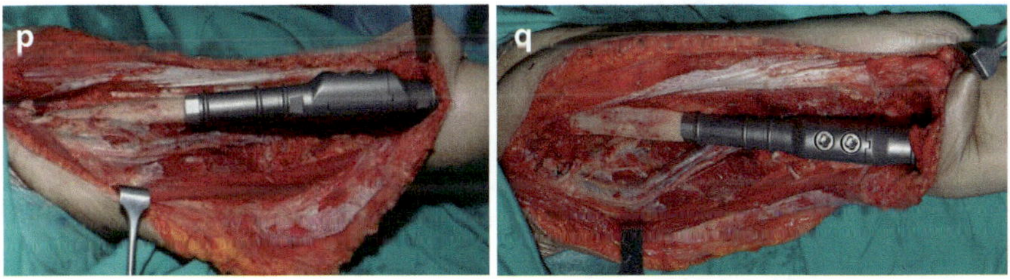

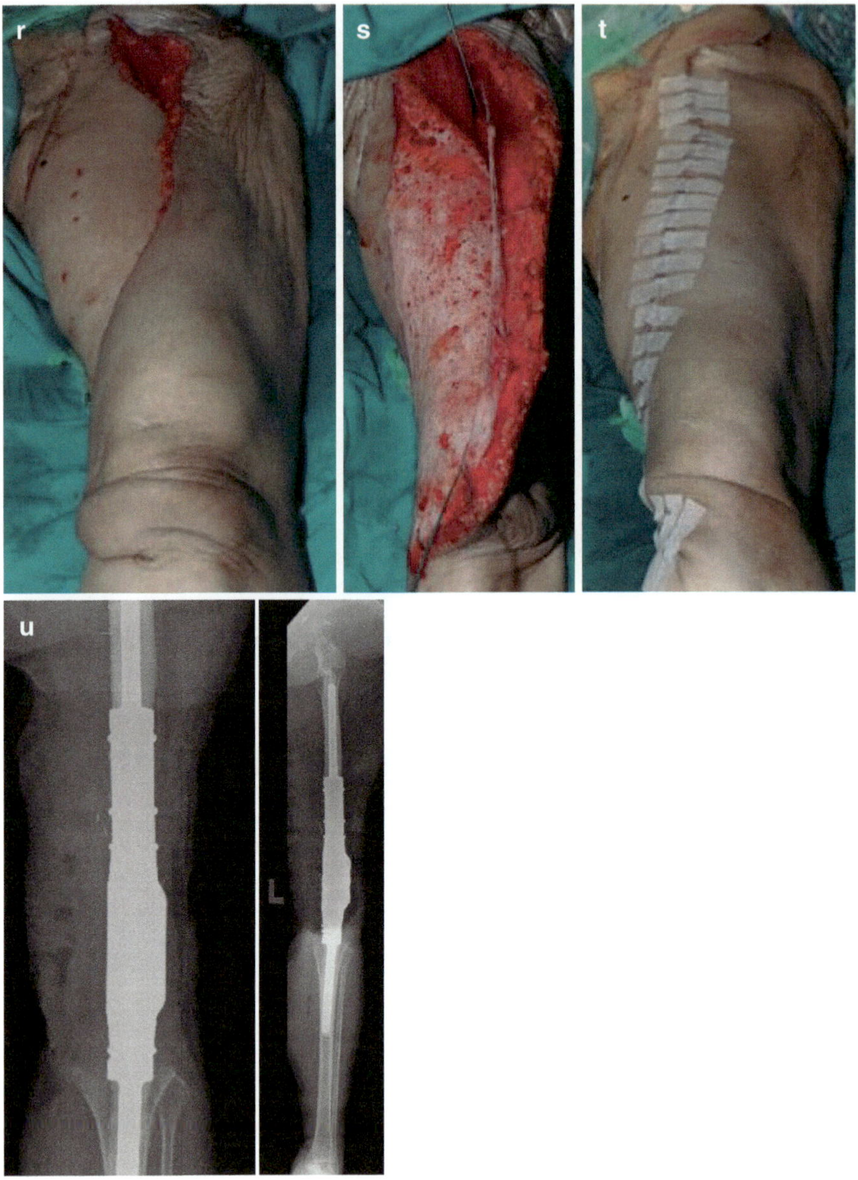

Remaining excessive skin flap was de epithelialized and overlap for closure to improve anterior contour and cosmesis. Knee arthrodesis by intercalary segmental prosthesis is an option after resection of a bone tumour. It allows early pain-free ambulation and acceptable quality of life. Early radiotherapy can be instituted without risk of reconstruction failure (Fig. 10r–u).

Suggested Reading

1. Abed YY, Beltrami G, Delcroix L, Balatri A, Capanna R. Quadriceps muscle reconstruction with free functioning latissimus dorsi muscle flap after oncological resection. Microsurgery. 2009;29(3):189–98.
2. Angelini A, Henderson E, Trovarelli G, Ruggieri P. Is there a role for knee arthrodesis with modular endoprostheses for tumor and revision of failed endoprostheses? Clin Orthop Relat Res. 2013;471:3326–35.
3. Karakousis CP. Tumor of the anterior thigh. In: Atlas of operative procedures in surgical oncology. Springer Science; 2015. p. 311–22.
4. Enneking WF, Shirley PD. Resection-arthrodesis for malignant and potentially malignant lesions about the knee using an intramedullary rod and local bone grafts. JBJS. 1977;59(2):223–36.
5. Ferguson PC, Griffin AM, O'Sullivan B, Catton CN, Davis AM, Murji A, Bell RS, Wunder JS. Bone invasion in extremity soft-tissue sarcoma. Cancer. 2006;106:2692–700.
6. Innocenti M, Abed YY, Beltrami G, Delcroix L, Balatri A, Capanna R. Quadriceps muscle reconstruction with free functioning latissimus dorsi muscle flap after oncological resection. Microsurgery. 2009;29(3):189–98.
7. Kulaylat MN, Karakousis CP. Modified anterior compartment resection of the thigh. Int Surg. 2007;92(5):266–71.
8. Malawer M, James C, Wittig, Sugarbaker P. Quadriceps resection. In: Musculoskeletal cancer surgery. Walter Kluwer Lippincott William & Wilkins; 2012. p. 297–306.
9. Nguyen CM, Ratanshi I, Giuffre JL, Buchel EW, Hayakawa TEJ. The technique of utilizing a single gracilis functional muscle transfer to restore quadriceps function following sarcoma surgery. Plast Aesthet Res. 2019;6:31.
10. Rowell PD, Ferguson PC, Tsoi KM, Nevin JL, Novak R, Griffin AM, Wunder JS. Endoprosthetic reconstruction for lower extremity soft tissue sarcomas with bone involvement. J Surg Oncol. 2023;128(4):660–6. https://doi.org/10.1002/jso.27300.
11. Pritsch T, Malawer MM, Wu C-C, Squires MH, Bickels J. Functional reconstruction of the extensor mechanism following massive tumor resections from the anterior compartment of the thigh. Plast Reconstr Surg. 2007;120(4):960–9.
12. Samargandi R, Benhenneda R, Rosset P, Bisson-Patoue A, Le Nail LR. Buried de-epithelialized flap: an original solution to fill dead space after sarcoma resection in the thigh. Surgical technique and results of 12 cases. Orthop Traumatol Surg Res. 2023:103748.

Posterior Thigh Resection

Wan Faisham Nu'man Bin Wan Ismail,
Syurahbil Abdul Halim, Norazman Mat Zin, Sahran Yahaya,
and Nawaz Hussain Mohamed Amir

Introduction

The posterior thigh consists of the semitendinosus, semimembranosus, biceps femoris and hamstring part of the adductor magnus muscle. The sciatic nerve runs between the medial and lateral hamstrings. Preservation is mandatory for motor and sensory function of the lower limbs. Wide resection of either muscle or entire compartment is possible without significant morbidity.

Surgical Anatomy

- Preoperative evaluation includes assessment of the compartment muscles involved and its correlation to their origin, the ischial tuberosity and linea aspera for bone infiltration.
- The sciatic nerve is covered by thick epineurium. Epineural dissection and preservation is possible with adequate quality margin. The common perineal nerve branch can be pushed by the tumour, and proximal exploration is necessary to prevent injury during resection.

W. F. N. B. W. Ismail (✉)
Prince Court Medical Center, Kuala Lumpur, Malaysia

Orthopaedic Oncology Reconstructive Unit, Universiti Sains Malaysia,
Kubang Kerian, Kelantan, Malaysia

S. A. Halim · N. M. Zin · S. Yahaya
Orthopaedic Oncology Reconstructive Unit, Universiti Sains Malaysia,
Kubang Kerian, Kelantan, Malaysia

N. H. M. Amir
KPJ Ipoh Specialist Hospital, Ipoh, Perak, Malaysia

A. Puri, W. F. N. B. W. Ismail (eds.), *Atlas of Orthopedic Oncology Volume 1*,
https://doi.org/10.1007/978-981-95-8958-6_4

- The biceps femoris inserted on the lateral fibula is in close proximity with the peroneal nerve. Exploration of the nerve and identification of the involved structures is important to achieve quality margins.
- The medial hamstring is inserted in the anserinas bursae tibia and blended with the posterior medial capsule and at risk for tumour extension.

Assessment

An MRI evaluation to identify whether partial resection myomectomy or complete resection of the entire compartment of posterior thigh is required.

- Detailed evaluation of the sciatic nerve and surgical relation with the tumour extension.
- Direct infiltration to the hamstring part of the adductor magnus and another adductor compartment.
- Retro gluteal space origin of the hamstring in proximal tumour extension, surgical planning to release the gluteus maximus insertion for complete evaluation and visualisation of the proximal tumour and ischium are important for clear margins.
- The popliteal space and its correlation with the femoral vessels and posterior capsule in distally situated tumours.

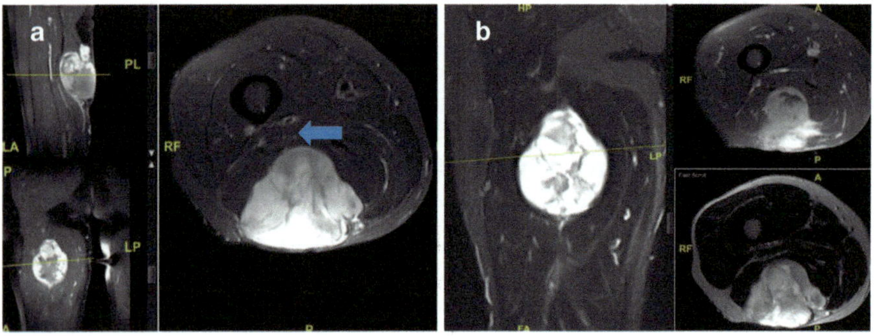

MRI of middle thigh posterior compartment sarcoma involving the semimembranosus and biceps femurs muscle with deep fascia and skin infiltration. The sciatic nerve was spared. Relation of tumour with the sciatic nerve is best seen on T2 image with contrast for evaluation of infiltration and oedema (Fig. 1a and b).

- Sciatic nerve

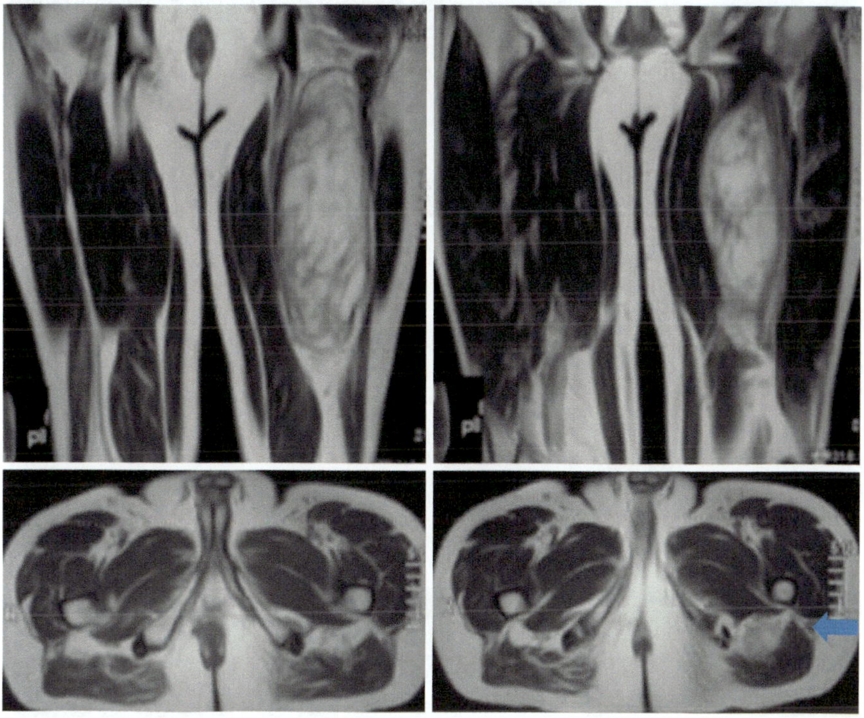

Proximal posterior thigh sarcoma with retro gluteal extension attached to its origin and in close proximity with the gluteus maximus muscle (Fig. 2).

- Retro gluteal tumour extension

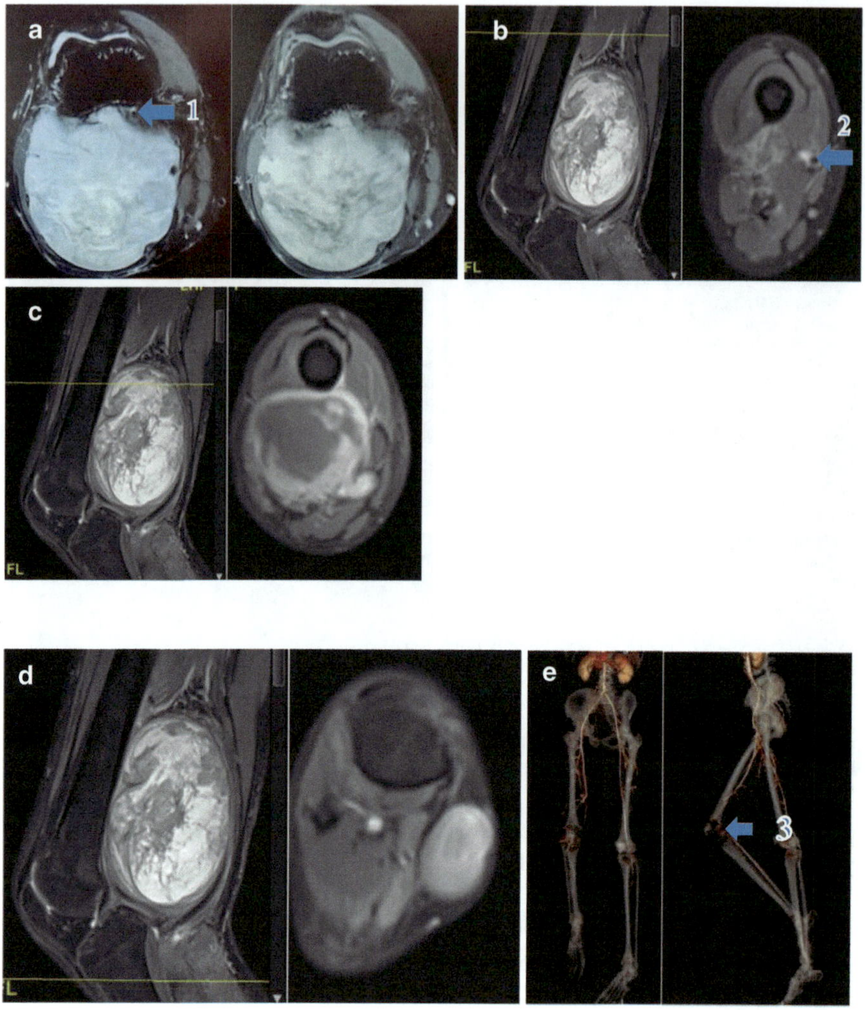

Distal tumour in the biceps femoris muscle closely attached to the posterior knee capsule. Assessment of popliteal vessels and tibial nerve is important for limb salvage or amputation (Fig. 3a–e).

1. Tumour infiltrated posterior capsule
2. Femoral vessel
3. Filling defect popliteal artery with collateral

Surgical Steps

- Patient is placed in the prone position for elevating fasciocutaneous flap and visualisation of the entire posterior thigh from the medial to lateral border of the hamstring.
- In proximally located tumours, the incision is curved laterally to release the gluteus maximus attachment for proper visualisation of the ischium.
- The sciatic nerve lies between the biceps femoris and medial hamstring and can be explored from the medial border by creating a plane and elevating the entire tumour with normal tissues. It rarely needs to be sacrificed. In close proximity to the tumour, epineural dissection of the nerve is possible with negative margins.

Resection of the entire hamstring is well tolerated, and patient is still able to flex the knee with action of the sartorius, gracilis and both the gastrocnemius muscles.

Posterior Thigh Resection

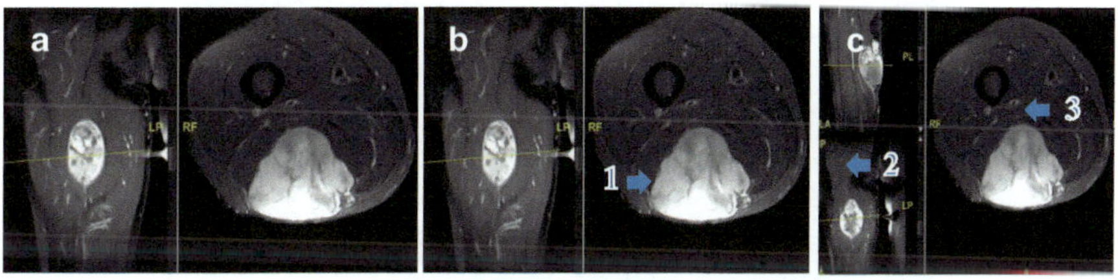

Heterogeneous sarcoma arising from the posterior compartment with skin involvement and oedema. Sciatic nerve is preserved and away from tumour margin. The superior border is below the gluteus maximus insertion (Fig. 4a–c). However, elevation of this muscle is sometimes necessary for achieving a clear superior margin.

1. Biceps femoris
2. Adductor magnus
3. Sciatic nerve

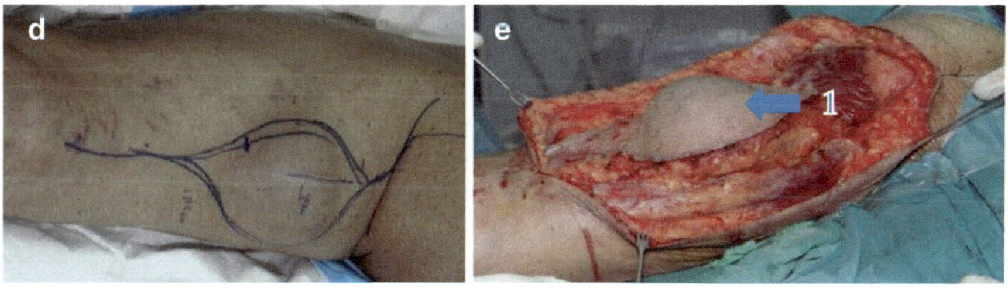

Skin and the subcutaneous tissue were resected together with the tumour to achieve margin (Fig. 4d and e). The tumour in the bicep femoris was attached to the semimembranosus and approached between the muscular plane of semitendinosus and adductor magnus. Wide margin was achieved by resecting 5 cm superior and inferior to the involved muscle (Fig. 4f–h).

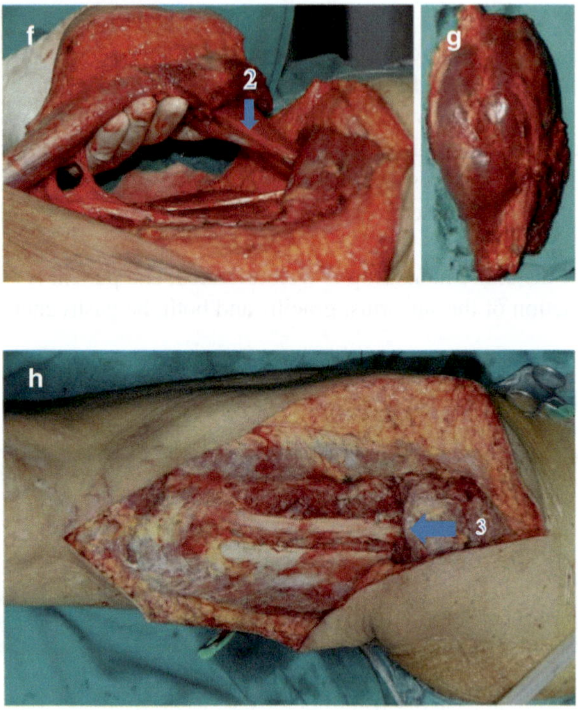

1. Biopsy scar and skin involvement removed as margin
2. Biceps femoris, semimembranosus and semitendinosus
3. Sciatic nerve

Exploration of the sciatic nerve from the lateral side up to the level of ischium to achieve superior 5 cm margin. Lateral attachment of the gluteus maximus has to be released for visualisation of the superior border.

Proximal Posterior Thigh Sarcoma

High-grade sarcoma involving the lateral compartment of the biceps femoris and semimembranosus with proximal extension to the ischial tuberosity. The sciatic nerve was spared (Fig. 5a–h).

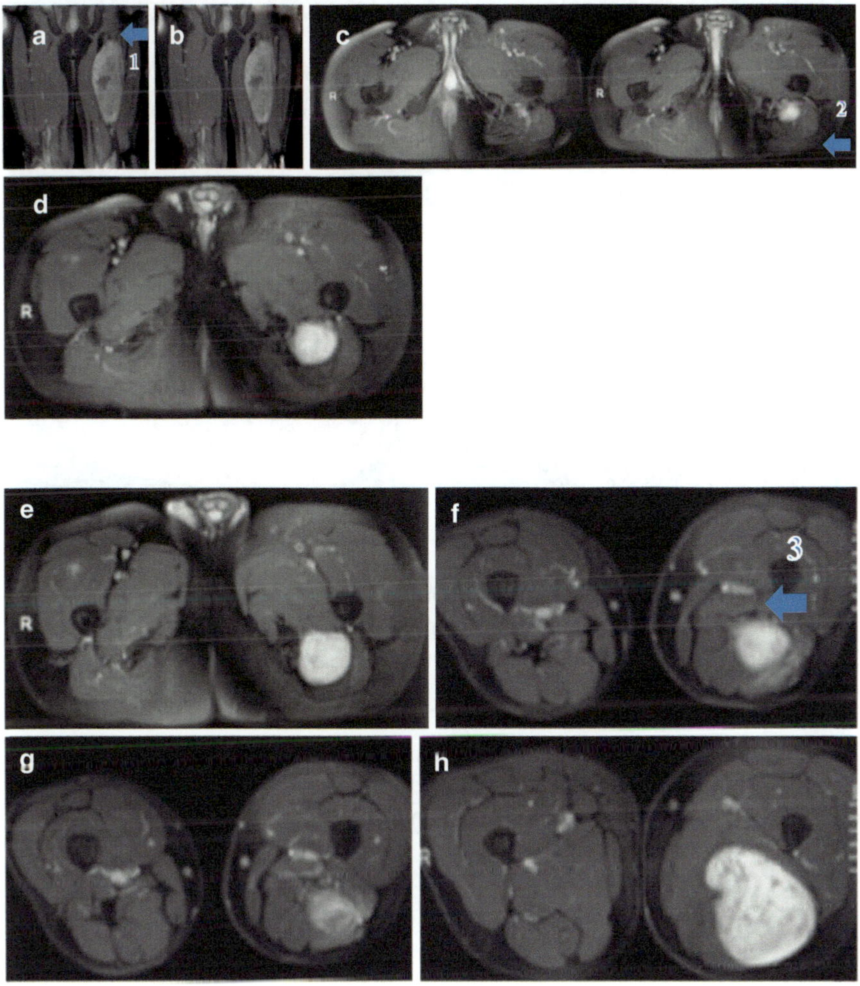

1. Ischial tuberosity—hamstring origin
2. Gluteus maximus
3. Sciatic nerve

Mobilisation of the gluteus maximus from its attachment for complete evaluation of ischial tuberosity. The medial and lateral plane of the hamstring is developed for complete compartment resection. The sciatic nerve is explored laterally after creating a plane of the biceps femoris from the lateral intermuscular septum. The entire tumour is mobilised medially and superior margin resection is at the ischial tuberosity and distal margin based on the MRI distal extension with resection of 5 cm normal muscle (Fig. 5i–l).

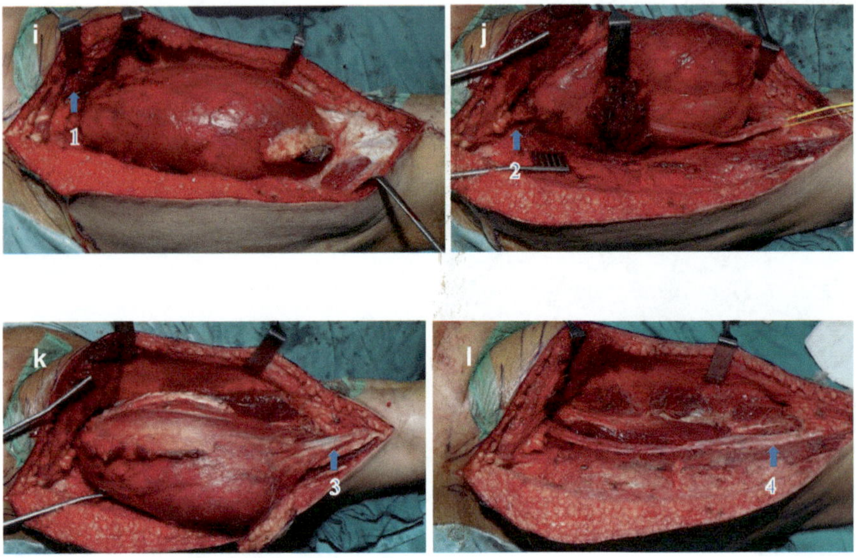

1. Gluteus maximus detached from femoral insertion
2. Ischial tuberosity—origin of hamstring
3. Semitendinosus and semimembranosus
4. Sciatic nerve

High-grade sarcoma requires more extensive compartmental resection. The gluteus maximus attachment must be released for superior exploration of the sciatic nerve and detachment of the hamstring from its origin.

Total Compartment Resection of Posterior Thigh

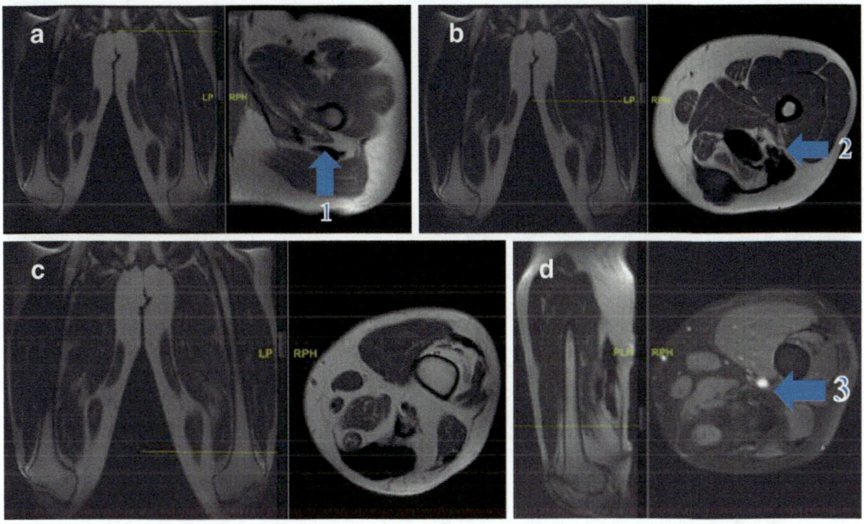

Liposarcoma involving the entire posterior compartment of the thigh with superior extension almost to the hamstring origin and inferiorly to the popliteal region (Fig. 6a–d). Exploration of the sciatic nerve is mandatory for removal of the entire posterior compartment. It can be done by detaching the gluteus maximus superiorly through a lateral approach and by elevating the short head biceps from the lateral inter-muscular septum. The peroneal branch of sciatic nerve can be identified from popliteal region by cutting of biceps femoris tendon and elevation of the muscle from lateral intermuscular septum. Finally, the medial hamstring is cut with adequate margin and elevated superiorly until origin at the ischial tuberosity (Fig. 6e–i).

1. Gluteus maximus with tumour at the hamstring origin
2. Sciatic nerve
3. Popliteal artery

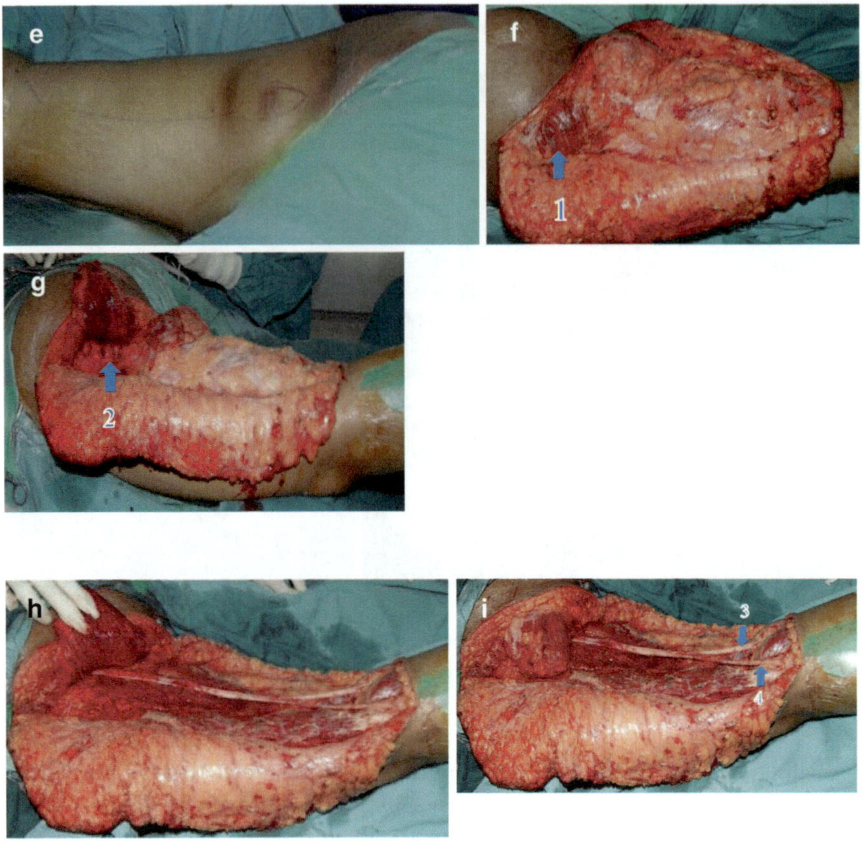

1. Gluteus maximus
2. Hamstring origin—ischial tuberosity
3. Peroneal nerve
4. Tibial nerve

Adductor Posterior Resection

Liposarcoma can present late with massive involvement of the adductor and posterior compartment. The femoral vessels are usually preserved. However, the sciatic nerve can be trapped within the tumour. Exploration of the femoral vessels and total adductor and posterior compartment resection and radiotherapy will minimise the risk of recurrence.

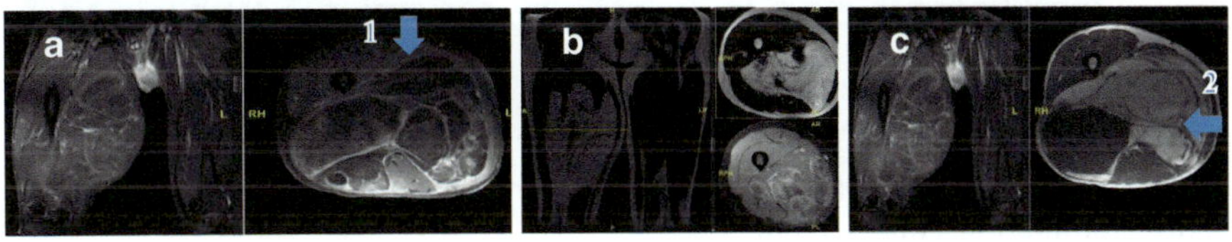

The entire posterior and adductor compartment shows signal changes due to involvement and infiltration by liposarcoma (Fig. 7a–c). Complete resection of the adductor and hamstring is mandatory to achieve clear oncological margin. The superficial femoral vessels are in close proximity to the tumour and have to be explored to prevent injury (Fig. 7d and e).

1. Superficial femoral artery
2. Heterogeneous signal intensity of liposarcoma in adductor and posterior compartment

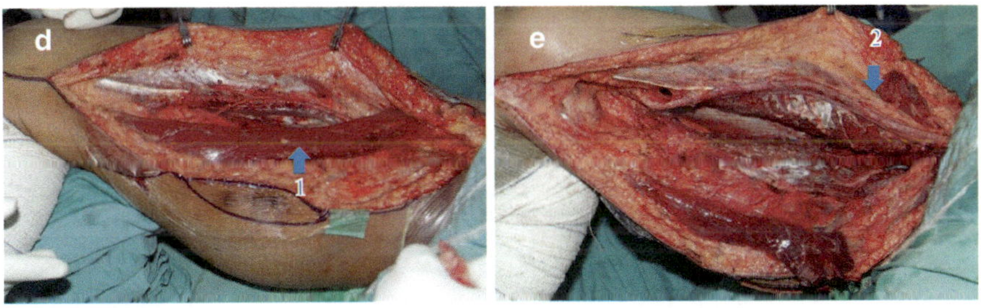

The adductor origin is detached after the superficial femoral vessels are secured and deep profunda vessels are ligated. The sciatic nerve is explored at the popliteal area following detachment of the medial hamstring and gastrocnemius muscle. In low-grade sarcoma, controlled marginal exploration of the nerve between the hamstring muscle plane can be done (Fig. 7f and g). In high-grade sarcoma, resection of the sciatic nerve is necessary with significant distal leg and foot morbidity.

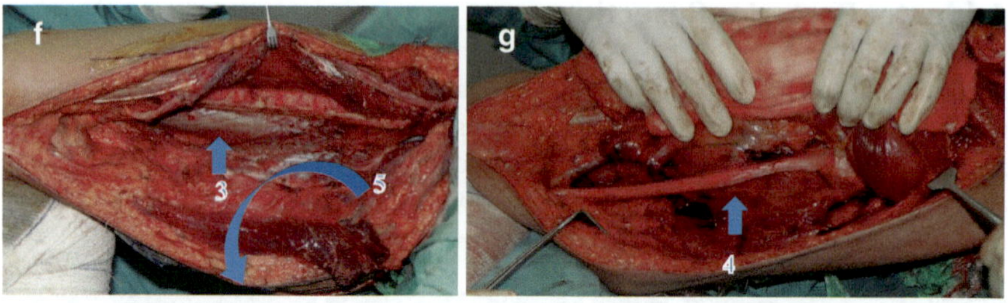

1. Sartorius
2. Superficial femoral vessels
3. Lateral intermuscular septum
4. Sciatic nerve
5. Adductor and posterior compartment mobilised medially after detached proximal origin

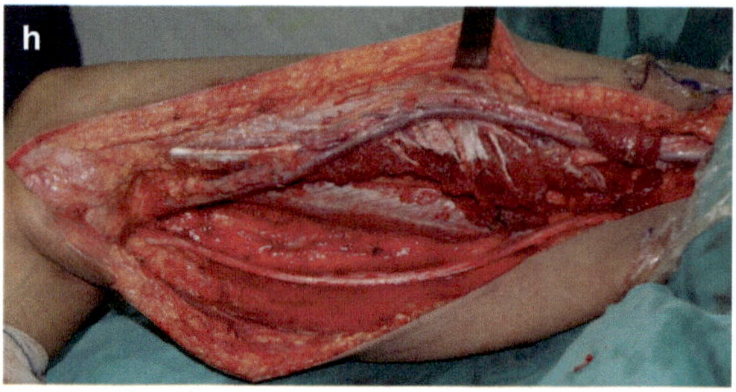

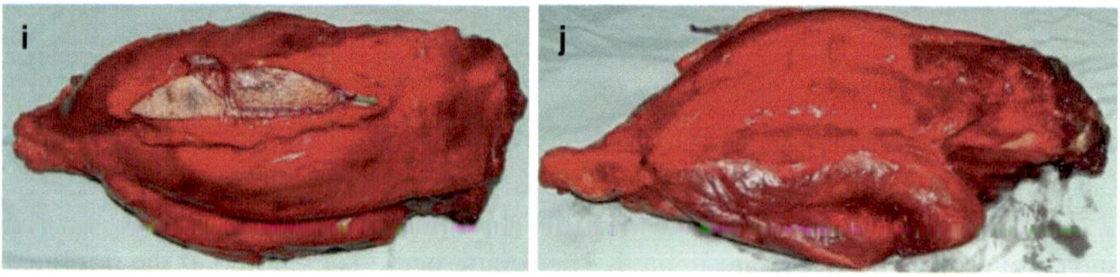

The entire posterior and adductor compartment is resected. The sciatic nerve is left intact and explored within the inter-muscular plane of the hamstring (Fig. 7h–j).

Large Adductor Posterior Compartment

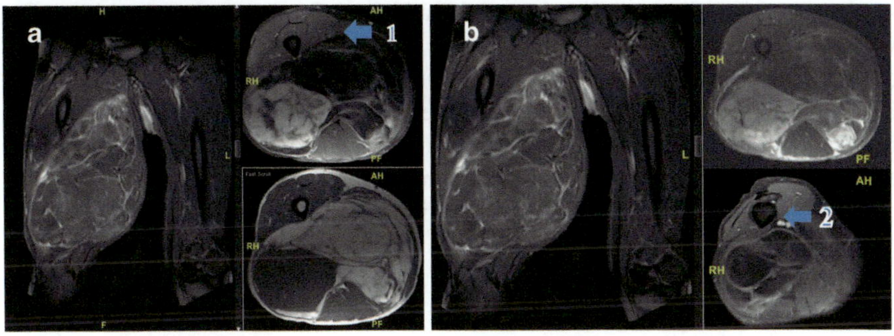

A case of liposarcoma that delayed surgical treatment due to asymptomatic slow growing mass. Involvement of the entire adductor and posterior compartment from origin to insertion, which requires total compartmentectomy for adductor and posterior involvement (Fig. 8a and b).

1. Proximal superficial femoral artery
2. Distal superficial femoral artery

An MRI assessment of tumour extension might be difficult due to massive tumour extension. Complete compartmentectomy resection was planned for optimum oncological clearance. The medial compartment is mobilised to the linea aspera and lateral inter-muscular septum after ligation of the profunda femoral vessel. The entire superficial femoral artery was explored from the inguinal ligament to the popliteal artery. The distal attachment of the adductor magnus is detached from the distal femur for complete mobilisation. The entire adductor muscle group was detached from the linea aspera in similar pattern for complete adductor resection. Exploration proceeded further laterally to the lateral inter-muscular septum by mobilising the short head of the biceps (Fig. 8c and d).

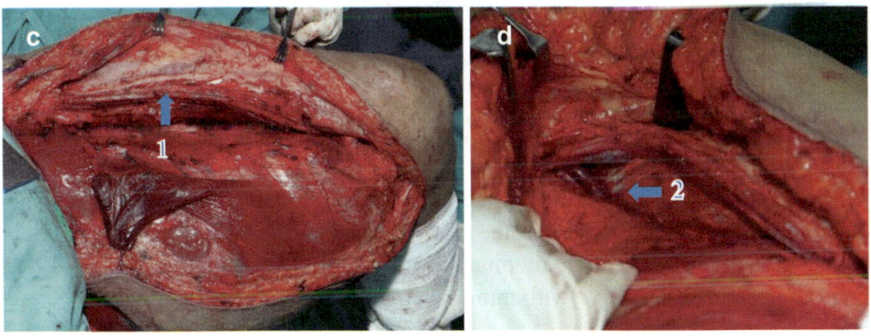

The sciatic nerve is explored from the popliteal fossa posterior to popliteal artery. Mobilisation of the hamstring to the lateral inter-muscular septum and superior and inferior mobilisation of the adductor from its origin and insertion will expose the entire adductor and posterior compartment. The sciatic nerve is attached to the main tumour bulk in between the septum of the hamstring. Exploration through the septum with epineural dissection can be done with minimal contamination. Care must be taken to prevent excessive tension to the sciatic nerve during exploration. Maintaining the biceps femoris origin and attachment during this procedure will minimise sciatic nerve tension and neuropraxia (Fig. 8e and f).

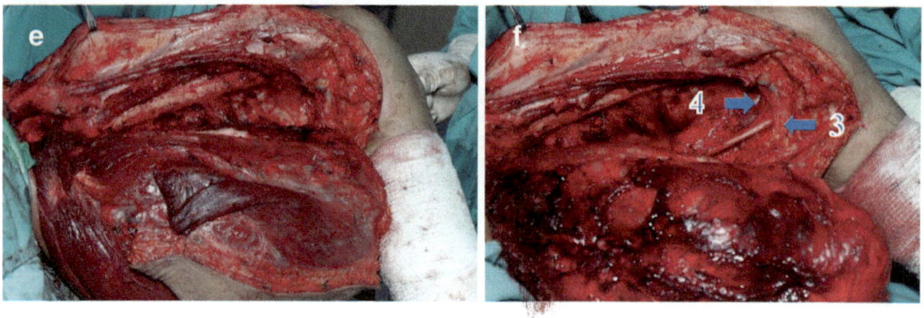

1. Superficial femoral vessels
2. Profunda femoral vessels
3. Tibial nerve
4. Peroneal nerve
5. Sciatic nerve

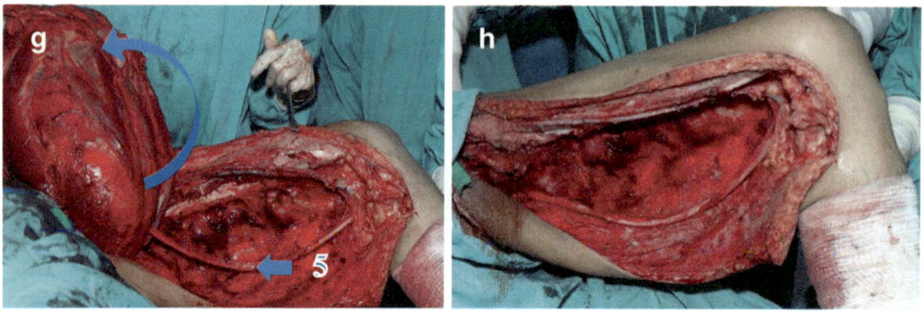

The sciatic nerve can sometimes be trapped within tumour compartment in long-standing lipomatous sarcomas of the adductor and posterior compartment. Intermuscular septum dissection and epineural release after securing the proximal and distal can preserve the nerve with minimal contamination (Fig. 8g and h).

Complete resection of the entire adductor and posterior compartment of the thigh. Ambulation function is expected to be good with presence of thigh quadriceps and knee flexion by gravity during walking and with presence of medial and lateral gastrocnemius muscles.

Suggested Reading

1. Karakousis CP. Tumor in the posterior thigh. In: Atlas of operative procedures in surgical oncology. Springer Science; 2015. p. 329–34.
2. Hussein Sweiti, Noor Tamimi, Fabian Bormann, Markus Divo, Daniela Schulz-Ertner, Marit Ahrens, Ulrich Ronellenfitsch, Matthias Schwarzbach. Limb-salvage surgery of soft tissue sarcoma with sciatic nerve involvement. Sarcoma. 2018:6483579.
3. Jairo Bascetta, Luis Alemán, Héctor Malavé, Gregorio Orta, José Gómez. Resection of the posterior thigh compartment and modification of the surgical technique for bulky tumors. Adv Med Eng Interdiscipl Res. 2023;1(2)
4. Kulaylat MN, King B, Karakousis CP. Posterior compartment resection of the thigh for soft-tissue sarcomas. J Surg Oncol. 1999;71(4):243–5.
5. Malawer M, Wittig JC, Sugarbaker P. Hamstrings muscle group (posterior thigh) resection. Operative technique. In: Orthopaedic surgical oncology. Lippincott Williams &: Wilkins, A Wolters Kluwer; 2012. p. 311–7.
6. Malawer M, Sugarbaker P. Resection of the posterior compartment of the thigh. In: Musculoskeletal cancer surgery. Springer; 2004.
7. Tamimi NN. Results of limb-sparing surgery of soft tissue sarcoma of the lower extremity with sciatic nerve involvement (Doctoral dissertation). 2020. https://doi.org/10.11588/heidok.00027695.
8. Williams MA, Athanasou N, Gibbons CL, Cosker TD. The management and outcome of large volume liposarcomas encasing the sciatic nerve. J Plast Reconstr Aesthet Surg. 2022;7(5):1537–42.

Subsartorial Sarcoma

Wan Faisham Nu'man Bin Wan Ismail

Sarcoma of the sartorial canal is complex and involves multi-compartment muscles that are in close proximity to the femoral vessels and saphenous nerves. Resection of the multiple compartment muscle with good margin around the femoral vessels is important for oncological clearance. Vessel resection and reconstruction are inevitable when the tumour invades and encircles the vessels.

Surgical Anatomy

- The sartorial canal is a tight space in the medial thigh bordered by the sartorius, vastus medialis and floor by the adductor magnus and longus.
- The superficial femoral artery enters the canal surrounded by thick fibrous fascia and exits through the adductor hiatus.
- The saphenous nerve and nerve to the vastus medialis run together with the femoral vessel and supply the muscle. The saphenous nerve exits below the sartorius proximal to the adductor hiatus.

W. F. N. B. W. Ismail (✉)
Prince Court Medical Center, Kuala Lumpur, Malaysia

Orthopaedic Oncology Reconstructive Unit, Universiti Sains Malaysia, Kubang Kerian, Kelantan, Malaysia

A. Puri, W. F. N. B. W. Ismail (eds.), *Atlas of Orthopedic Oncology Volume 1*, https://doi.org/10.1007/978-981-95-8958-6_5

Assessment

- Muscle compartment involvement and its length are important for proper planning of the resection, surgical margin and approach.
- Tumours encircling the entire vascular structures need resection and preoperative preparation of reconstruction.
- Assessment of venous thrombosis and direct tumour invasion are mandatory as venous resection improves oncological clearance.

Surgical Steps

- An extensile approach from the superior part of the femoral canal to the medial knee epicondyle for clearance of the adductor hiatus is needed.
- Tumour arising from the sartorial canal can distort the normal vascular anatomy and needs proximal and distal exploration for control.
- Vessel sheaths are opened away from tumour extension to minimise contamination and achieve quality margins.
- In cases where the entire sheath is encircled by the tumour, resection of the femoral vessels is inevitable.
- The femoral vein can be sacrificed without significant morbidity. Care must be taken to preserve the saphenous vein for superficial drainage in case femoral vein is sacrificed.

Benign Subsatorial Tumour

Sartorius muscle tumour in close proximity to femoral neurovascular through its entire course. Lipoblastoma of the sartorius muscle and is in close proximity to the femoral vessels in the proximal part Distal part of the tumour infiltrated the adductor magnus and needed resection for clearance (Fig. 1a–e).

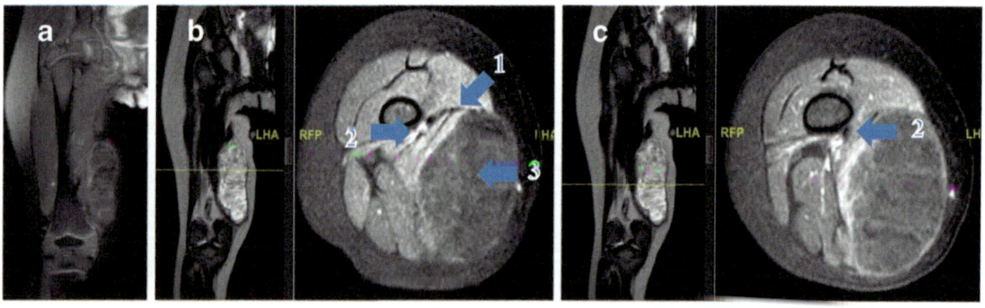

- 1. Sartorius
- 2. Femoral neurovascular
- 3. Adductor magnus

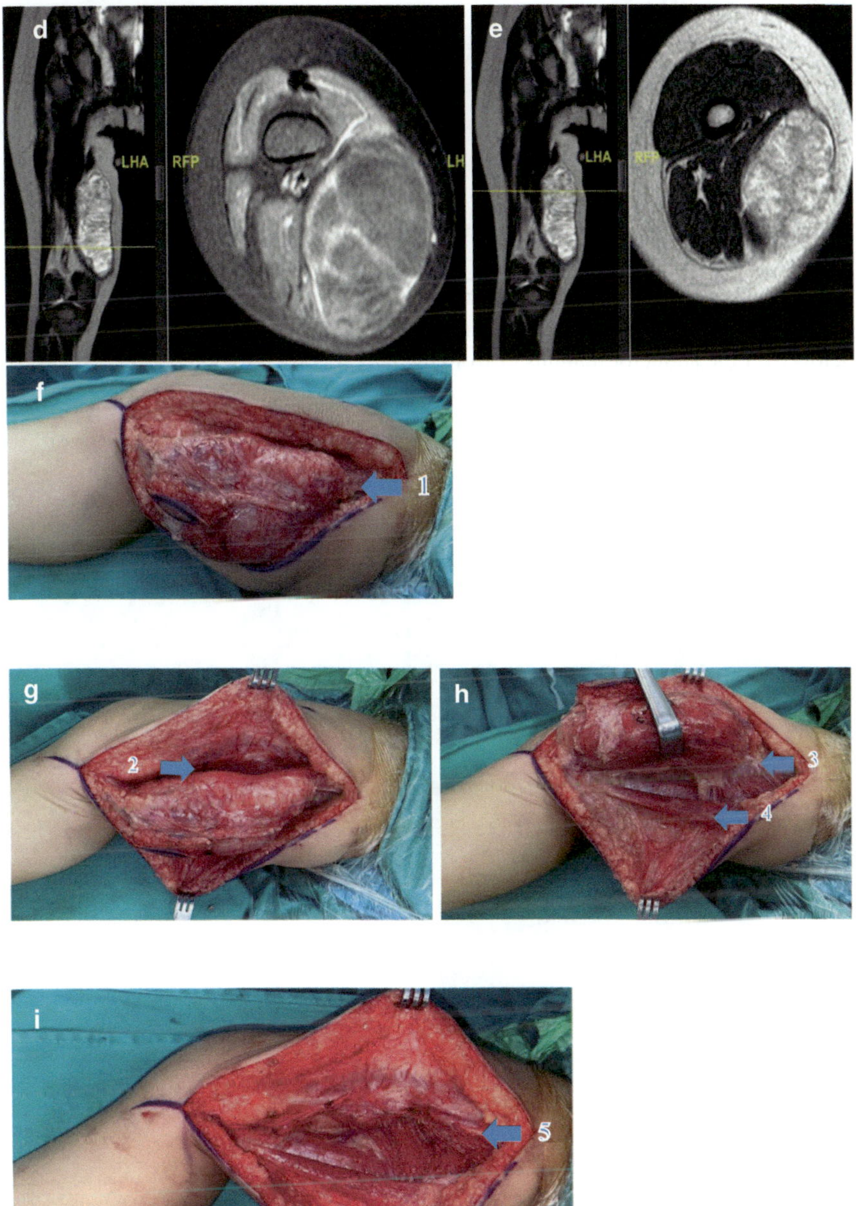

Step-by-step surgical technique resection of sartorius with partial adductor magnus (Fig. 1f–i).

1. Sartorius muscle
2. Plane of vastus medialis to subsartorial space
3. Adductor magnus
4. Gracilis tendon
5. Femoral vessels in intact sheath

Subsatorial Sarcoma with Vastus Medialis Involvement

Subsatorial tumour involves the sartorius muscle and vastus medialis and is in close proximity to the adductor magnus. The femoral vessels are better approached from below over the adductor magnus or from the lateral border after elevating the vastus medialis.

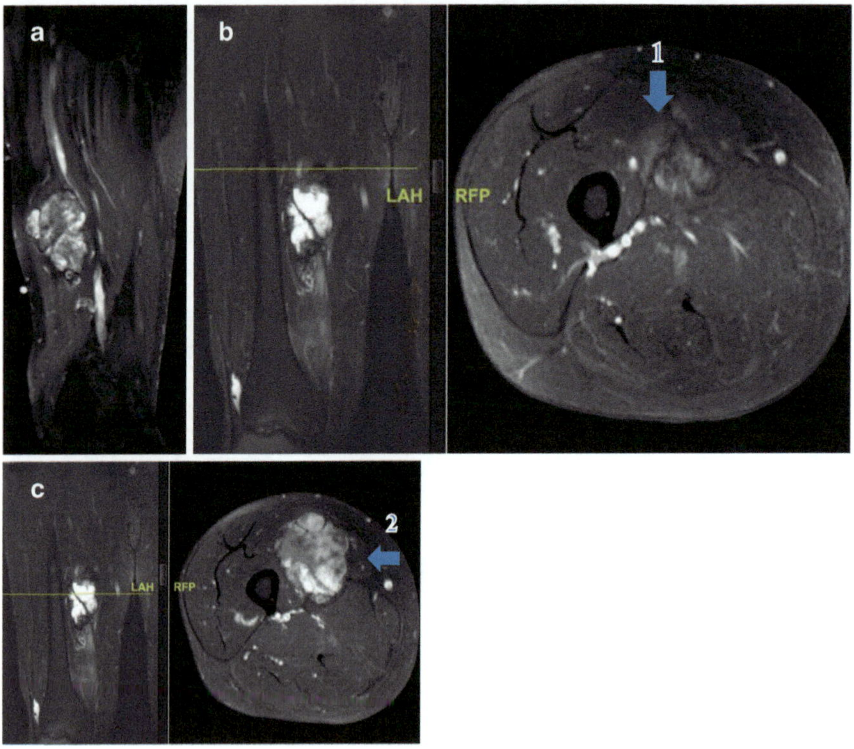

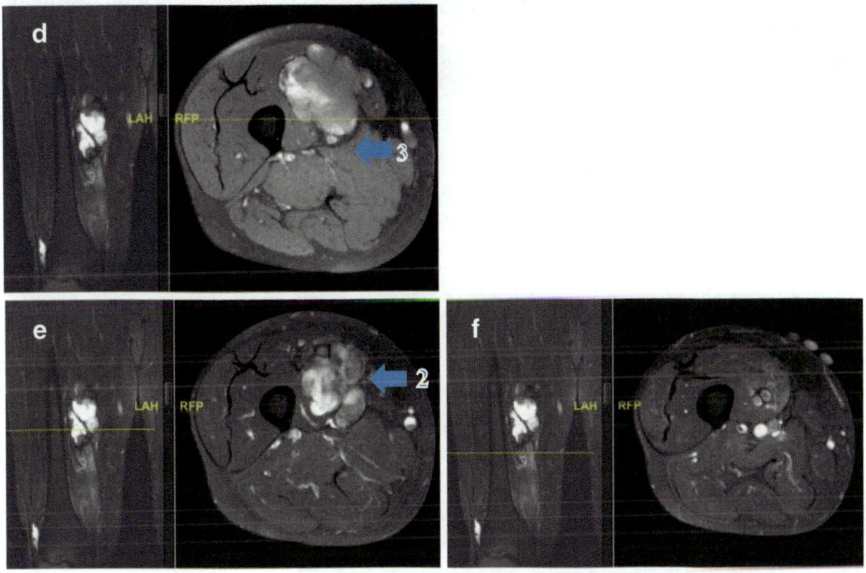

1. Vastus medialis
2. Sartorius—poor plane demarcation of vastus medialis and sartorius
3. Femoral vessels

MRI assessment of the subsartorial sarcoma and its correlation with the femoral vessels is important for surgical approach of the vascular sheath for oncological margin (Fig. 2a–f). In this case, the femoral vessels can be explored and released after clearance of the adductor, vastus medialis and intermedius margin.

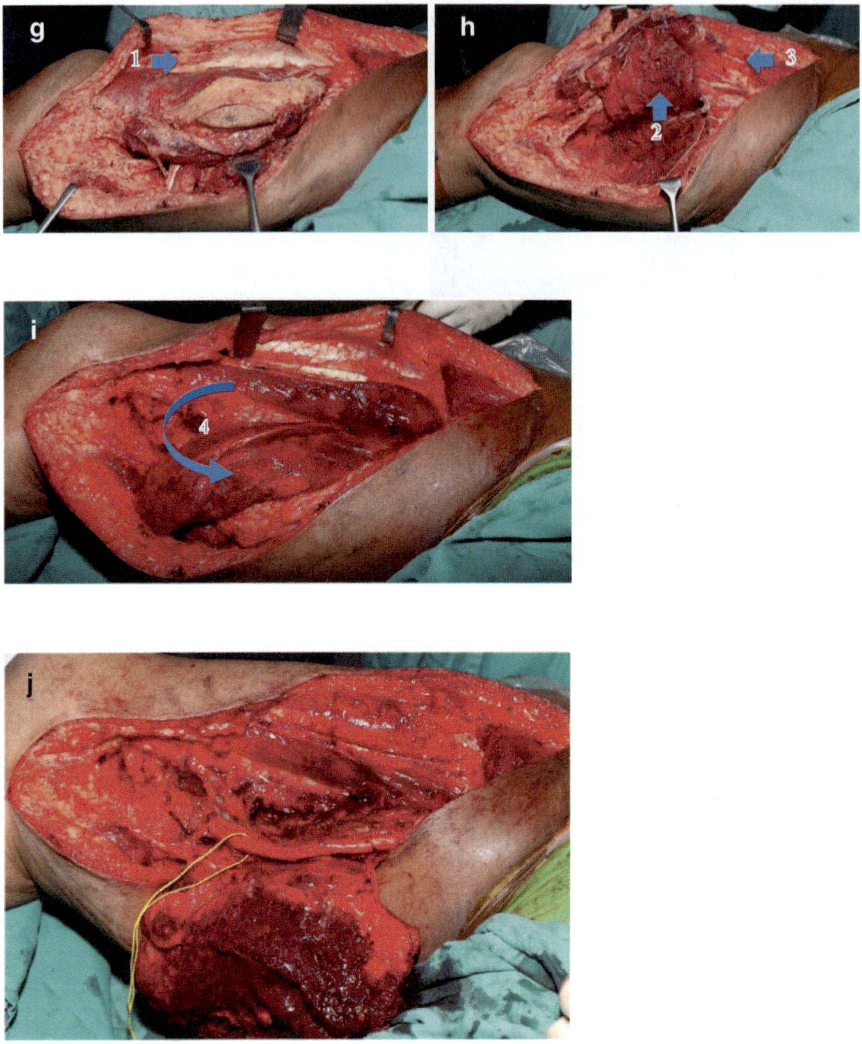

The vastus medialis and intermedius are resected with cuff of tissue from tumour margin to the periosteum layer. The entire tumour is mobilised medially by exposing the femoral sheath. The femoral vessels are cleared from the sheaths for better quality margin (Fig. 2g–j).

1. Vastus medialis
2. Adductor magnus
3. Femoral vessels within the sheaths
4. Entire vastus medialis and intermedius detached from rectus femoris and femoral periosteum

The femoral neurovascular bundle in the sub sartorial canal is closely attached to the tumour; however, it can be released after opening the vascular sheath from below. The adductor magnus, vastus medialis and intermedius muscles are partially resected with cuff of normal tissue for wider surgical margin. The entire tumour is detached together with fascia covering the femoral vessels from the medial border of the vastus medialis for better quality margins.

Subsartorial Sarcoma with Resection of Femoral Artery

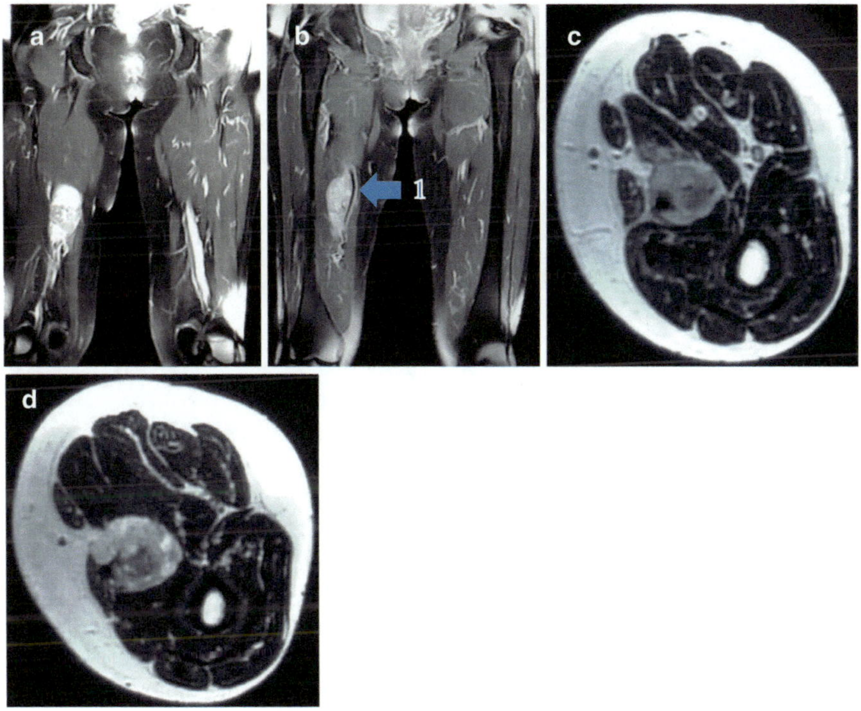

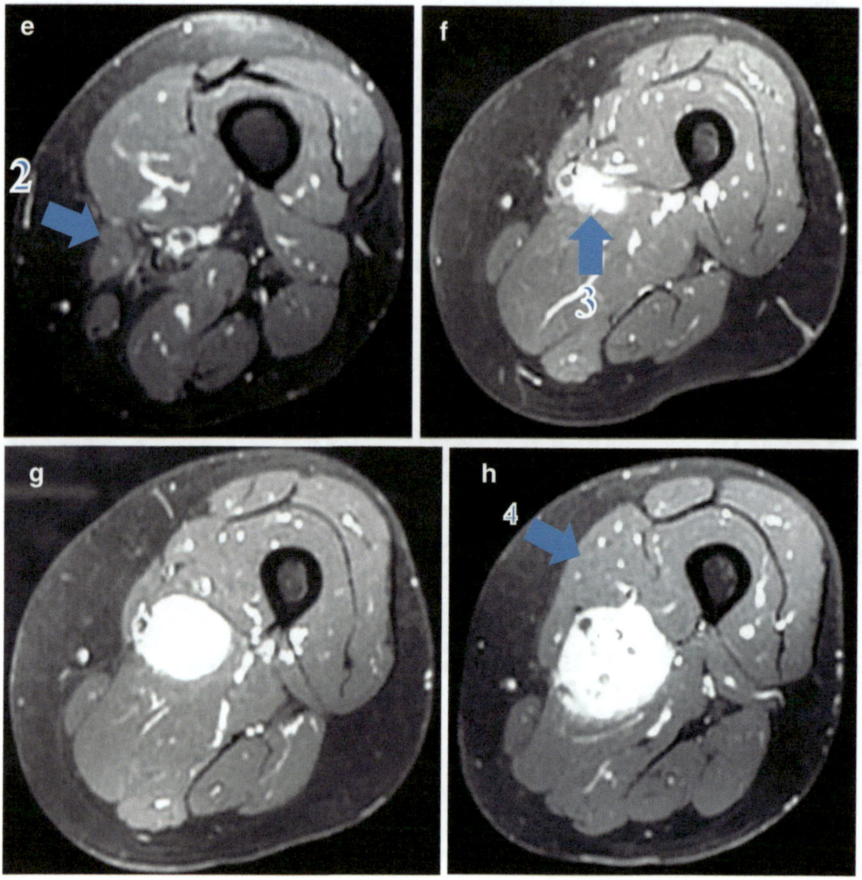

Subsartorial sarcoma involving the adductor magnus and vastus medialis muscle usually will encase the femoral vessels. In cases where entire vessels are within the tumour, the vessels will need to be resected together with the tumour to achieve wide margin surgery. An MRI and MR angiography showed that the vessels were within the tumour (Fig. 3a–h).

1. Femoral vessels
2. Sartorius
3. Adductor magnus
4. Vastus medialis

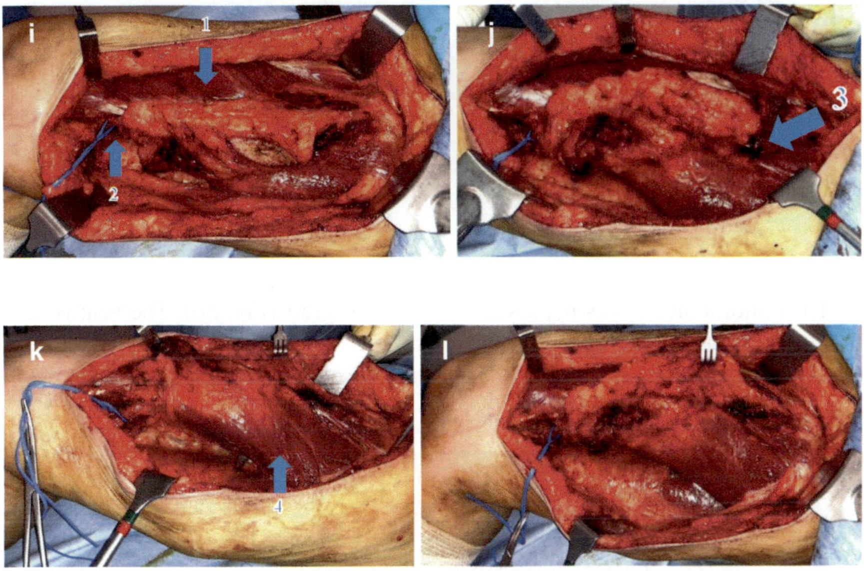

1. Vastus medialis
2. Adductor opening—distal femoral vessels
3. Sartorius—proximal femoral vessels
4. Adductor magnus

The femoral vessels at the mid-thigh were encased and resected in total with the cuff of normal muscle. The proximal and distal femoral vessels were explored in the subsatorial canal and over the adductor hiatus. A medial flap was created over the vastus medialis for a better oncological margin resection. The compartment of the adductor magnus was detached from the distal tendon attachment over the adductor hiatus with 5 cm margin superiorly from the proximal tumour border. A cuff of vastus medialis muscle covering the tumour margin was removed together with femoral neurovascular bundle (Fig. 3i–n).

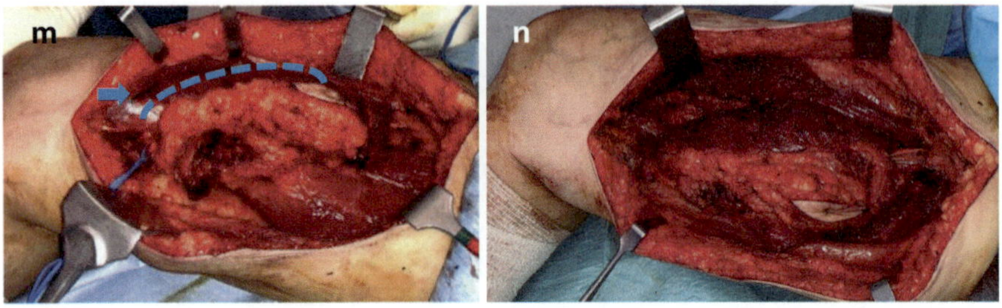

The femoral artery was bypassed with a PTFE graft (Fig. 3o). The vein is normally not bypassed due to good anastomosis over the profunda venous system and superficial saphenous system. The distal limb was evaluated for an hour for acute swelling prior to final closure.

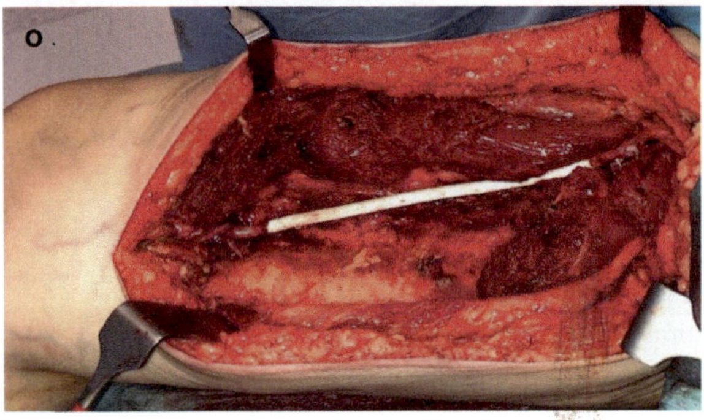

Vascular Tumour with Femoral Popliteal Artery Reconstruction

Subsartorial and popliteal vascular tumour of multiple arteriovenous malformation complicated with recurrence after multiple endovascular intervention. MRI revealed long segment vascular tumour extending from distal femur to the popliteal region involving perivascular fat tissue and surrounding skin (Fig. 4a–f).

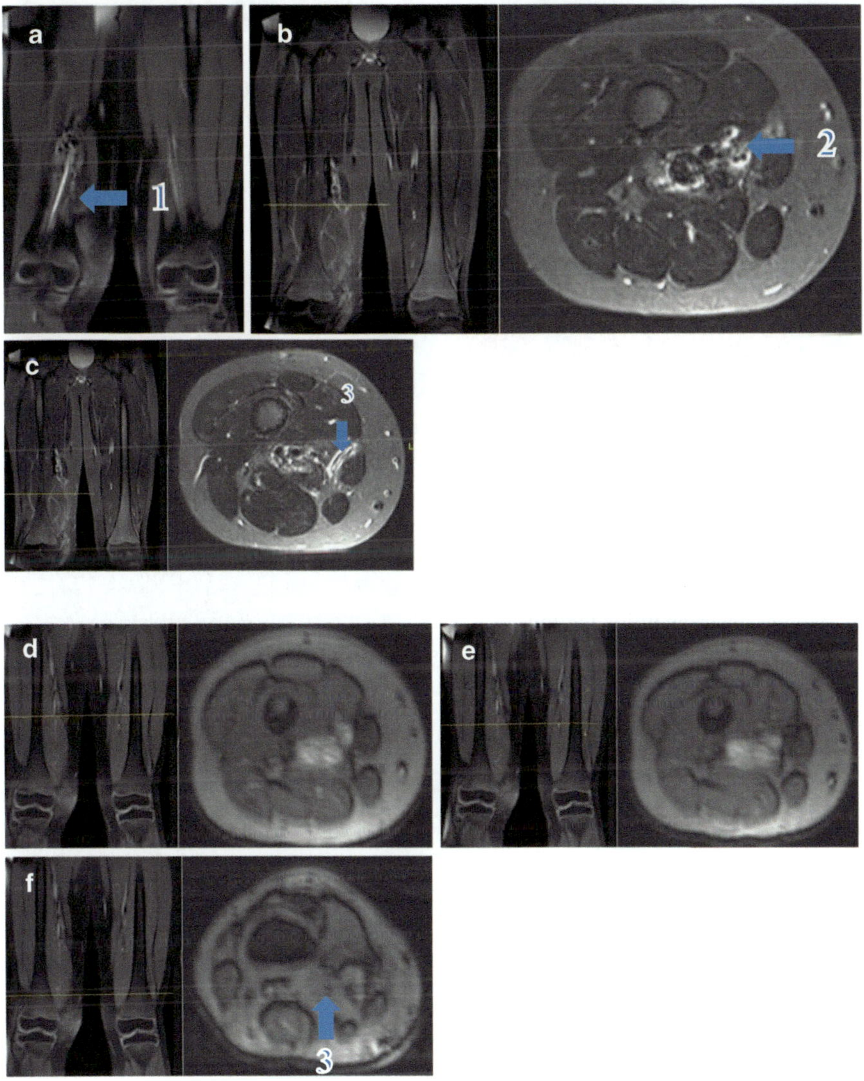

1. Femoral vessels
2. Involvement of sartorius muscle
3. Perivascular fat tissue

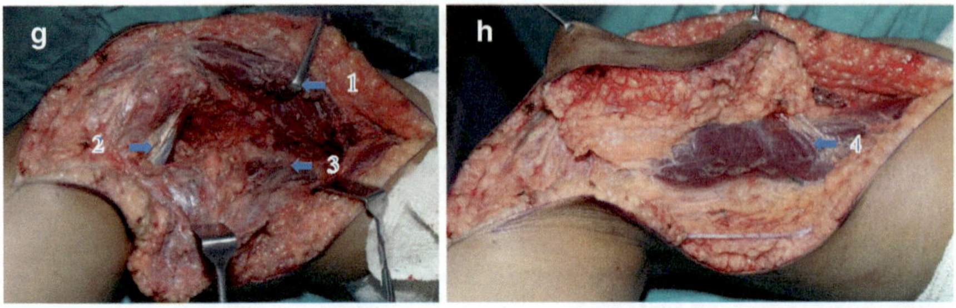

Plane between vastus medialis and medial muscular septum created, the adductor magnus tendon insertion at the distal femur detached to mobilise the femoral sheath together with sartorius muscle. Popliteal fossae explored from medial side and entire arteriovenous malformation removed together with surrounding fat tissue (Fig. 4g–j).

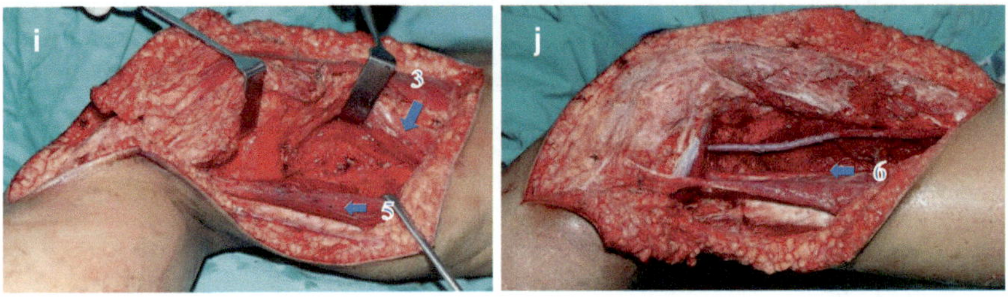

1. Vastus medialis
2. Medial gastrocnemius tendon
3. Adductor magnus with femoral vessels mobilises medially
4. Sartorius muscle
5. Gracilis muscle
6. Sciatic nerve

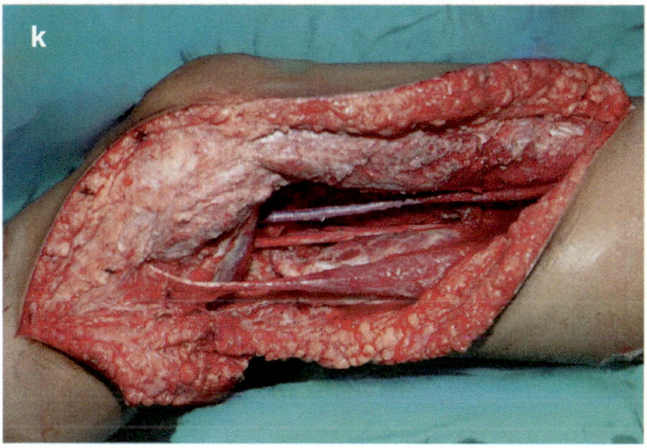

The femoral artery was bypassed with reverse saphenous vein graft (Fig. 4k).

Suggested Reading

1. Bickels ASJ, Tov TB, Malawer MM. Primary tumors of the sartorial canal: limb sparing resection of soft-tissue sarcomas arising in a unique location. Curr Orthop Pract. 2009;20:416–22.
2. Karakousis CP. Tumor of the anterior thigh. Tumour along the femoral vessels atlas of operative procedures in surgical oncology 311–322. Springer Science; 2015.
3. Matsushita M, Kuzuya A, Mano N, et al. Sequelae after limb- sparing surgery with major vascular resection for tumour of the lower extremity. J Vasc Surg. 2001;33:694–9.
4. Sternheim A, Bickels J, Ben-Tov T, Malawer MM. Space sarcomas: extra compartmental soft tissue tumors of the lower extremities a systematic approach to sarcomas of the femoral triangle, sartorial canal, and popliteal space. J Surg Oncol. 2009;99(5):281–91.
5. Singh DK, Jalan D, Narwani A, Kumar N, Rustagi A, Saifi AS, Singh U, Kaur S, Nischal, N. Assessment of neurovascular bundle involvement by an extremity sarcoma on MRI: a critical decision for sarcoma surgeon. Skeletal Radiol. 2025;54(9):1803–10.

Popliteal and Leg Sarcoma

Wan Faisham Nu'man Bin Wan Ismail

Popliteal sarcoma arises from the attachment of the muscle and tendon around the back of the knee. Close proximity to the popliteal vessels and tibial nerve needs a careful preoperative assessment and meticulous surgical technique to achieve quality margin for sarcoma resection.

Surgical Anatomy

- Popliteal fossa is a diamond- shaped structure bordering the biceps femoris, semimembranosus and semitendinosus superiorly and gastrocnemius head inferiorly.
- The femoral arteries enter the space from the adductor magnus opening and join the sciatic nerve.
- The popliteal artery is traced from the adductor opening through its course until trifurcation and peroneal tibial junction for its involvement. It lies directly behind the posterior capsule of the knee joint. Branches of the geniculate arteries must be carefully evaluated and ligated to prevent bleeding.
- The peroneal nerve exits deep in the lateral gastrocnemius head and biceps femoris.

W. F. N. B. W. Ismail (✉)
Prince Court Medical Center, Kuala Lumpur, Malaysia

Orthopaedic Oncology Reconstructive Unit, Universiti Sains Malaysia, Kubang Kerian, Kelantan, Malaysia

A. Puri, W. F. N. B. W. Ismail (eds.), *Atlas of Orthopedic Oncology Volume 1*,
https://doi.org/10.1007/978-981-95-8958-6_6

Assessment

Sarcoma of the popliteal fossae will displace the neurovascular structures. Assessment of its structures is crucial for salvaging limbs.

- The anatomical origin of the tumour and extension must be identified to plan the surgical approach and margin.
- The popliteal artery is traced in detail through its course for its involvement.
- The superior extension, particularly the head of the gastrocnemius and popliteal loose adipose tissues, must be evaluated for wide oncological margin.
- Distal extension of tumour should be measured and planned for quality of margin.

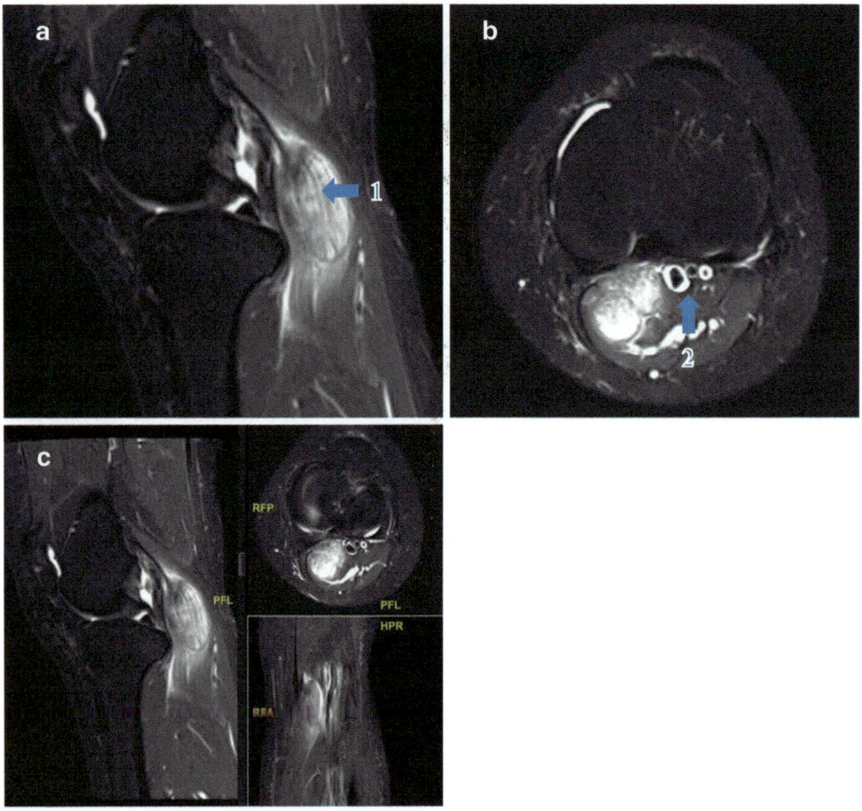

The MRI showed a tumour arising from medial gastrocnemius muscle with local oedema of the tendon to the femoral origin distally and in close proximity with the popliteal artery and vein (Fig. 1a–c).

1. Medial gastrocnemius tendon and muscle
2. Popliteal artery and tibial nerve

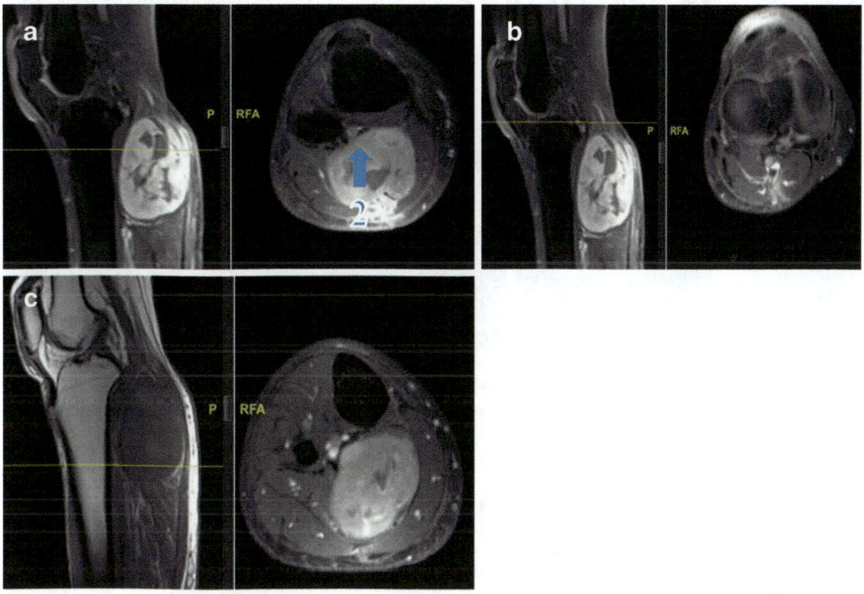

Larger tumour arising from the soleus with poor zone demarcation of both the head of gastrocnemius and centre infiltration. The superior border of the gastrocnemius was infiltrated, and the surrounding popliteal fat tissue showed evidence of oedema. The popliteal neurovascular was spared (Fig. 2a–c).

Resection of Proximal Medial Gastrocnemius and Soleus Muscle

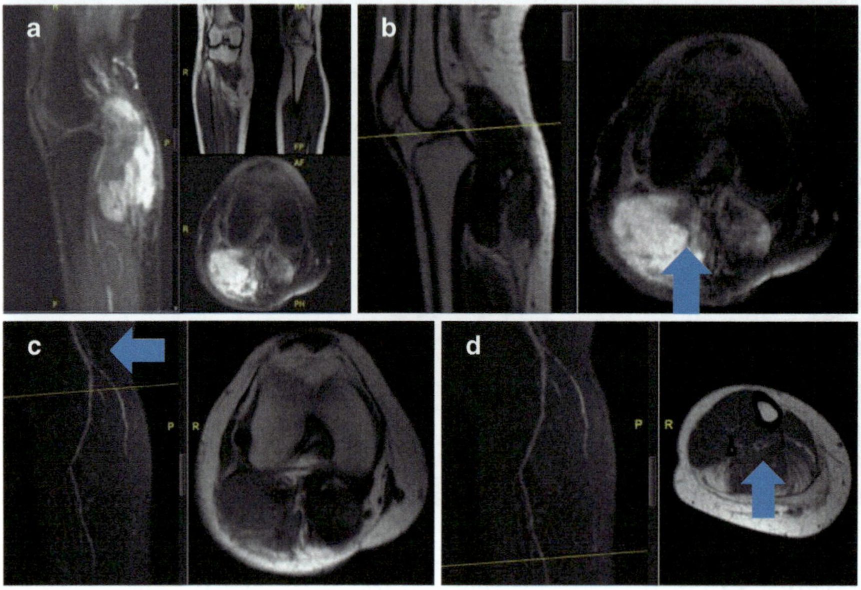

A case of sarcoma involving the proximal medial gastrocnemius extension to part of the medial soleus. The neurovascular was spared and laterally displaced (Fig. 3a–d).

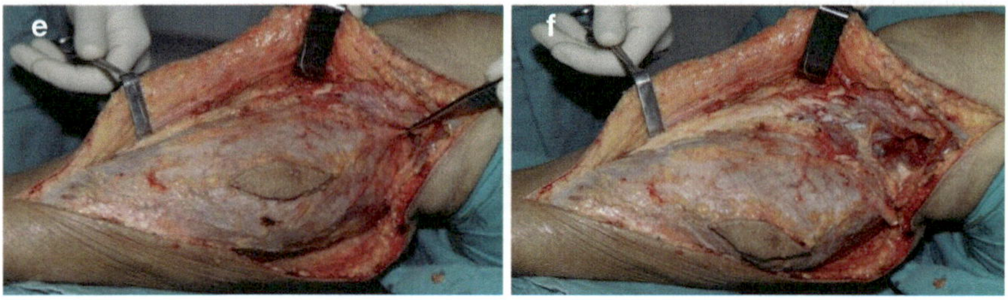

The tumour was approached medially by creating a flap to the medial tibial for identification of the soleal line. The entire tendon attached to the anserinus bursae proximally detached for exposure of medial gastrocnemius origin for quality margin (Fig. 3e and f).

1. Soleal line
2. Popliteal vessels exposure after detached gastrocnemius tendon
3. Tendon attachment to the anserinus bursae detached

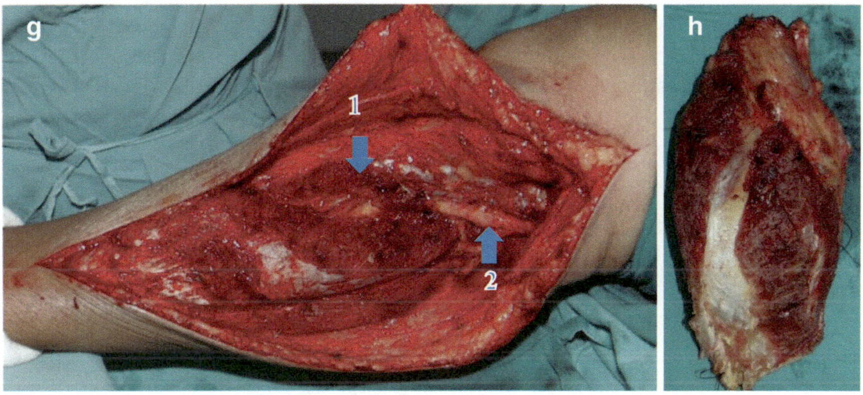

The entire medial gastrocnemius muscle was resected together with the proximal soleus for wide margin surgery. The popliteal and posterior tibial vessels were well visualised and spared (Fig. 3g and h).

1. Soleal line
2. Tibial nerve and popliteal vessels

Resection of Popliteal Gastrocnemius Soleus

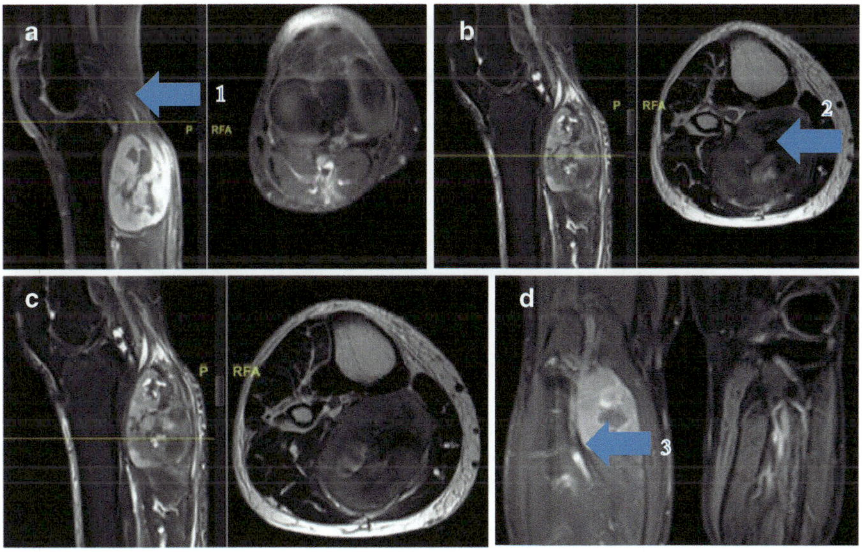

Larger tumour arising from the soleus muscle with poor zone demarcations of both the gastrocnemius muscles and displacing the neurovascular structures (Fig. 4a–d).

1. Medial gastrocnemius tendon attachment
2. Soleus
3. Popliteal trifurcation

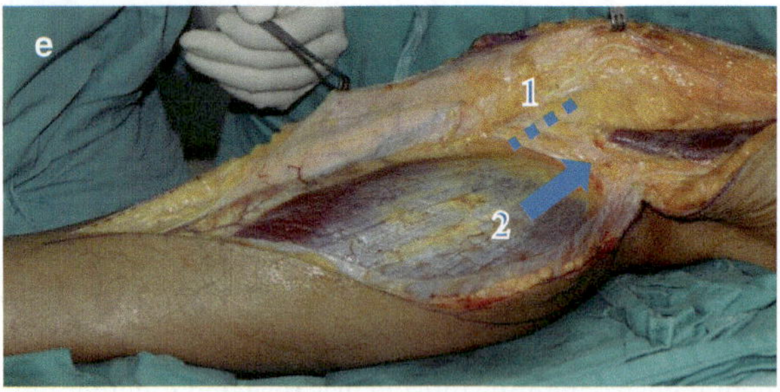

The anserinus tendon was detached from the medial tibial for medial exploration. The medial gastrocnemius head was detached from its insertion and soleus muscle was freed from the soleal line and subsequently detached from the medial fibula border. Care must be taken to prevent injury to the peroneal artery along the fibula. The attachment of the soleus over lateral fibula was finally detached after distal resection to prevent injury to the neurovascular structures (Fig. 4e and f).

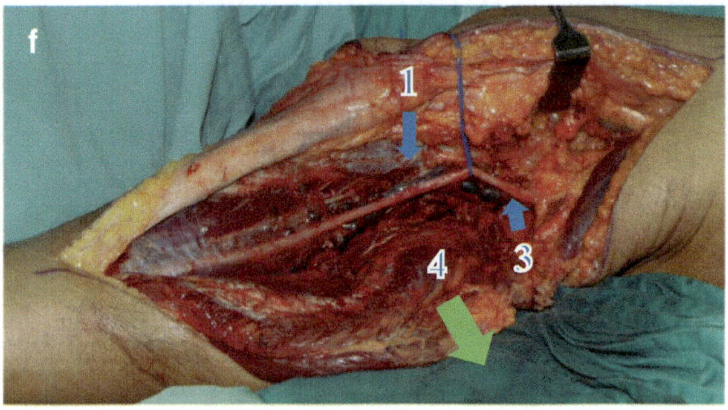

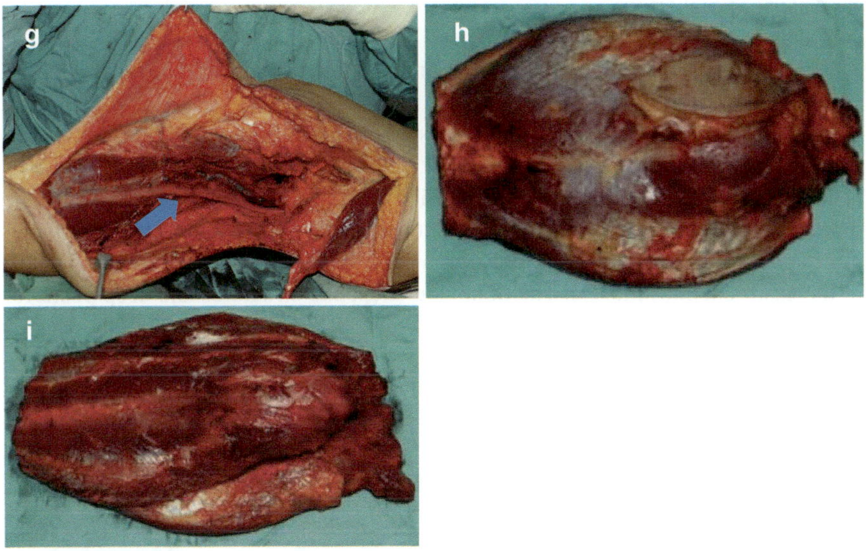

Finally, the gastrocnemius head was detached, and the popliteal fossae fat was removed together after exploration of the popliteal artery and major trifurcation branches (Fig. 4g–i).

1. Soleal line
2. Sartoris, gracilis and semitendinosus tendon
3. Popliteal vessels and tibial nerve
4. Both gastrocnemius head and soleus mobilise medially after exploration of neurovascular structures (green arrow)

Posterior Middle Compartment Resection

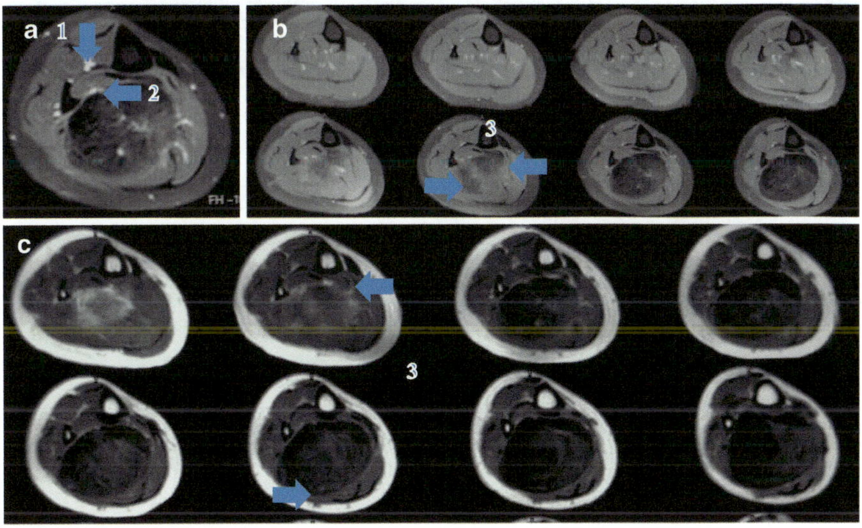

1. Anterior tibial artery
2. Displaced posterior tibial vessels
3. Poor plane demarcation with both medial and lateral gastrocnemius

Mid-leg resection is less demanding as the neurovascular structure is confined within the fascia of the deep compartment. The oncological anatomical boundaries is more definite. The superior and inferior resection margins are based on the tumour's grade and extension. The entire superficial compartment of the gastrocnemius and soleus was involved. There was a poor plane demarcation with both heads of the gastrocnemius muscle. The tibial neurovascular structures and deep posterior compartment were spared (Fig. 5a–c).

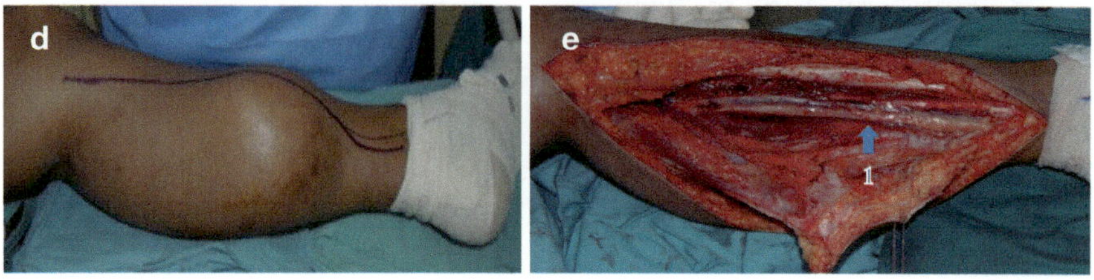

Exploration of the medial neurovascular structures and ligation of the vessels to medial and lateral gastrocnemius head. The fibula attachment of the soleus was detached. Care must be taken to identify and protect the peroneal vessels, which are in close proximity to the fibula (Fig. 5d and e).

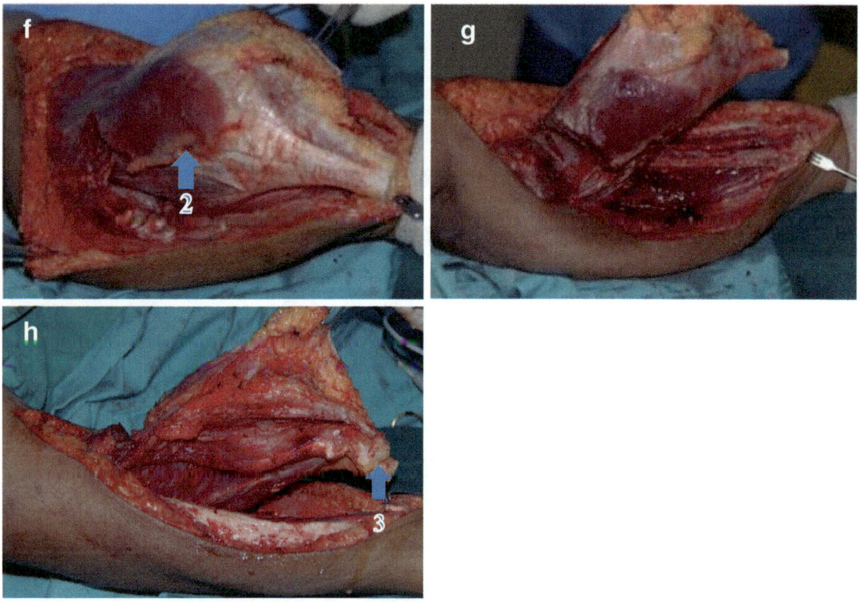

The distal margin over the Achilles tendon was identified and detached. A proximal margin of at least 3 cm from superior tumour over the gastrocnemius was preserved for bulk and leg cosmesis (Fig. 5f–h).

1. Posterior tibial vessels and nerve
2. Both medial and lateral gastrocnemius
3. Achilles tendon

Resection of Lateral Compartment Leg

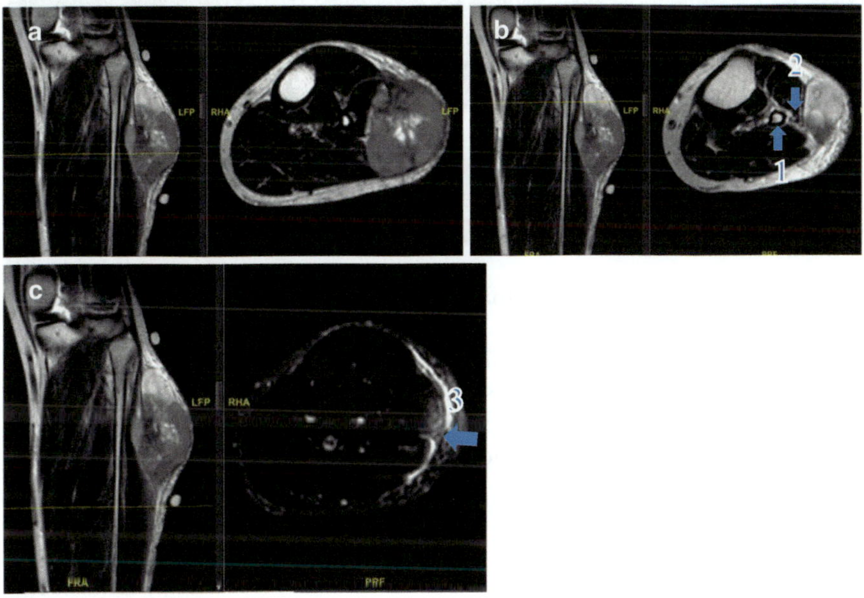

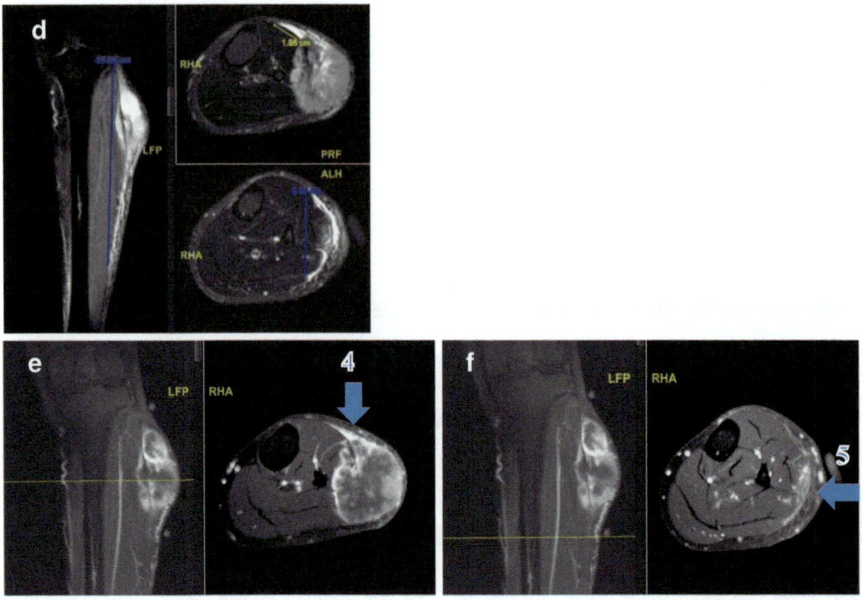

Soft tissue sarcoma arising from proximal anterolateral compartment will affect the peroneal compartment, anterior and superficial posterior, especially the lateral gastrocnemius and soleus. The peroneal nerve must be carefully evaluated on an MRI for involvement and preoperative disability consultation and preparation of a cable nerve graft. The deep posterior compartment and posterior neuromuscular structure must be carefully evaluated for bigger tumour involvement (Fig. 6a–f).

1. Fibula
2. Peroneal artery
3. Soft tissue and skin oedema
4. Superior tumour tail with extensive skin oedema "infiltration"
5. Gadolinium-enhanced image confirmed tail involvement but limited distal extension

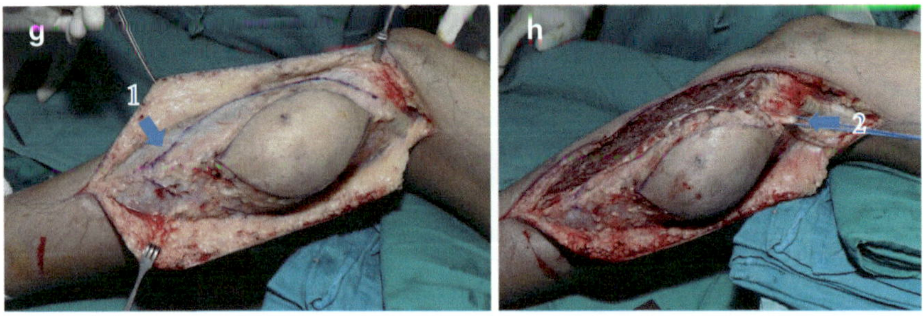

Sarcoma involving the entire peroneal compartment with poor zone demarcation with extensor hallucis anteriorly and lateral gastrocnemius and soles posteriorly. The peroneal nerve cannot be traced at the level neck of the fibula. However, the deep posterior structures and neuromuscular structures were not involved.

1. Mark for resection of fascial and tumour border (Fig. 6g)
2. Peroneal nerve protected (Fig. 6h)
3. Lateral border fibula
4. Soleus muscle
5. Lateral gastrocnemius flap—covers fibula and peroneal nerve

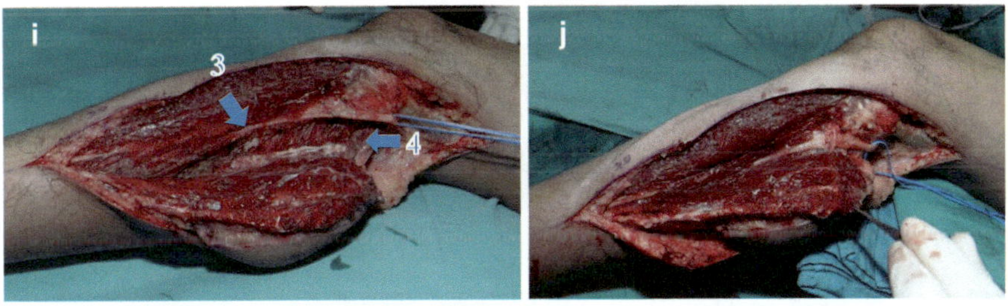

Anterior and posterior skin flap and part of the subcutaneous tissue, which showed infiltration, are included in the wide margin of the fascia. The peroneal nerve and its branch to the anterior compartment are explored. The superior part of the extensor hallucis longus was included as part of the oncological margin (Fig. 6i and j).

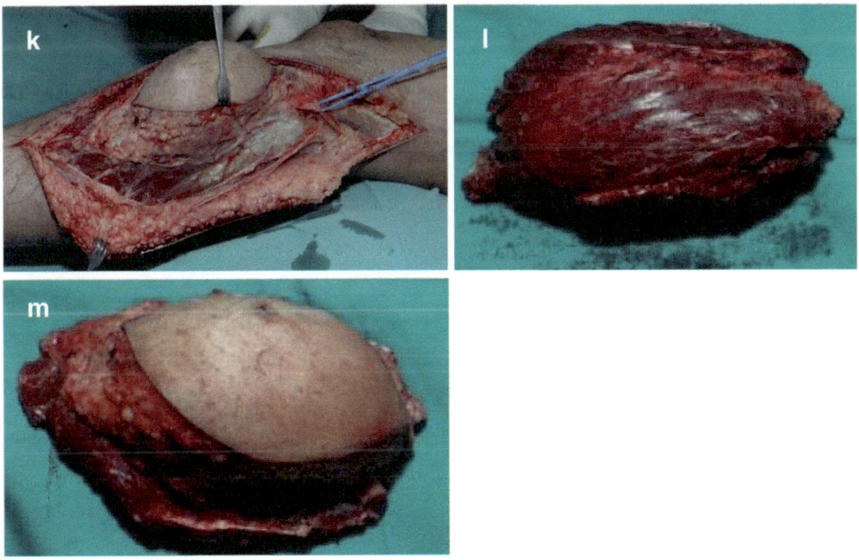

Lateral border of the soles was detached from the fibula attachment for evaluation for free cuff of normal oncological margin. A posterior skin flat over the gastrocnemius muscle was created for cuff of normal tissue surgical margin. The muscle was transected from the posterior for final resection (Fig. 6k–n).

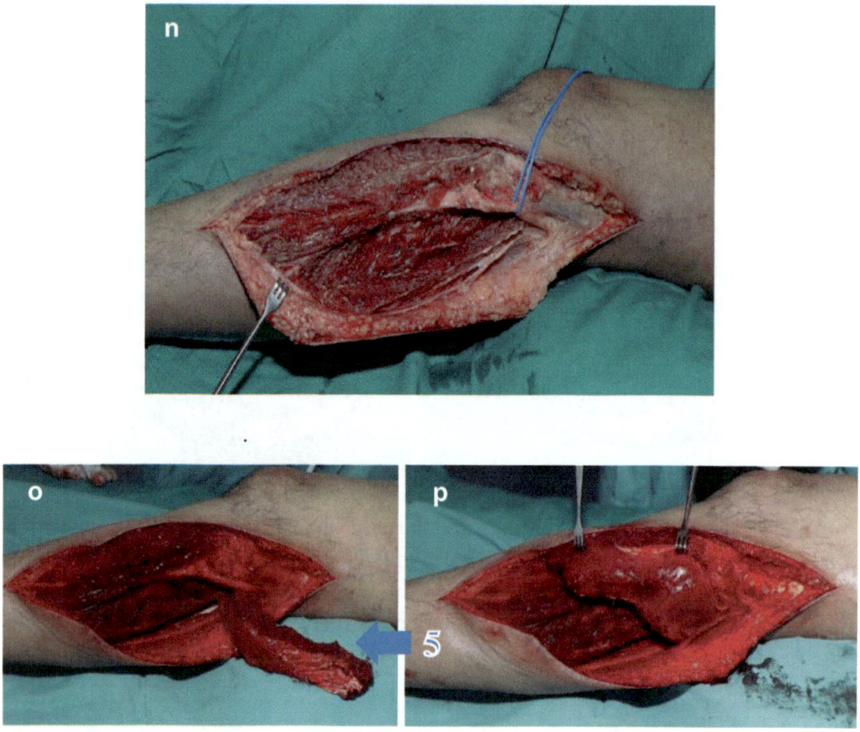

Remnant of medial gastrocnemius muscle was mobilised to cover the lateral defect (Fig. 6o and p).

Sarcoma with Osseous Involvement

Sarcoma with anterior tibial cortex erosion and circumferentially attached to the anteromedial cortex is best to resect together with tibial hemicorticotomy to achieve good oncological margin (Fig. 7a–e).

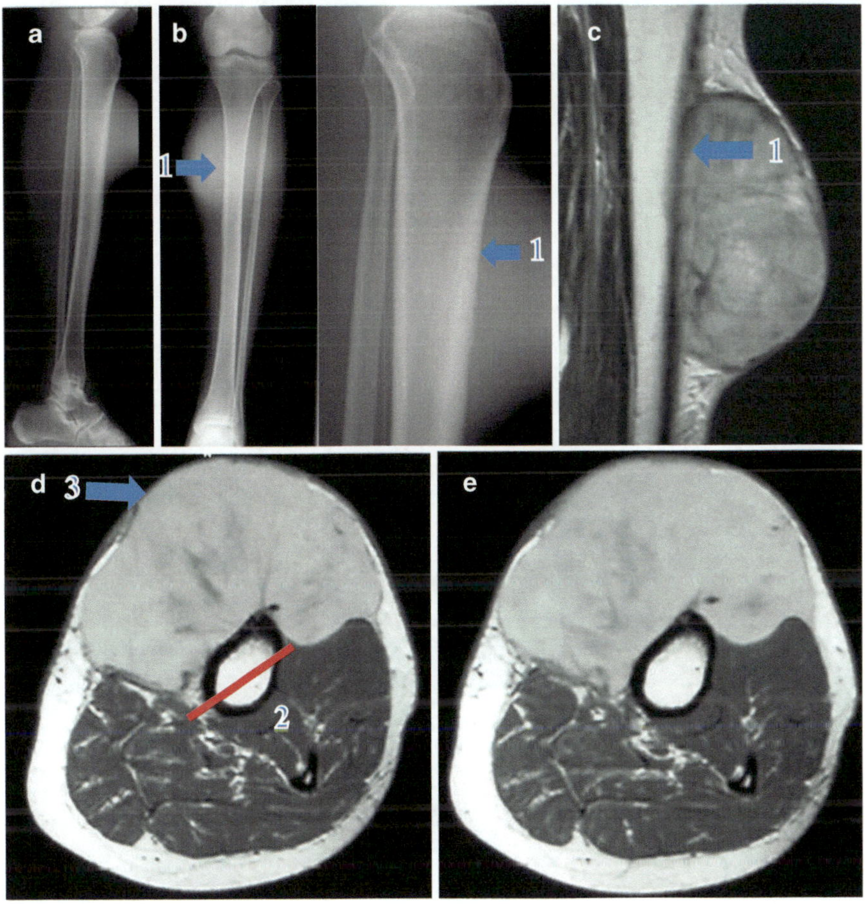

1. Antero-medial cortex erosion
2. Plan corticotomy
3. Skin infiltration

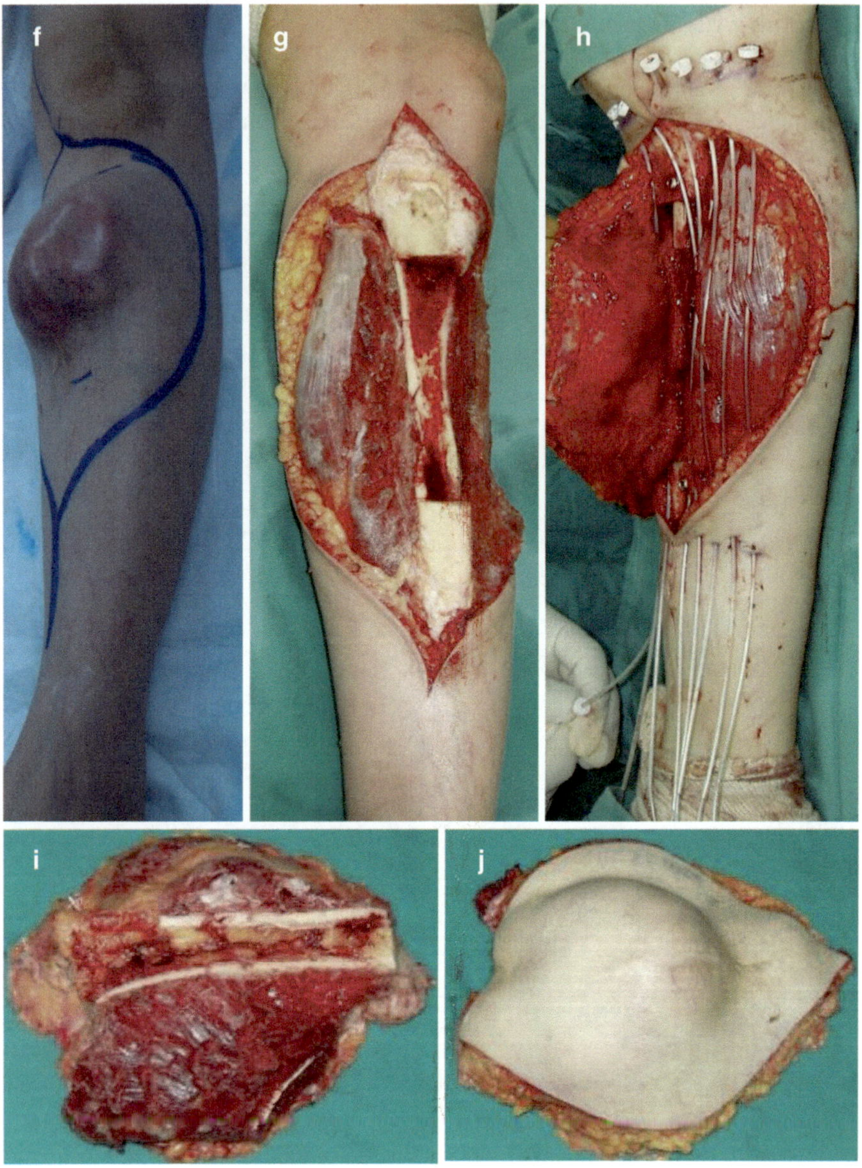
f
g
h
i
j

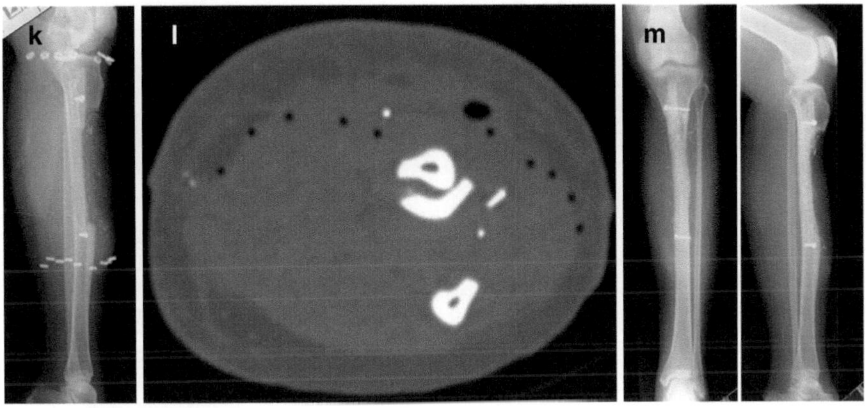

A combination wide margin surgery, vascularised tissue reconstruction and localised brachytherapy and adjuvant radiotherapy able to control local aggressive disease (Fig. 7f–j). The fibula showed good hypertrophy, even though local radiation was given to minimised local recurrence (Fig. 7k–m).

Suggested Reading

1. Huh WW, Guadagnolo BA, Munsell MF, Patel S, Lewis VO. Soft tissue sarcomas of the popliteal fossa: a single-institution retrospective review. Cancer. 2011;117(12):2728–34.
2. Turcotte RE, Ferrone M, Isler MH, Wong C. Outcomes in patients with popliteal sarcomas. Can J Surg. 2009;52(1):51–5.
3. Pritsch T, Bickels J, Winberg T, Malawer MM. Popliteal sarcomas: presentation, prognosis, and limb salvage. Clin Orthop Relat Res. 2007;455:225–33.
4. Rüdiger HA, Beltrami G, Campanacci DA, Mela MM, Franchi A, Capanna R. Soft tissue sarcomas of the popliteal fossa: outcome and risk factors. Eur J Surg Oncol. 2007;33(4):512–7. Epub 2006 Dec 15
5. Paolo Spinnato, Roberta Clinca. MRI tail sign in soft-tissue sarcoma. Radiology. 2021;299(2):276.

Resection Soft Tissue Sarcoma: Upper Limb

Biceps Resection and Motorised Muscle Transfer

Wan Faisham Nu'man Bin Wan Ismail

Introduction

Biceps sarcoma is very rare. Resection of the entire anterior arm compartment will lead to loss of elbow flexion and significant morbidity. Functional muscle transfer utilising a rotational latissimus dorsi flap or free vascularised motorised transfer is indicated for flexion function of the elbow.

Surgical Anatomy

The anterior compartment consists of the biceps brachii, brachialis and coracobrachialis muscle and is supplied by the musculocutaneus nerve that pierces the coracobrachialis in the upper arm.

- The biceps are composed of the short and long head, which originate from the coracoid process and supraglenoid tubercle of the scapula, and are inserted in the radial tuberosity.
- The brachialis muscle originated from the lower half of the humerus and is inserted at the coracoid process of the ulna. It is prime elbow flexor and is supplied by the musculoskeletal and radial nerves.
- The musculocutaneous nerve piercing the coracobrachialis and long head of the biceps is important for motorised muscle group transfer for elbow flexion.

W. F. N. B. W. Ismail (✉)
Prince Court Medical Center, Kuala Lumpur, Malaysia

Orthopaedic Oncology Reconstructive Unit, Universiti Sains Malaysia, Kubang Kerian, Kelantan, Malaysia

A. Puri, W. F. N. B. W. Ismail (eds.), *Atlas of Orthopedic Oncology Volume 1*,
https://doi.org/10.1007/978-981-95-8958-6_7

- The brachial artery crosses laterally and lies above the brachialis muscle accompanied by the median nerve before piercing the pronator teres below the elbow and dividing into radial and ulnar arteries. Evaluation of the brachial artery and median nerve is important, especially in distally based sarcoma.

Assessments

An MRI evaluation of the anterior arm compartment aims to determine the following structures:

- Superior extension of the tumour and correlation with the coracobrachialis, pectoralis major insertion and deltoid muscle.
- Relation of the tumour with major neurovascular bundles.
- Involvement of the brachialis muscle and relation with the brachial artery and median nerve for distal compartment sarcoma.
- The lateral triceps are bounded by thick lateral septum and rarely involved. However, the distal part of the deltoid must be evaluated for tumour extension.

Surgical Steps

- Exploration of the medial neurovascular structures and mobilisation from the short head biceps are needed. Coracobrachialis muscle preservation is based on local infiltration.
- The distal part of the brachial artery and median nerve is explored by mobilising the distal biceps after resection of the tendon stump.
- Musculoskeletal nerve must be identified for motorised muscle transfer.

Soft Tissue Sarcoma of Anterior Compartment Arm

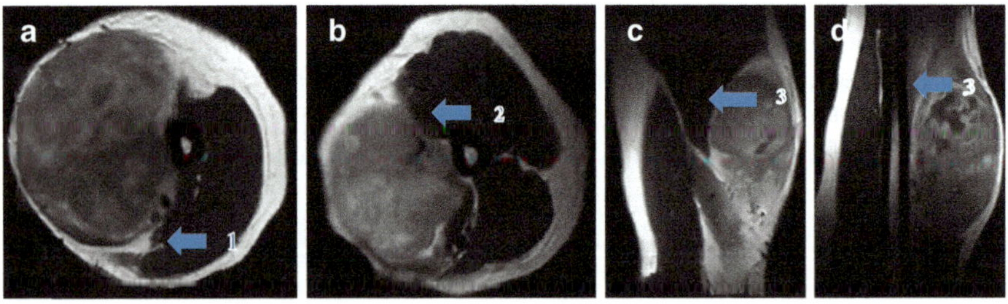

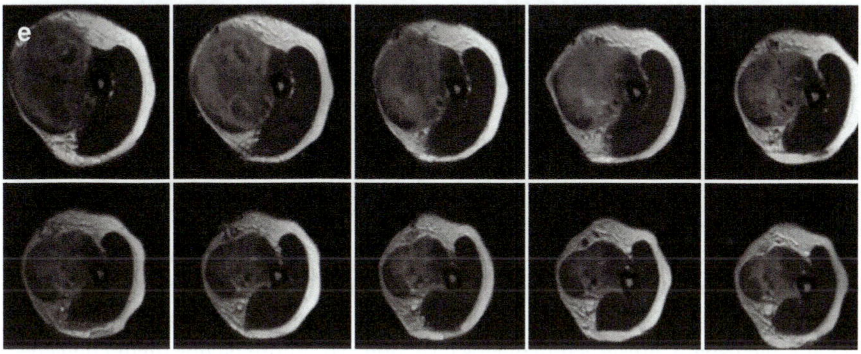

1. Medial neurovascular—brachial vessels, median, ulna and radial nerves
2. Lateral intermuscular septum
3. Deltoid—closely attached short head biceps
4. Series of MRI from shoulder to elbow for compartment evaluation (Fig. 1e)

Soft tissue sarcoma involving the entire biceps and coracobrachialis that displaced the medial neurovascular structures. The median nerve and brachial artery were spared (Fig. 1a–d).

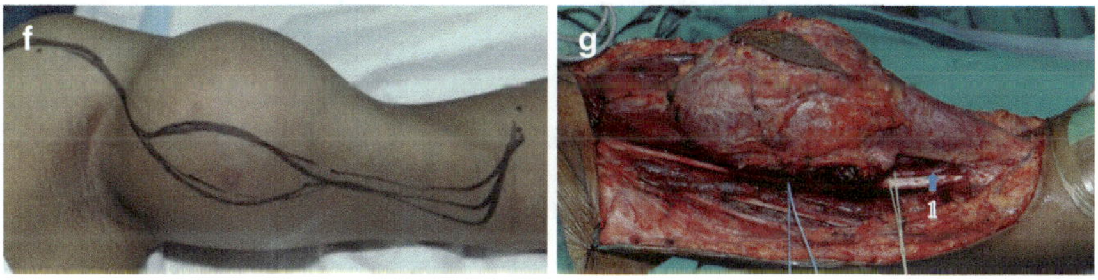

The medial neurovascular structures and intermuscular septum are exposed for medial surgical margin of the biceps. The musculocutaneous nerve pierces the coracobrachialis. The long head of the biceps is explored and identified as a donor for motorised muscle group transfer for elbow flexion. Remnant of the proximal and distal biceps tendon is preserved for reconstruction of elbow flexion (Fig. 1f–k).

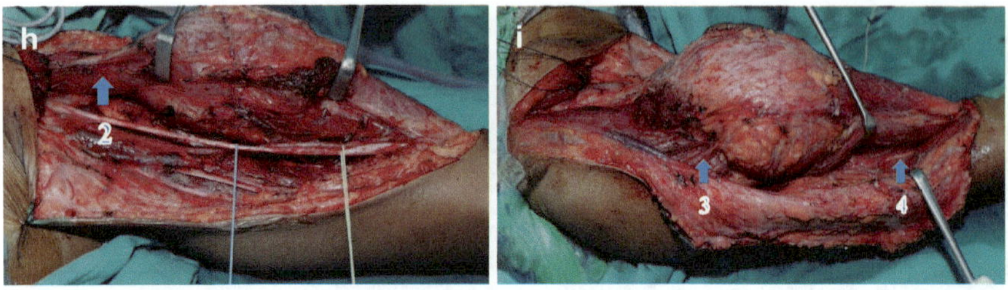

Lateral septum identified by creating a skin flap to the lateral border of the brachialis and triceps. The radial nerve is protected between the brachialis and brachioradialis and usually preserved in biceps resection. The entire biceps finally detached from the anterior humerus.

1. Median nerve and brachial artery
2. Long head of biceps
3. Deltoid border attached to straight head of biceps and brachialis
4. Radial nerve

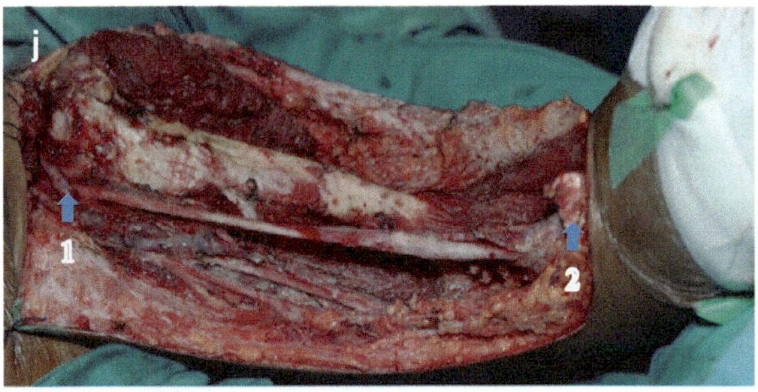

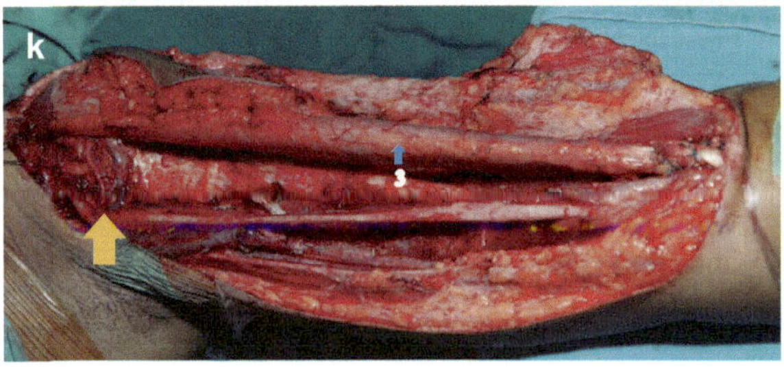

1. Stump of musculocutaneous nerve as motorised donor gracilis flap (Fig. 1j)
2. Stump of biceps tendon (Fig. 1j)
3. Gracilis flap

The gracilis muscle is a long strap muscle with sizable distal tendon supplied by the long neurovascular pedicle. It is a frequently used muscle for elbow flexion in delayed reconstruction plexus injuries. The size was matched with the biceps, especially when the skin was preserved during resection. Furthermore, the gracilis is a slender muscle and fits nicely in the anterior compartment and is easy for correct tension during reconstruction. The anterior branch of the obturator nerve that supplies the gracilis is hooked to the donor of the remnant musculocutaneous nerve (Fig. 1k and l).

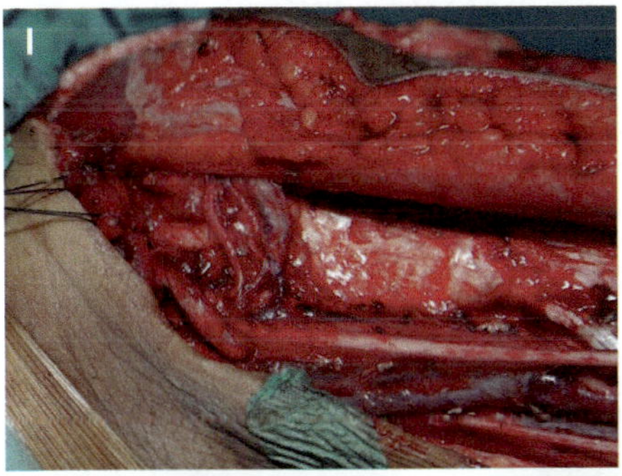

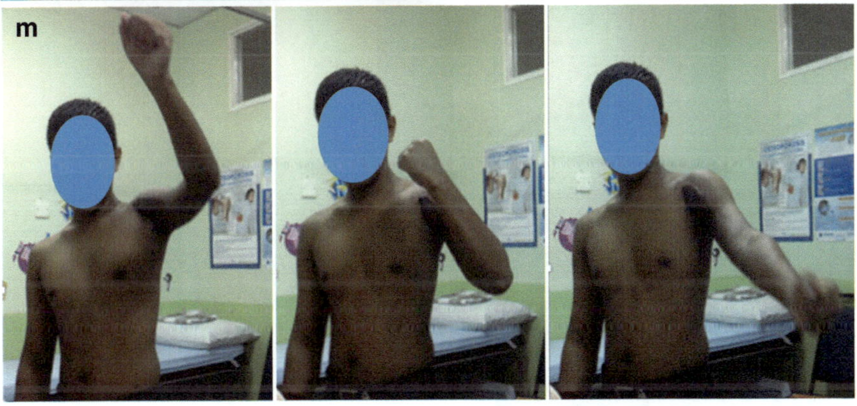

Function of elbow flexion of MRC grade 4/5–6 months after surgery (Fig. 1m).

Aggressive Fibromatoses of the Biceps

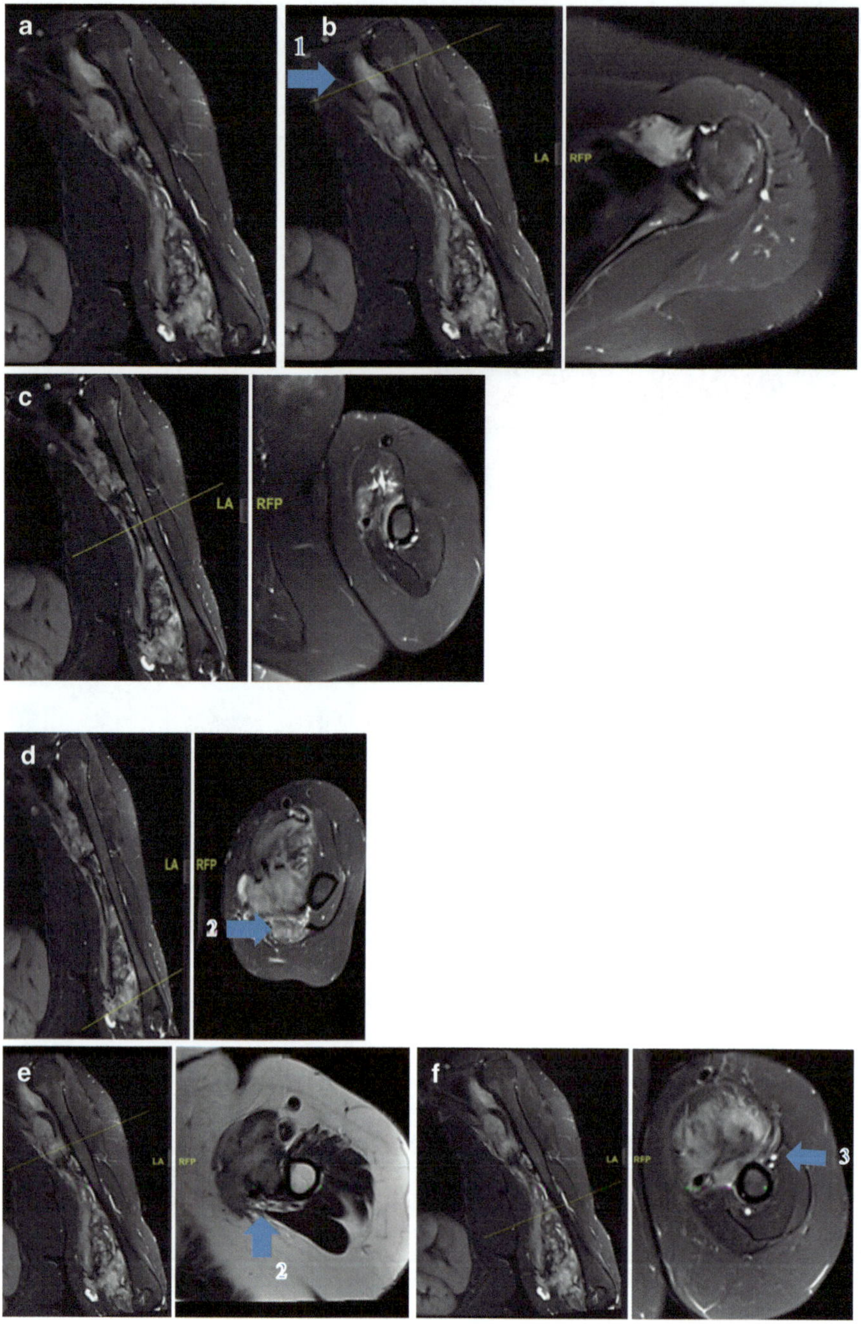

Infiltrative type of fibromatoses involving the entire anterior compartment of the arm, including the biceps and brachialis muscle. The proximal part of the biceps at the coracoid process was involved and needed to be cleared for good surgical margin. The medial neurovascular structure was in proximity with the tumour and the distal brachial artery was trapped within the tumour (Fig. 2a–f).

1. Coracoid process—origin of long head biceps
2. Brachial vessels trapped within the tumour
3. Lateral intermuscular septum

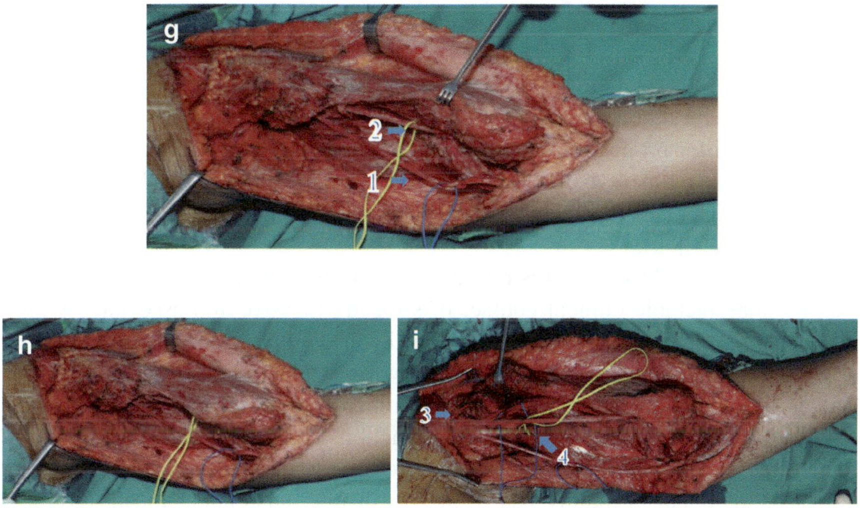

1. Ulna nerve
2. Median nerve with brachial artery
3. Musculocutaneous nerve
4. Radial nerve

Exploration of the ulnar and median nerve through the medial inter-muscular septum and mobilising it from the medial edge of the tumour mass. The lateral border of the brachial and radial nerve is identified for lateral margin of the resection. The brachial artery and vein were resected and bypassed. The brachial artery was trapped within the tumour mass and planned for resection to minimise the contamination and reverse saphenous bypass. Care must be taken to maintain all superficial vein drainage and deep venous system of the profundi to minimise forearm and hand swelling (Fig. 2g–i).

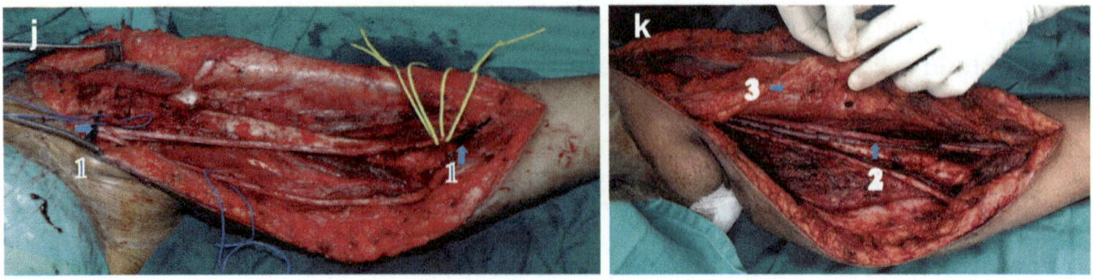

1. Brachial artery stump
2. Reverse saphenous vein graft bypass
3. Rotational latissimus dorsi flap

Motorised rotational latissimus dorsi is an option for replacement of the biceps muscle group for elbow flexion. The thoracodorsal artery and nerve are preserved and mobilised for proper sitting, alignment and tension of the latissimus doors for optimum flexion function of the elbow. The latissimus dorsi muscle and tendon were tagged in tension to the coracoid process and remnant of the biceps tendon and brachialis (Fig. 2j–k).

Desmoid-type fibromatosis is a rare benign fibroblastic proliferation characterised by unpredictable clinical course. It is locally invasive and associated with a high local recurrence rate and no established consensus for the treatment is available as of today. Due to the specific infiltrative growth pattern, surgical resection is needed to achieve negative margins. Recurrence of disease poses more fibrosis-restricted joint motion and impaired limb function. Conservative strategy is chosen in majority of patient with close monitoring of disease progression. The cut-off for an active treatment is mainly based on growth rate, anatomical localisation and worsening of function. Preservation of function became a priority either medical treatment, local radiotherapy or wide margin surgery is decided. If surgery is considered as an option, additional radiotherapy should always be considered to minimise the risk of local relapse.

This case highlighted a rare progression following intralesional surgery of desmoid fibromatoses of the flexor compartment of arm that causes limitation of elbow and shoulder function. Aggressive surgery with good-quality margin and preservation of major nerve is important to minimise disability. Local radiation is mandatory to minimise local recurrence.

Acknowledgement The author thanks Professor Wan Azman Wan Sulaiman, Professor Arman Zaharil Mat Saad and Professor Ahmad Sukari Halim from the plastic reconstructive unit at Universiti Sains Malaysia and MSU Medical Centre, Management and Science University, for their contributions and team member for managing the patients. All plastic reconstructive and microsurgery surgical procedures were performed by the team members.

Suggested Reading

1. Karakousis CP. Tumor in the anterior compartment of the arm atlas of operative procedures in surgical oncology. Springer Science; 2015. p. 37–40.
2. Engelhardt TO, Alghamdi HG, Wallmichrath J, Holzbach T, Dürr HR, Giunta RE. Handchir. Free gracilis flap for anatomic reconstruction after limb-sparing sarcoma resection. Mikrochir Plast Chir. 2015;47(2):111–7.
3. Koulaxouzidis G, Simunovic F, Bannasch H. Soft tissue sarcomas of the arm—ocosurgical and reconstructive principles within a multimodal, interdisciplinary setting. Front Surg. 2016;3:12.
4. Kim JY, Youssef A, Subramanian V, Rogers BA, Pollock RE, Robb GL, Chang MDW. Upper extremity reconstruction following resection of soft tissue sarcomas: a functional outcomes analysis. Ann Surg Oncol. 11(10):921–92.
5. Muramatsu K, Ihara K, Doi K, Yoshida K, Iwanaga R, Hashimoto T, Taguchi T. Functional neuro-vascularized muscle transfer for oncological reconstruction of extremity sarcoma. Surg Oncol. 2012;21:263e268.
6. Payne CE, Hofer SO, Zhong T, Griffin AC, Ferguson PC, Wunder JS. Functional outcome following upper limb soft tissue sarcoma resection with flap reconstruction. J Plast Reconstr Aesthet Surg. 2013;66(5):601–7.
7. Saint-Cyr M, Langstein HN. Reconstruction of the hand and upper extremity after tumour resection. J Surg Oncol. 2006;94(6):490–503.
8. Kasper B, Baumgarten C, Garcia J, Bonvalot S, Haas R, Haller F, Hohenberger P, et al. An update on the management of sporadic desmoid-type fibromatosis: a European consensus initiative between sarcoma PAtients EuroNet (SPAEN) and European organization for research and treatment of cancer (EORTC)/soft tissue and bone sarcoma group (STBSG). Ann Oncol. 2017;28(10):2399–408.

Deltoid Resection

Wan Faisham Nu'man Bin Wan Ismail

Introduction

Complete resection of a deltoid sarcoma is rarely performed and is thought to compromise shoulder abduction. Loss of the deltoid muscle in isolation with normal rotator cuff results in fairly normal shoulder function in daily activity, including overhead movement. However, abduction strength is weaker for strenuous activity. In general, muscle transfer to enhance shoulder abduction is rarely performed following this procedure.

Surgical Anatomy

The deltoid muscle has multipennate origins from the lateral third clavicle, acromion process and spine of the scapulae.

- It is supplied by the axillary nerve, which exits in the quadrangular space below the lower border of teres minor together with the axillary vessels.
- It passes around the posterior humerus on the deep surface of the deltoid muscle.
- The axillary nerve and vessels must be protected and maintained in partial deltoid resection for vascularity and function.
- Insertion of the deltoid is in close proximity to the long head of the biceps, brachialis and lateral head of the triceps. All these structures must be carefully evaluated for tumour involvement.

W. F. N. B. W. Ismail (✉)
Prince Court Medical Center, Kuala Lumpur, Malaysia

Orthopaedic Oncology Reconstructive Unit, Universiti Sains Malaysia, Kubang Kerian, Kelantan, Malaysia

A. Puri, W. F. N. B. W. Ismail (eds.), *Atlas of Orthopedic Oncology Volume 1*,
https://doi.org/10.1007/978-981-95-8958-6_8

Assessment

An MRI evaluation is aimed to determine the following structures (Fig. 1a–f):

- Origin of the deltoid at the clavicle, acromion and scapulae spine and its close proximity with the tumour for local infiltration
- Correlation of deep tumour with the proximal humerus, shoulder joint and supraspinatus, infraspinatus, and subscapularis attachment
- The proximal triceps muscle can be infiltrated with large posterior deltoid tumour and needs to be included in the margin
- The distal multipennate attachment and course of the radial nerve for distally based deltoid sarcoma

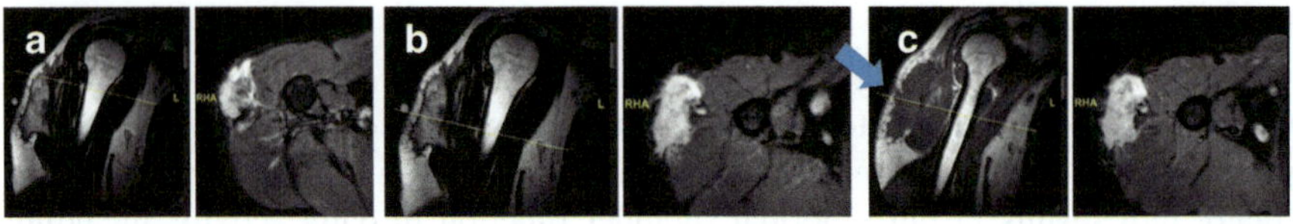

Sarcomas involving the anterior and middle portions of the deltoid with skin infiltration. Biopsy scar and skin with fascia must be included in the resection margin for oncological clearance.

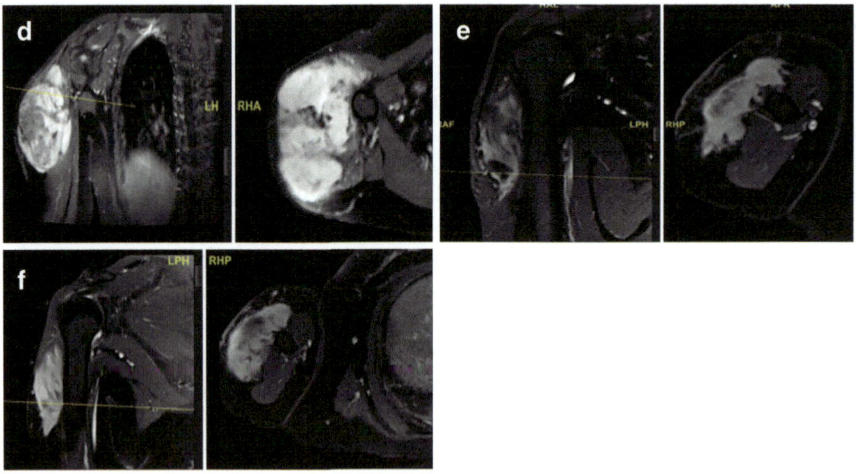

Sarcomas involving the entire deltoid that are still confined within the compartment need a complete resection for clearance.

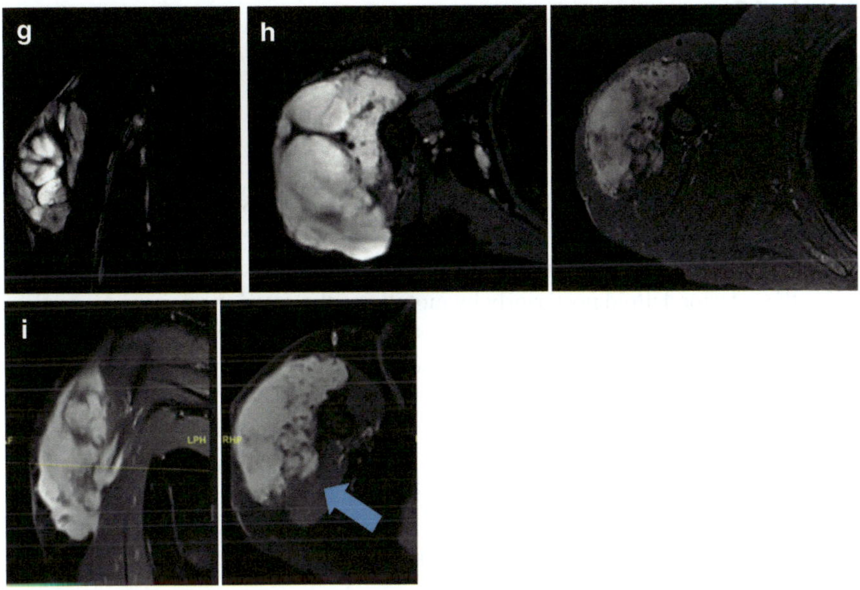

Sarcomas involving proximal deltoid with infiltration of the triceps need a complete resection with the long head of the triceps for complete clearance. Proximity with the proximal humerus with no bony infiltration and periosteum of proximal humerus must be included as surgical margin (Fig. 1g–i).

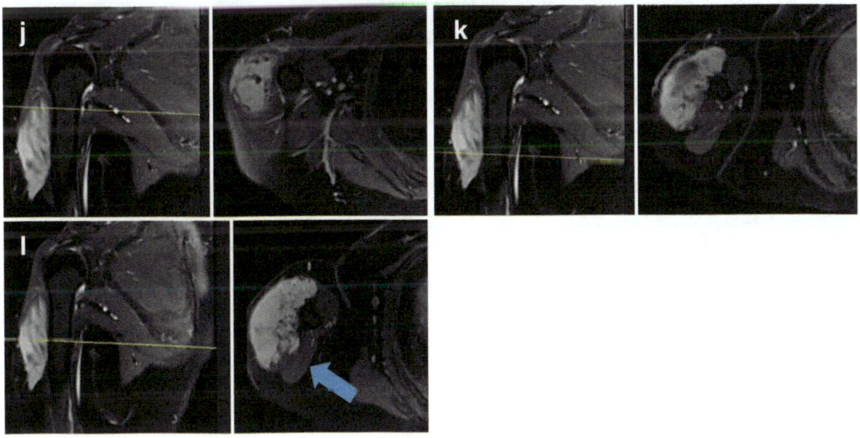

Distal deltoid sarcoma in close proximity to the lateral triceps and profunda humeral artery. The radial nerve needs to be mobilised and cleared prior resection (Fig. 1j–l).

Surgical Steps

For complete total deltoid resection:

- Create a medial and lateral flap for entire deltoid muscle visualisation and cover the entire acromion, lateral clavicle and scapula spine.
- Create a plane at the deltopectoral approach and mobilise the cephalic vein medially.
- Detach the deltoid origin and create a space to the rotator cuff muscle and mobilise the anterior deltoid posteriorly by mobilising the anterior origin and insertion.
- The posterior circumflex humeral artery and axillary nerve is visualised after 2/3 of the anterior deltoid muscle is mobilised and needs to be protected and ligated.

Deltoid muscle resection can be partial, subtotal or total based on tumour extension and surgical margin. Subtotal excision indicates that more than half of the deltoid muscle is resected. Shoulder abduction function is usually preserved with minimal impairment provided the rotator cuff is spared. Simple closure with a large drain is important to prevent seroma. A flap is not necessary to improve function.

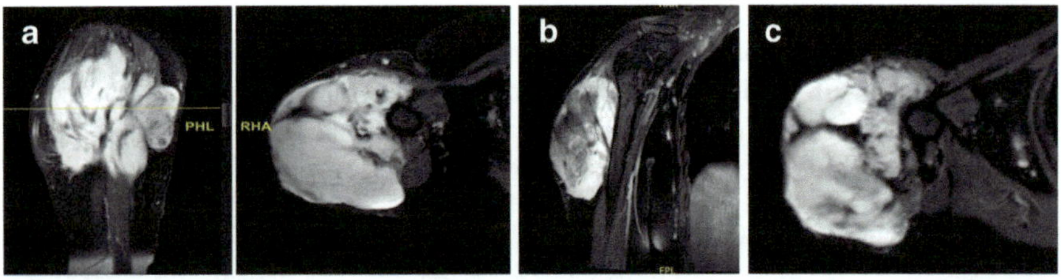

High-grade sarcoma with infiltrative margin needs a wider resection for good oncological margin (Fig. 2a–c).

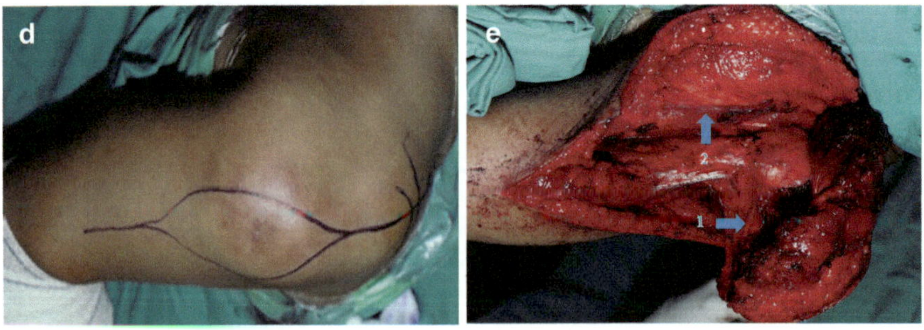

An anterior and posterior skin flap is created to visualise the entire deltoid. The intermuscular plane of the deltopectoral groove is identified by detaching the deltoid origin from the clavicle. The entire deltoid is detached over the acromion and scapular spine proximally. The insertion of the deltoid is multipennate and must also be detached from the humerus (Fig. 2d–f).

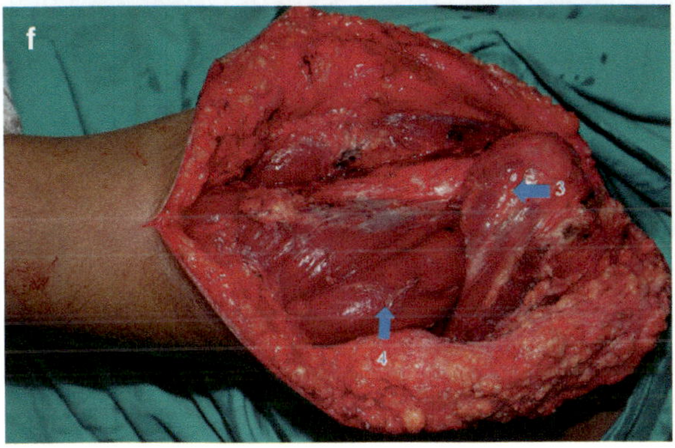

1. Posterior circumflex humeral artery
2. Pectoralis major—deltopectoral plane
3. Infraspinatus tendon attachment at greater tuberosity
4. Long head triceps

The posterior circumflex humeral artery must be ligated for homeostasis at the inferior border of the surgical neck of the humerus. The axillary nerve is sacrificed in total deltoid resection. The entire proximal humerus can be covered without muscle reconstruction with minimal disability.

Functional outcome after total deltoid resection, shoulder abduction function by supra and infraspinatus muscle (Fig. 2g–j).

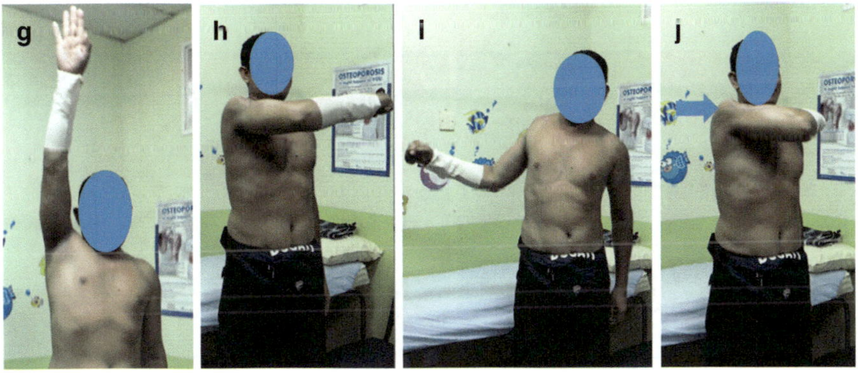

Partial Deltoid Resection

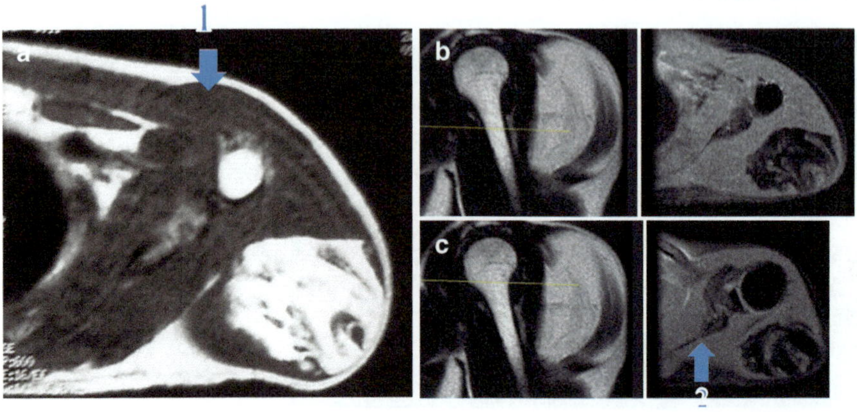

In low-grade sarcoma involving the posterior deltoid, partial deltoid resection with preservation of the anterior deltoid can be done by mobilising the deltoid attachment over the scapular spine and acromion (Fig. 3a–c).

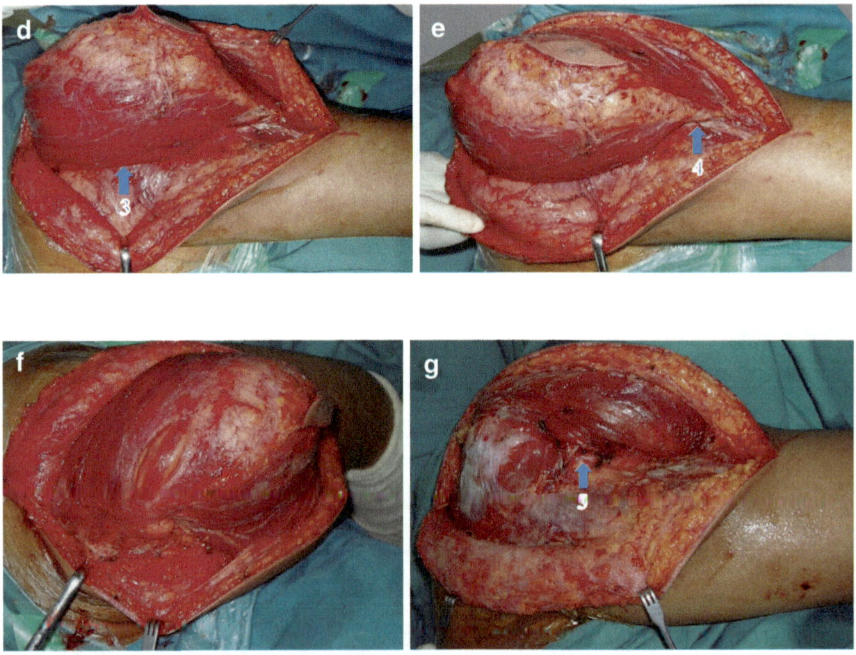

1. Deltopectoral groove
2. Scapular spine

3. Posterior border deltoid
4. Deltoid tuberosity
5. Branch posterior circumflex humeral artery

The origin of the deltoid over the scapular spine and acromion is detached before assessment of the margin for final resection (Fig. 3d–g).

Total Deltoid Resection with Lateral Triceps

Large sarcoma of the deltoid is abutting or usually infiltrates and involves the lateral triceps and lateral part of the brachialis muscle. The radial nerve crosses around the radial groove of the humerus and is at risk during resection. Distal exploration of the radial nerve is crucial prior to resection of the entire sarcoma (Fig. 4a–c).

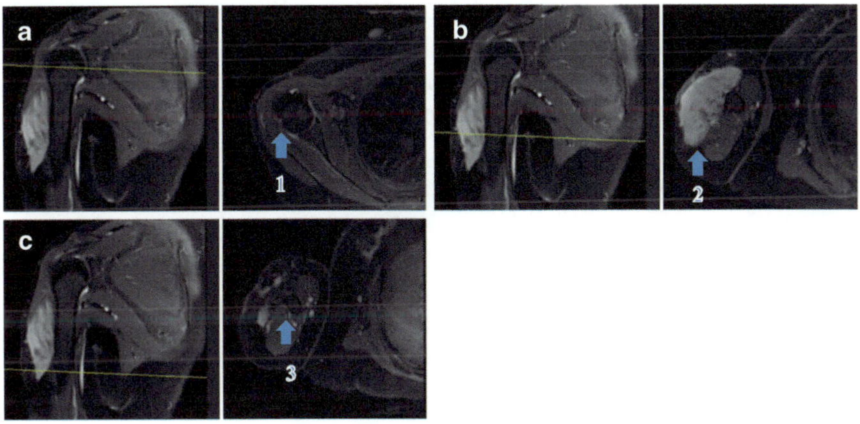

1. Rotator cuff not involved
2. Deltoid and lateral triceps—no clear plane
3. Profunda humerus artery—landmark for radial nerve

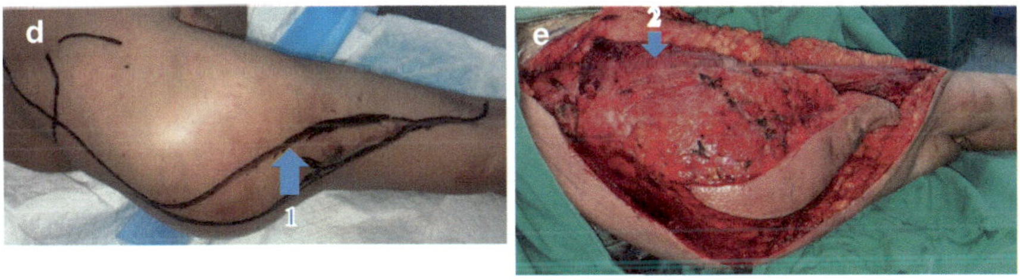

Exploration of the distal radial nerve and detachment of the biceps origin over the clavicle and acromion. The multipennate attachment is cleared from the bone from anterior to posterior. Part of the lateral brachialis muscle and lateral triceps are resected for better surgical margin (Fig. 4d and e).

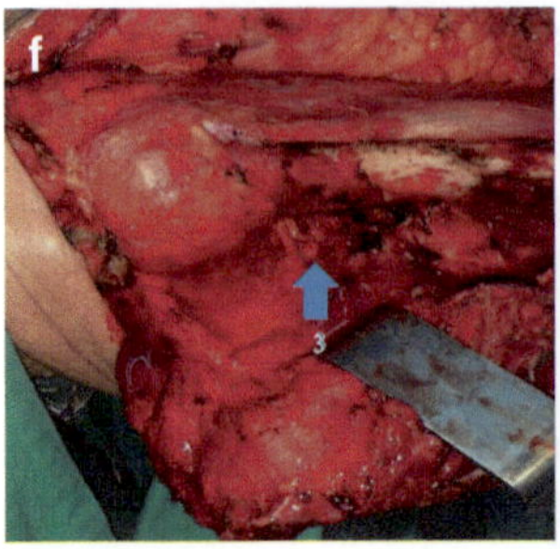

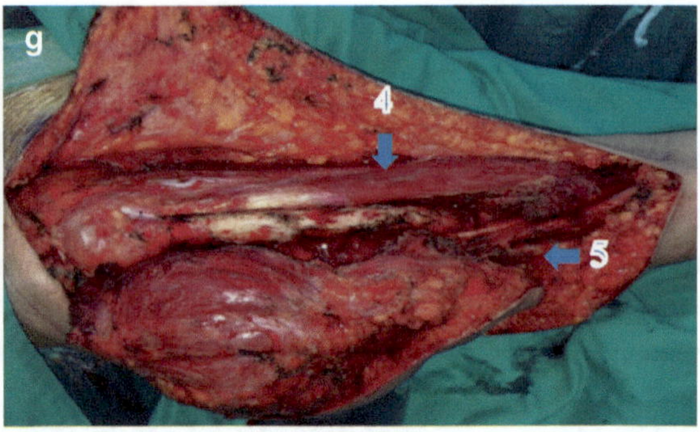

The posterior circumflex humeral artery and axillary nerve are identified at the surgical neck once all the tissue attachments to the humerus are cleared (Fig. 4f–h).

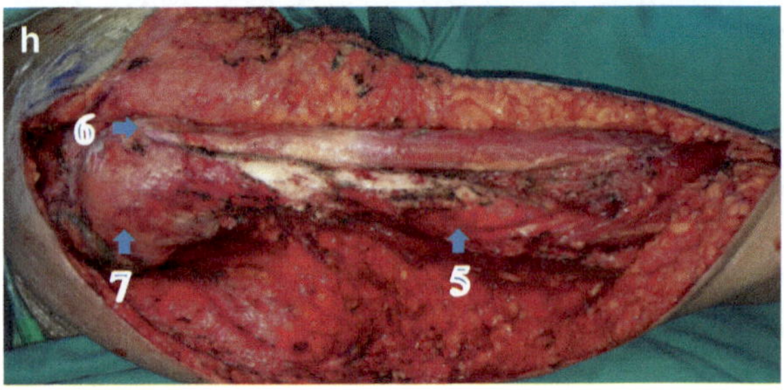

1. Skin infiltration by the sarcoma was remove and include as margin
2. Deltopectoral plane and biceps
3. Posterior circumflex humeral vessels
4. Biceps
5. Radial nerve
6. Bicipital groove greater tuberosity
7. Rotator cuff insertion

Resection of Entire Deltoid and Lateral Triceps

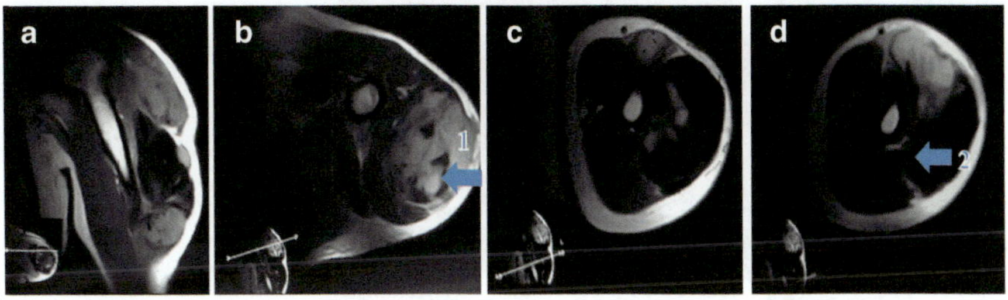

Deltoid sarcoma with extension to the lateral triceps can be in close proximity to radial nerve which is at risk of injury during resection (Fig. 5a–d). The tumour has to be mobilised entirely before epineural clearance of the radial nerve to minimise morbidity.

1. Entire deltoid tumour
2. Profunda humeral artery—anatomical landmark of radial nerve

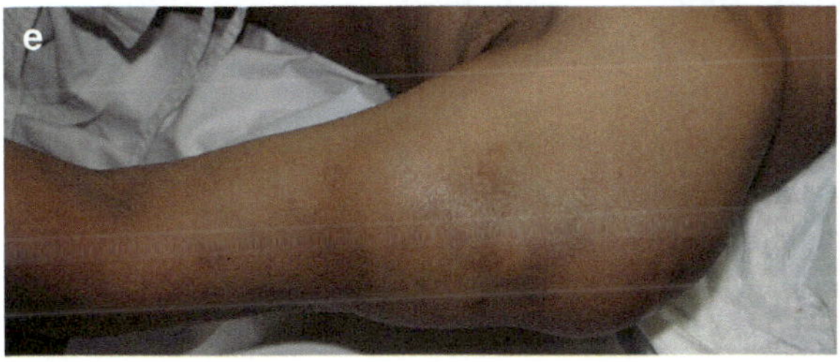

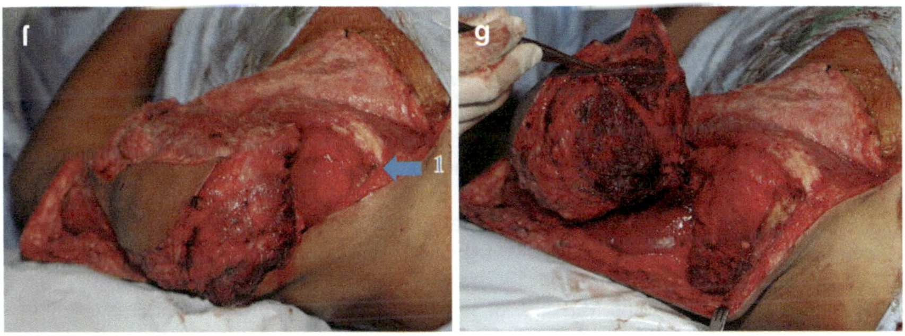

Mobilising the proximal tumour and exploration of the radial nerve distally and part of the lateral triceps is included in the resection margin (Fig. 5e–j).

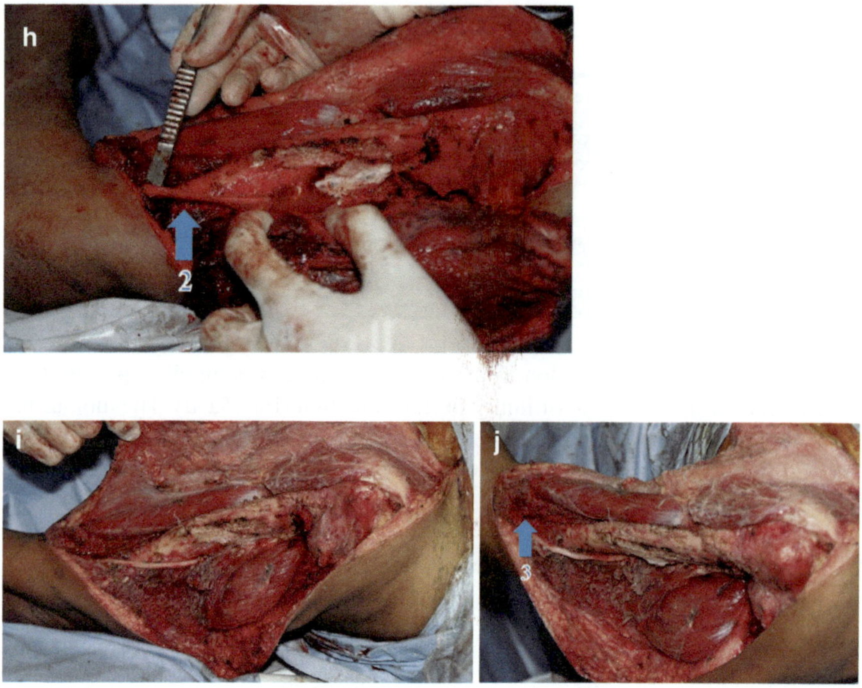

1. Deltoid origin detached from acromion
2. Epineural dissection of radial nerve
3. Remnant of brachialis muscle

Suggested Reading

1. Al Absi E, Karim T, Colterjohn N, Ghert M. A novel surgical approach to lipomatous tumours of the deltoid region. Sarcoma. 2010;49:5834.
2. Arteau A, Seeli F, Fuchs B. Complete deltoid resection in early childhood without muscle transfer results in normal shoulder function at long-term follow-up: a case report. J Med Case Rep. 2017;11(1):13–8.
3. Hamada S, Nishida Y, Takanari K, Ota T, Urakawa H, Ikuta K, Sakai T, Tsukushi S, Kamei Y, Ishiguro N. Functional evaluation following deltoid muscle resection in patients with soft tissue sarcoma. Jpn J Clin Oncol. 2020;50(7):772–8.
4. Mimata Y, Nishida J, Gotoh M, Akasaka T, Shimamura T. Limb function after excision of a deltoid muscle sarcoma. J Shoulder Elb Surg. 2013;22:e1–5.
5. Muramatsu K, Ihara K, Tominaga Y, Hashimoto T, Taguchi T. Functional reconstruction of the deltoid muscle following complete resection of musculoskeletal sarcoma. J Plast Reconstr Aesthet Surg. 2014;67(7):916–20.

Triceps (Posterior Arm) Resection

Wan Faisham Nu'man Bin Wan Ismail

Introduction

Upper extremities sarcoma poses a major challenge due to its complex anatomy for safe oncological clearance and high functional demand. The posterior compartment of the arm consists of the triceps brachii muscle, which has three origins. All three heads merge together to form a single tendon, inserted at the olecranon process. The oncological anatomical boundaries for resection are not well defined. In high-grade sarcoma, complete compartment resection is an option for adequate oncological clearance.

Surgical Anatomy

The triceps arises from three heads:

- The long head originating from the intra-glenoid tuberosity descends in front of the teres minor and behind the teres major.
- The lateral head originates between the insertion of the teres minor and posterior part of the deltoid tuberosity. It covers the radial nerve and profunda brachii vessels.
- The medial head arises from the back of the shaft of the humerus, distal to the groove of the radial nerve.

W. F. N. B. W. Ismail (✉)
Prince Court Medical Center, Kuala Lumpur, Malaysia

Orthopaedic Oncology Reconstructive Unit, Universiti Sains Malaysia, Kubang Kerian, Kelantan, Malaysia

A. Puri, W. F. N. B. W. Ismail (eds.), *Atlas of Orthopedic Oncology Volume 1*,
https://doi.org/10.1007/978-981-95-8958-6_9

The radial nerve passes to the posterior compartment of the arm together with the profunda brachii artery and descends to the radial groove between the medial and lateral heads of the triceps. The nerve passes the lateral inter-muscular septum between the brachialis and brachioradialis muscles.

Assessments

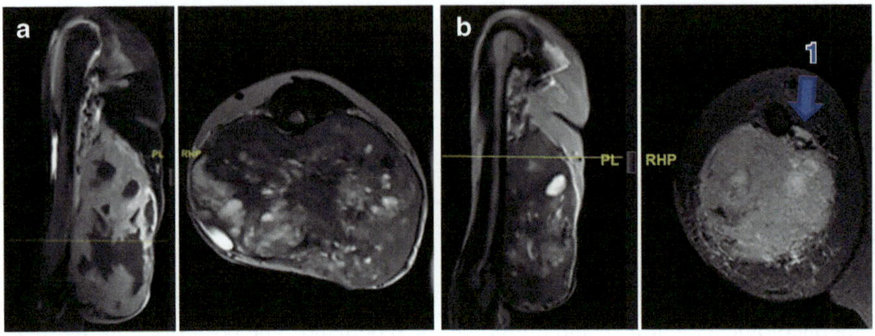

- Brachial artery with median and ulnar nerve

Sarcoma occupied the entire posterior compartment of the arm below the origin to the triceps tendon. The medial margin was in close proximity to the major neurovascular structures. The radial nerve and profunda humeral artery were trapped within the tumour mass (Fig. 1a and b).

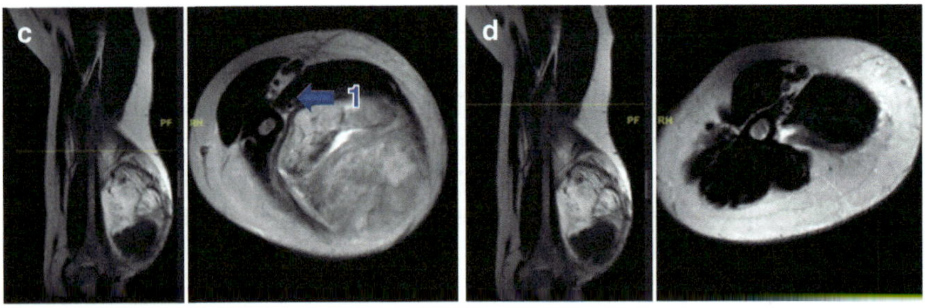

- Profunda humeral artery with radial nerve

Distal triceps sarcoma. The image showed the radial nerve accompanied by the profunda artery with good tissue boundaries with respect to the tumour (Fig. 1c and d).

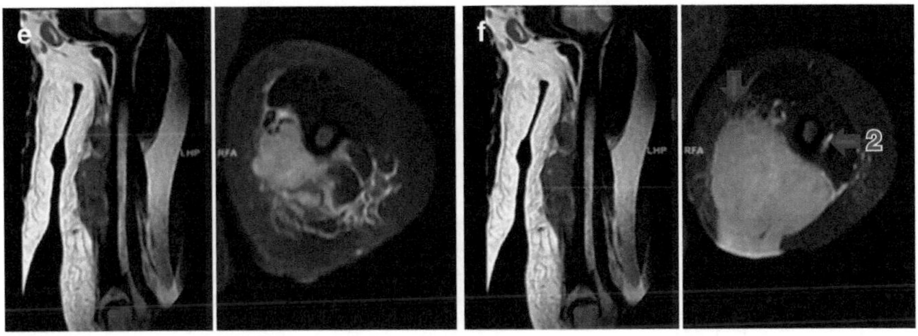

1. Medial neurovascular bundle
2. Profunda artery and radial nerve

Mid-arm posterior sarcoma with skin infiltration. However, the profunda can be traced with good boundaries (Fig. 1e and f).

Surgical Steps

Posterior arm compartment resection involving a proper evaluation of the tumour and correlation with:

- Origins of the three heads of the triceps and their relations to each other.
- Preservation of a portion of the triceps with an intact nerve supply will minimise morbidity and maintain extension at the elbow joint.
- Sacrifice of the radial nerve for oncological margin results in significant disability; however, the functional result is still superior to a high amputation of the arm.

Localised Lateral Triceps Resection

Low-grade tumour confined to lateral triceps can be removed completely with good oncological margins. Tracing the profunda humeral artery in contrasted MRI images indirectly for radial nerve is important for planning of surgical margin (Fig. 2a–d).

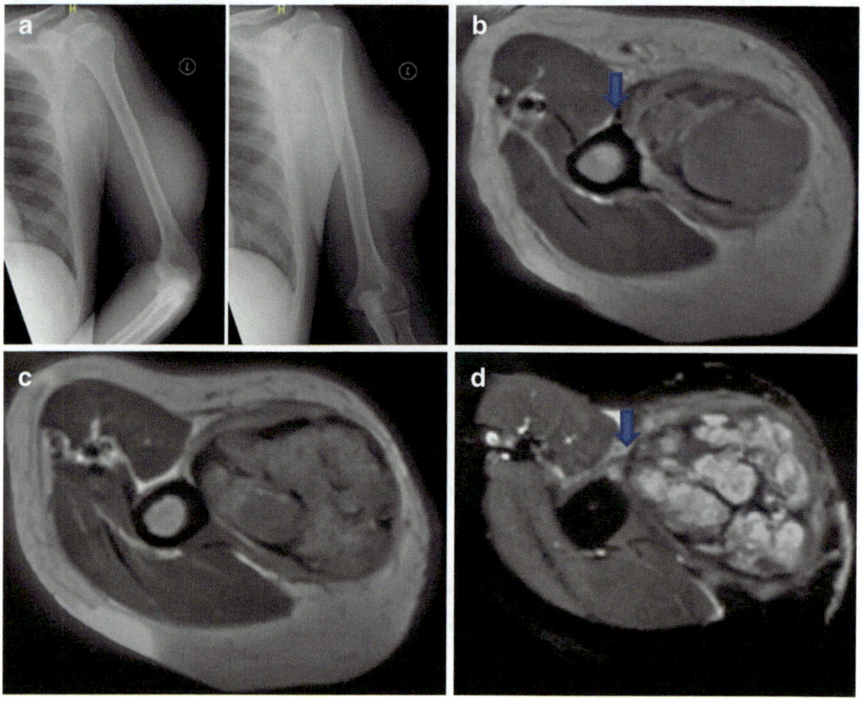

- Profunda brachial artery and radial nerve

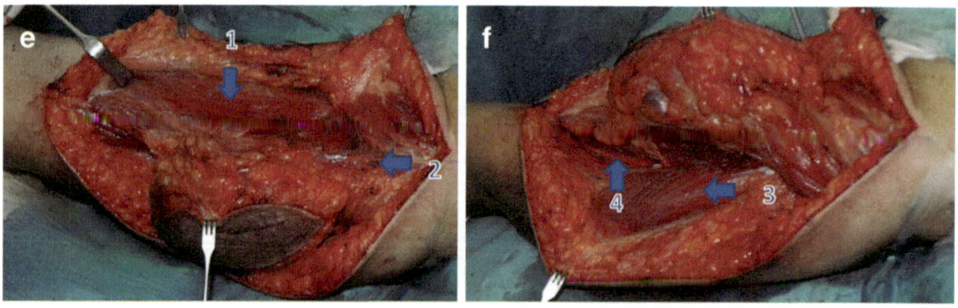

Anterior and posterior fasciocutaneous flaps created to identify lateral intermuscular septum between biceps and lateral triceps. Radial nerve explored through plane between brachialis and brachioradialis before it turns posteriorly between lateral and medial triceps plane. The upper border of lateral triceps attached to the deltoid tuberosity at the insertion of deltoid tendon (Fig. 2e–j)

1. Biceps
2. Lateral intermuscular septum
3. Medial triceps
4. Radial nerve

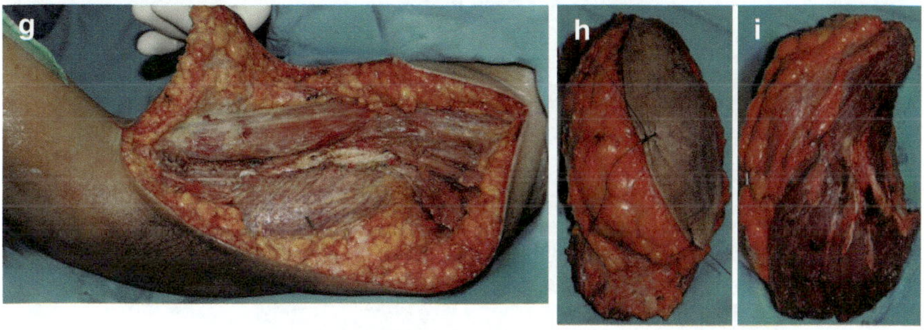

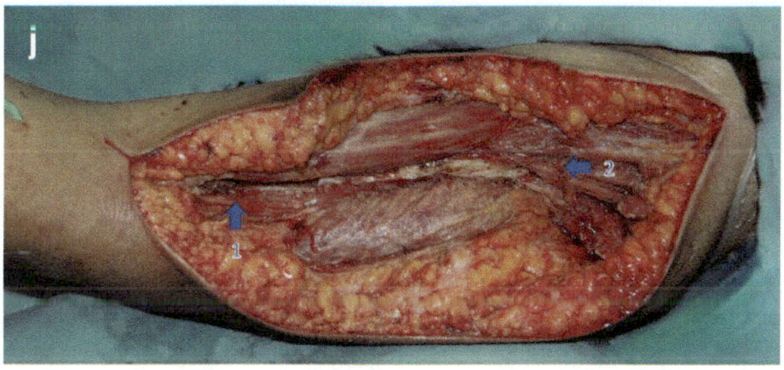

1. Radial nerve
2. Deltoid tuberosity

Resection of Total Triceps Compartment

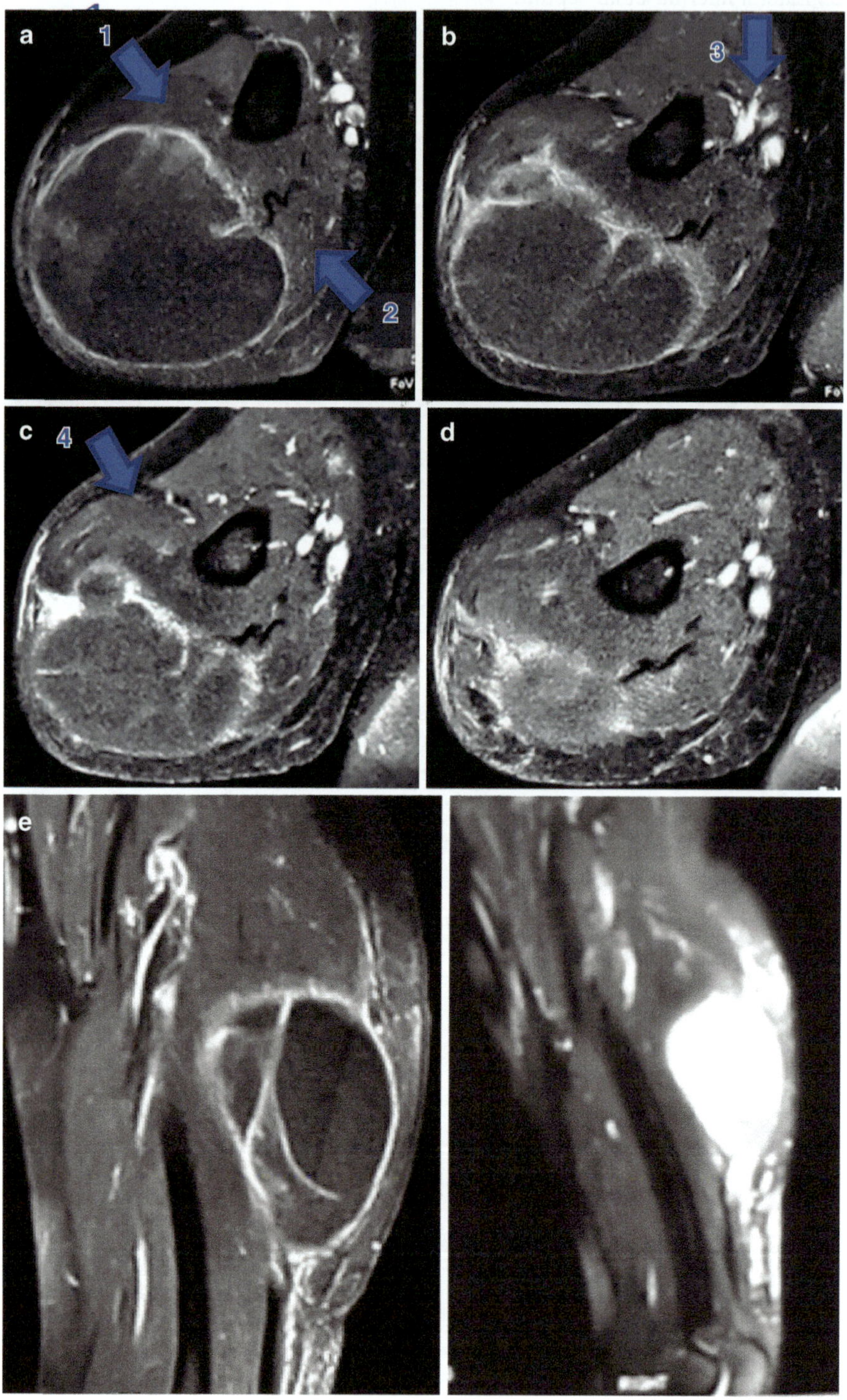

High-grade sarcoma with cystic degeneration and intra-tumoral bleeding and oedema of the entire posterior compartment of the arm. The deep structures of medial and lateral head were spared. The radial nerve can be explored without compromising the surgical margin (Fig. 3a–e)

1. Lateral head triceps
2. Medial head triceps
3. Brachial artery and major nerve—median and ulna
4. Profunda humeral artery with radial nerve

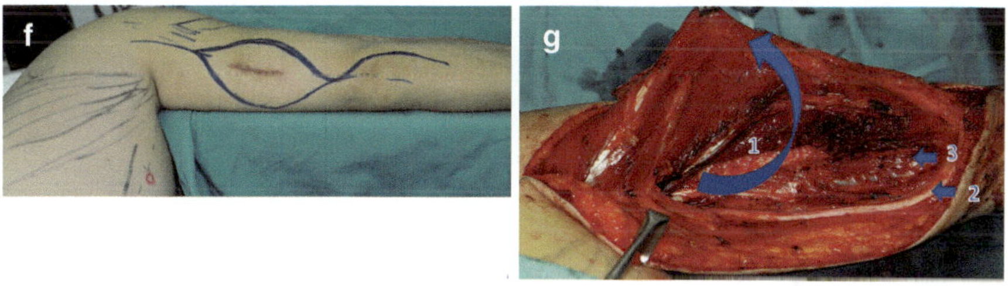

1. Medial exploration of ulna nerve and elevation medial triceps from medial intermuscular septum
2. Ulna nerve
3. Medial intermuscular septum

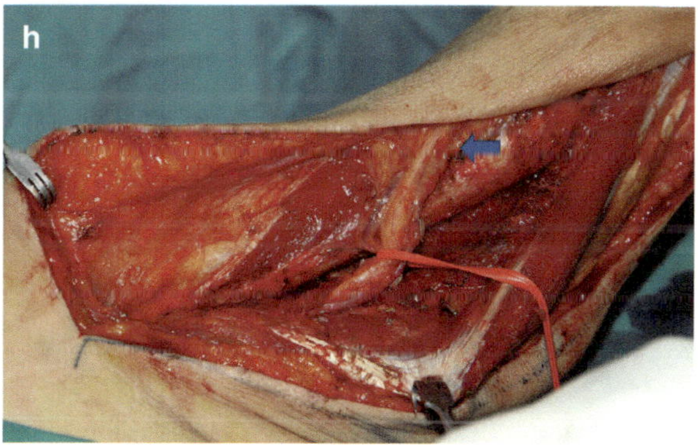

- Radial nerve with profunda humeral artery

Exploration of the ulnar nerve over the medial intermuscular septum and proximal and distal exploration of the radial nerve to prevent injury during complete compartment resection. The entire triceps can be removed without reconstruction. Gravity helps extend the elbow and biceps provide for elbow flexion (Fig. 3f–k).

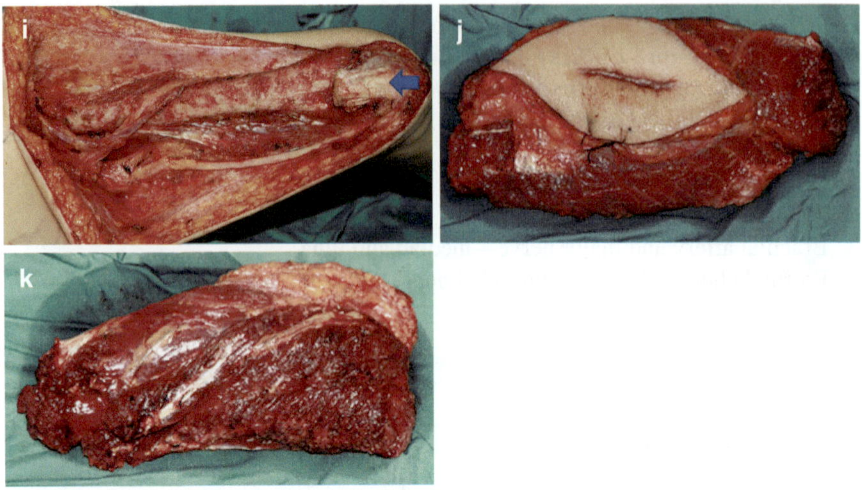

- Remnant triceps tendon

High-Grade Sarcoma with Nerve Epineural Dissection

Sarcoma involving the entire posterior compartment will ocasionally include the ulnar nerve within the involved medial margin. Epineural exploration after securing the surgical margin and isolating the operated area will reduce contamination and minimise local recurrence. Postoperative radiotherapy is mandatory for this technique of radial and ulna nerve preservation.

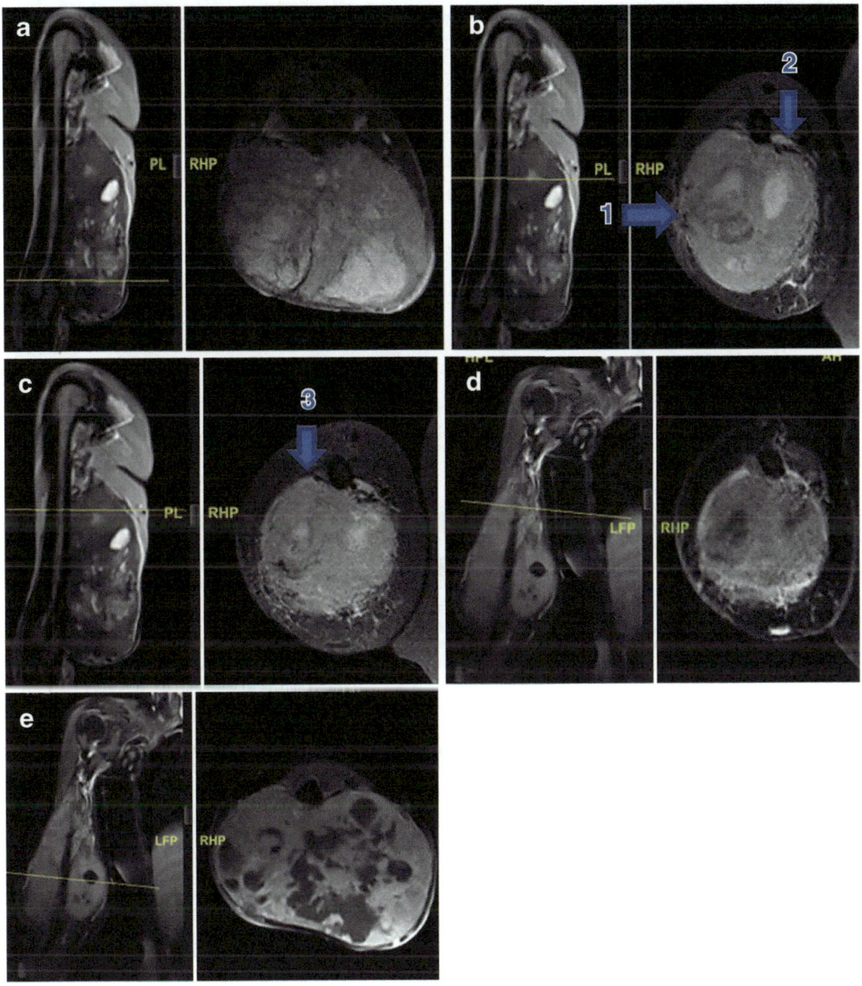

1. Skin infiltration must be included as margin
2. Brachial artery with major nerve—ulna and median nerve
3. Profunda humeral artery—radial nerve

MRI of high-grade sarcoma involving entire posterior arm compartment (Fig. 4a–e).

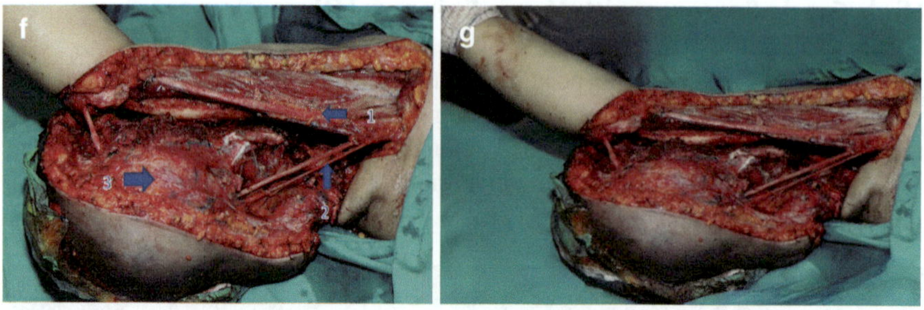

1. Brachial artery and median nerve
2. Ulna nerve trapped within the tumour margin
3. Entire triceps compartment resection

Epineural dissection and clearance of the nerve after the entire tumour mobilised and isolation from the surgical bed to minimise contamination (Fig. 4f–i).

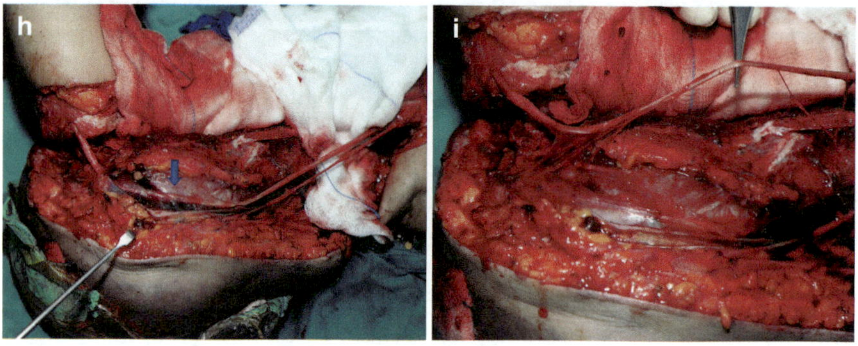

- Marginal margin with epineural dissection and clearance

Soft tissue defect can be reconstructed using a rotational latissimus dorsi flap. Motorised function is an option utilising the thoraco-dorsal nerve for elbow extension (Fig. 4j–l).

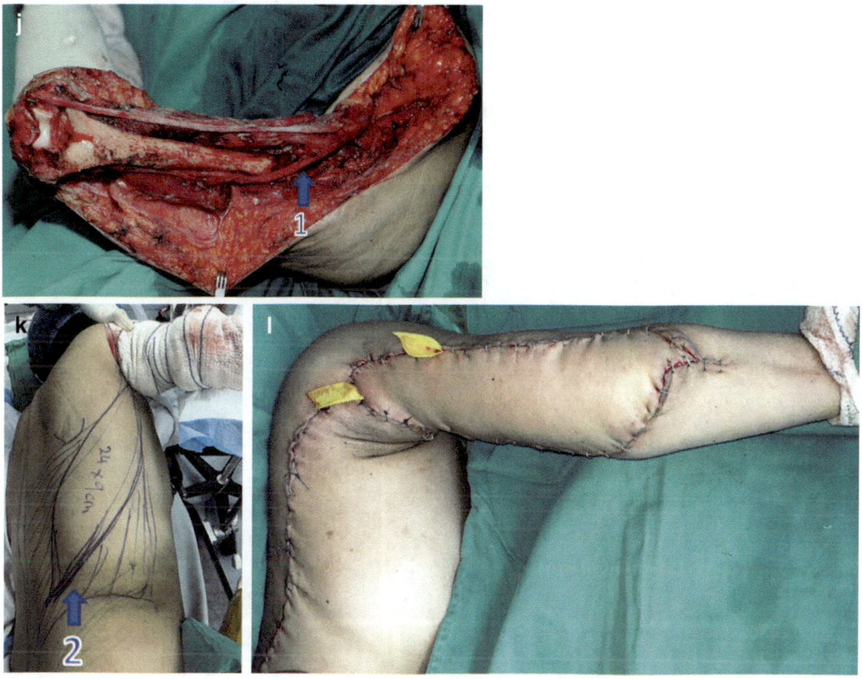

1. Radial nerve
2. Rotational latissimus dorsi flap

Recurrence Sarcoma of the Lateral Triceps with Brachialis Infiltration

Recurrent tumour over the triceps needs a more radical margin of the entire compartment for better oncological clearance.

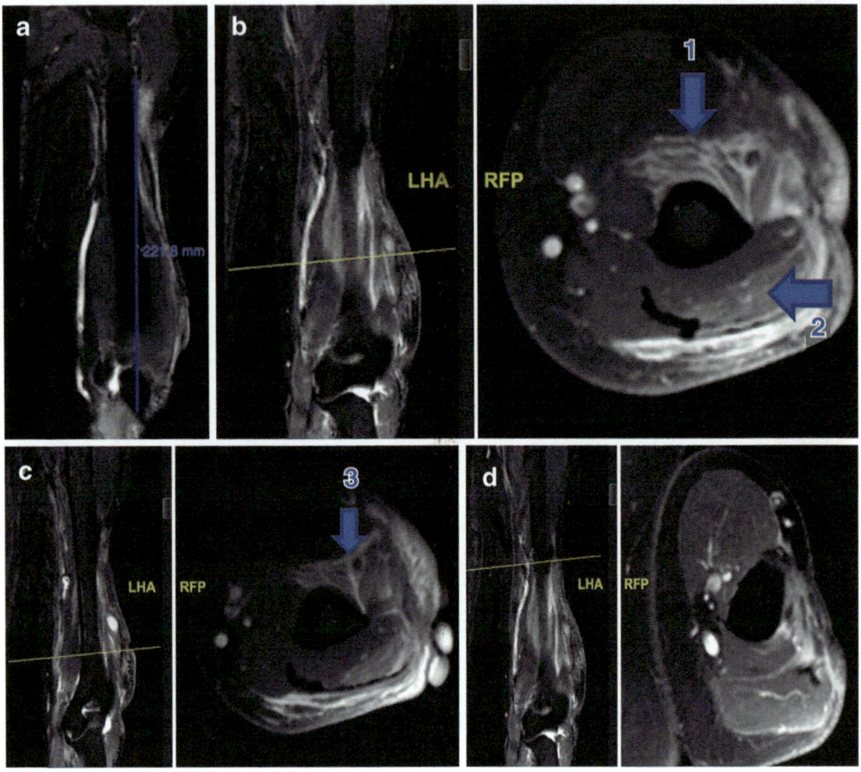

A recurrent sarcoma contaminating the entire posterior compartment and extending to the lateral part of the brachialis muscle. There is a clear plane with the biceps muscle. The medial neurovascular structures are not involved (Fig. 5a–d) The biceps muscle was elevated from the lateral border above the brachialis. The entire triceps was removed together with the brachialis for a more radical margin. The medial neurovascular structures were separated from medial triceps (Fig. 5e–g)

1. Triceps infiltration by recurrence sarcoma
2. Brachialis muscle involvement
3. Profunda humeral artery—radial nerve

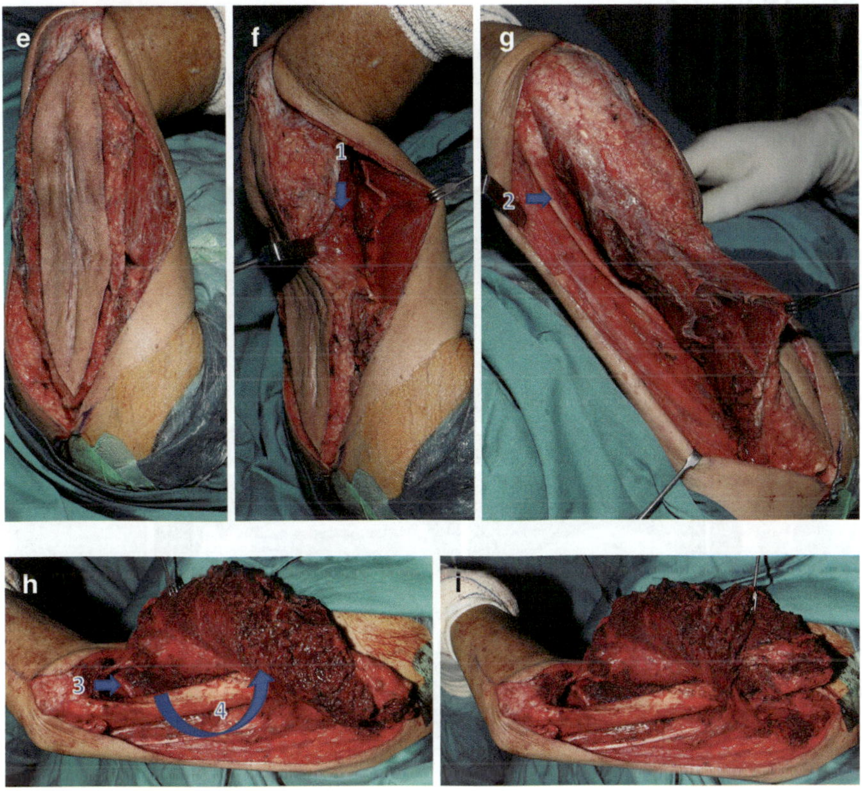

The entire posterior compartment was removed together with the lateral part of the brachialis by elevating the entire muscle from the periosteum (Fig. 5h–j). Motorised latissimus dorsi provides good coverage as well as extensor elbow function (Fig. 5k)

1. Brachialis muscle—anatomical plane with biceps muscle
2. Medial triceps and ulna nerve
3. Radial nerve
4. Elevation of entire triceps above periosteum together with brachialis muscle
5. Remnant triceps

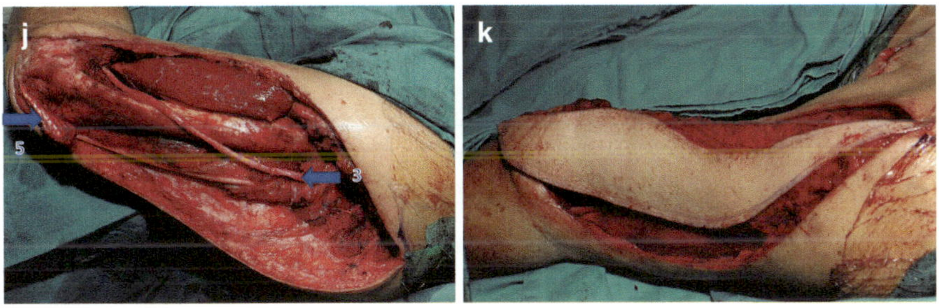

Distal Triceps Sarcoma

Distally based sarcoma over the triceps involving all the muscle compartments to the olecranon attachment. Exploration of the medial septum and ulnar nerve for medial margin and radial nerve laterally to minimise surgical injury and morbidity.

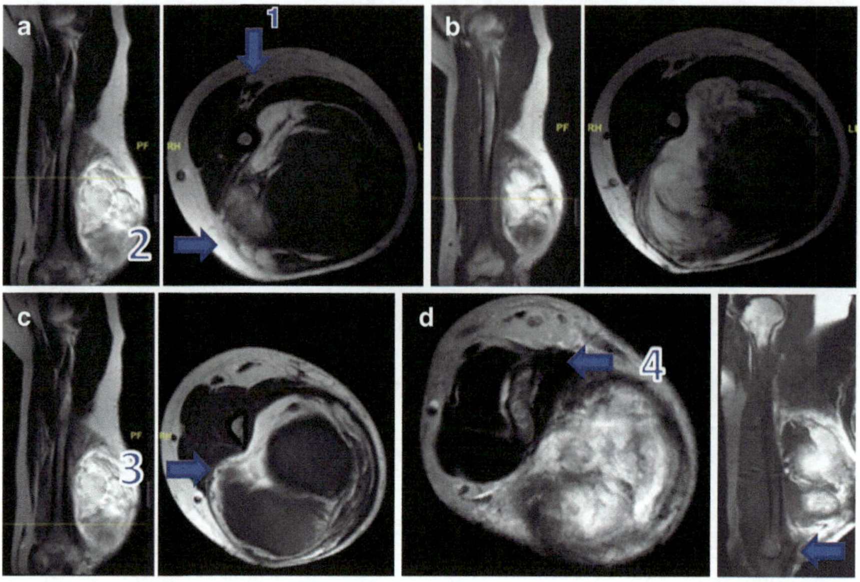

1. Brachial artery, median and ulna nerve
2. Radial nerve between brachioradialis and brachialis
3. Ulna nerve
4. Tip olecranon/triceps attachment

MRI evaluation of distal triceps sarcoma (Fig. 6a–d). Steps of surgical resection (Fig. 6e–g).

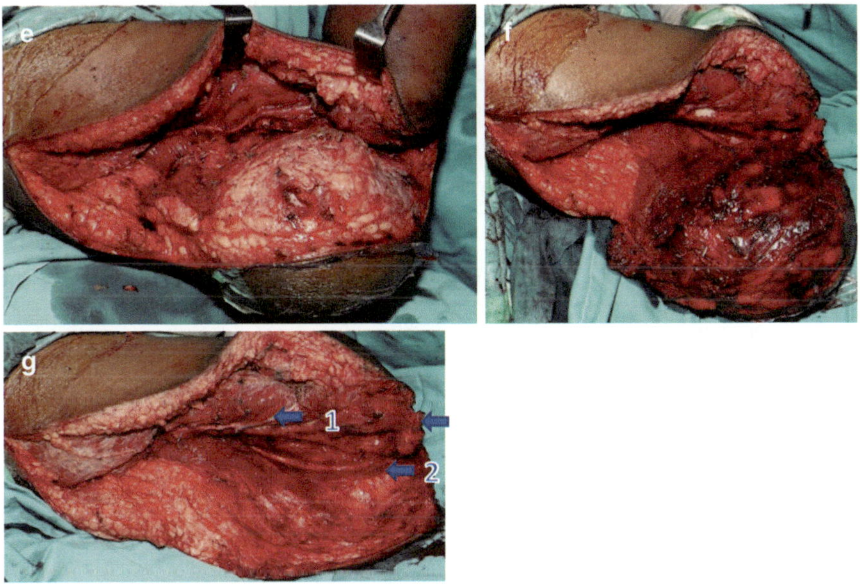

Reconstruction of the triceps continuity with an iliotibial band tendon graft is an option, provided the remnant of proximal tendon is adequate for secure fixation. Distal fixation to the olecranon is reinforced by imbrication by the extensor muscle origin of the forearm (Fig. 6h). Patient has active elbow extension function with good range of motion (Fig. 6I and j).

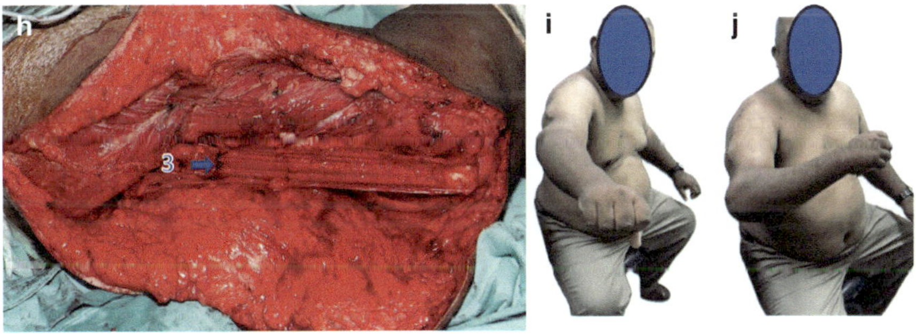

1. Radial nerve
2. Ulna nerve
3. Elbow extensors reconstruct with iliotibial band fascia

Acknowledgement The author thanks Professor Wan Azman Wan Sulaiman, Professor Arman Zaharil Mat Saad and Professor Ahmad Sukari Halim from the plastic reconstructive unit at Universiti Sains Malaysia and MSU Medical Centre, Management and Science University, for their contributions and team member for managing the patients. All plastic reconstructive and microsurgery surgical procedures were performed by the team members.

Suggested Reading

1. Arguello AM, Sullivan MH, Mills GL, Moran SL, Houdek MT. Pedicled functional latissimus flaps for reconstruction of the upper extremity following resection of soft-tissue sarcomas. Curr Oncol. 2023;30(3):3138–48.
2. Clancy R, Lim Z, Ravinsky RA, O'Neill A, Ferguson P, Wunder J. Use of a fascia lata autograft to reconstruct a large triceps tendon defect after en-bloc resection of a soft-tissue sarcoma: a case report. JBJS Case Connector. 2020;10(1):e0390.
3. Karakousis CP. Tumor in the dorsal aspect of the arm atlas of operative procedures in surgical oncology. New York: Springer Science; 2015. ISBN978-1-4939-1634-4
4. Muramatsu K, Ihara K, Doi K, Yoshida K, Iwanaga R, Hashimoto T, Taguchi T. Functional neuro-vascularized muscle transfer for oncological reconstruction of extremity sarcoma. Surg Oncol. 2012;21:263e268.
5. Lohman RF, Nabawi AS, Reece GP, Pollock RE, Evans GRD. Soft tissue sarcoma of the upper extremity a 5-year experience at two institutions emphasizing the role of soft tissue flap reconstruction. Cancer. 2002;15:94–8.

Axillary Tumour and Shoulder Girdle

Wan Faisham Nu'man Bin Wan Ismail

Introduction

The axillary and para scapulae shoulder girdle are complex areas with unique functions. A major neurovascular bundle supplies the upper limb and runs across the clavicle and main part of the axillary content. The shoulder girdle muscle, inserted mainly in the scapulae, accomplishes main shoulder function. Understanding the anatomical correlation to these structures and evaluating their involvement by the sarcoma are important for surgical and treatment planning. Surgical morbidity, quality of the surgery and margin and adjuvant treatment morbidity are important aspects of discussion prior to intervention.

Surgical Anatomy

The axilla is bound by the serratus anterior, latissimus dorsi, clavipectoral fascia and subscapularis. It is a pyramid-shaped space, and the axillary sheath is a fibrous sheath that encloses the axillary artery and three cords of the brachial plexus to form the neurovascular bundle.

The shoulder girdle consists of four rotator cuff muscles, including the supraspinatus, infraspinatus, teres minor, subscapularis and accessory girdle of the pectoralis major, minor, deltoids, trapezius and serratus anterior. These muscles are attached to the scapular surface and assist with abduction and external and internal rotation of the glenohumeral joint. Hence, understanding the attachment and function is important for predicting functional morbidity following sarcoma resection.

W. F. N. B. W. Ismail (✉)
Prince Court Medical Center, Kuala Lumpur, Malaysia

Orthopaedic Oncology Reconstructive Unit, Universiti Sains Malaysia, Kubang Kerian, Kelantan, Malaysia

A. Puri, W. F. N. B. W. Ismail (eds.), *Atlas of Orthopedic Oncology Volume 1*,
https://doi.org/10.1007/978-981-95-8958-6_10

Assessments

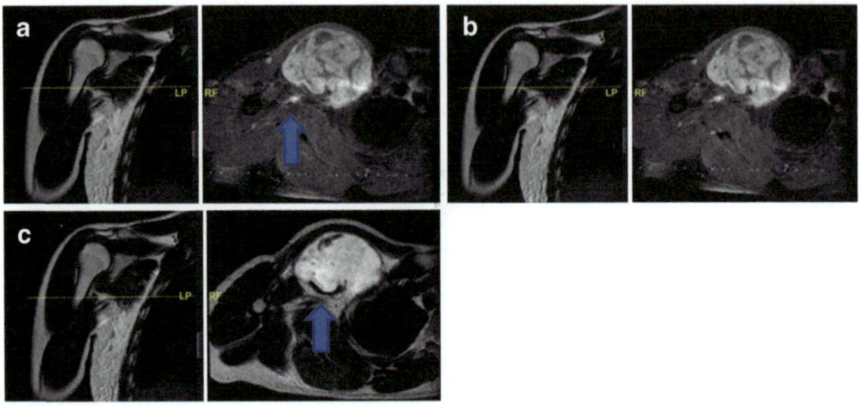

Pectoralis major muscle sarcoma involving the clavicle and sternum head. The axillary neurovascular structures are not involved. The brachial plexus is protected by the pectoralis minor (Fig. 1a–c).

- Axillary vessels
- Brachial plexus

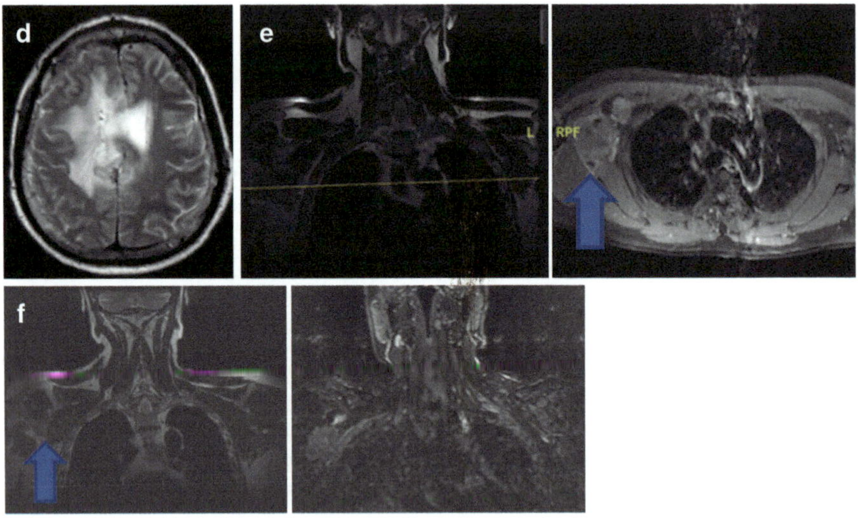

A case of neurofibromatosis with MPNSTS of the brachial plexus showing the entire infraclavicular area of the plexus was involved. The axillary artery and vein were trapped within the tumour mass. Resection would result in a flail limb with a narrow margin and would require vascular reconstruction and adjuvant radiotherapy (Fig. 1d–f).

- MPNST involved the entire brachial plexus

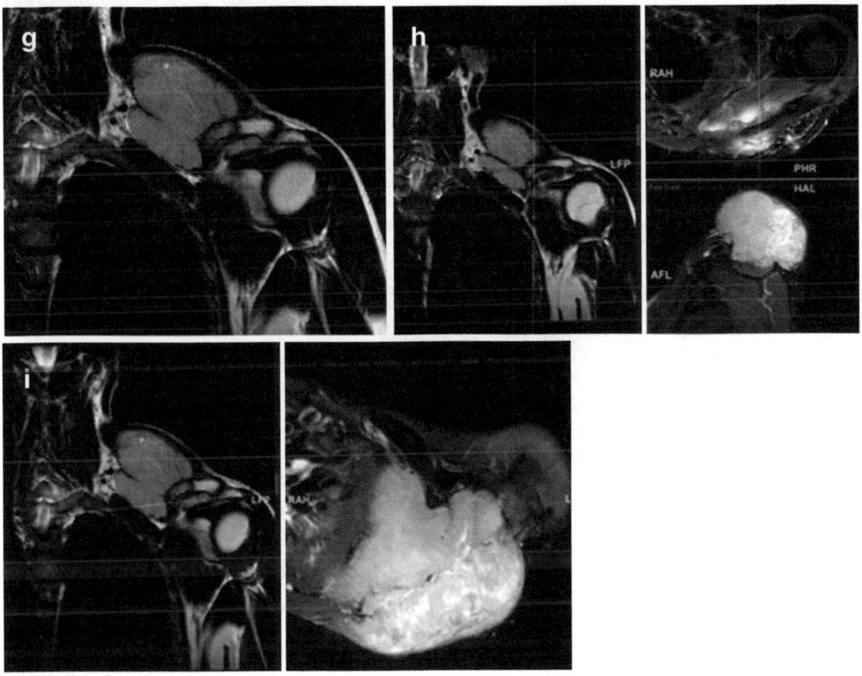

Complex sarcoma shoulder girdle involving the trapezius, levator scapulae, supraspinatus and encircling proximal part of the clavicle (Fig. 1g–i). Complex resection and functional morbidity are expected. Adjuvant radiotherapy is mandatory in view of narrow margin.

Surgical Steps of Different Regions of the Axillary and Shoulder Girdle

Superficial Axillary Sarcoma

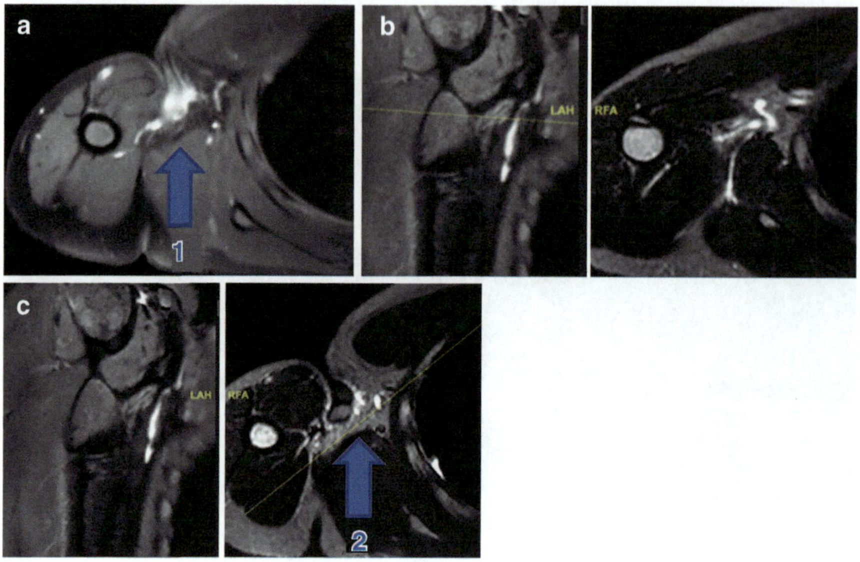

A case of sarcoma of the axillary region with previous excision biopsy of the skin with an involved margin. An MRI evaluation showed the surrounding oedema and multiple axillary nodes. The axillary sheath was preserved without contamination (Fig. 2a–c). Adequate skin, subcutaneous tissue, fascia, and axillary fat content with the nodes were removed for quality margins. Subsequent histopathology revealed that the nodes were reactive without infiltration (Fig. 2d–h)

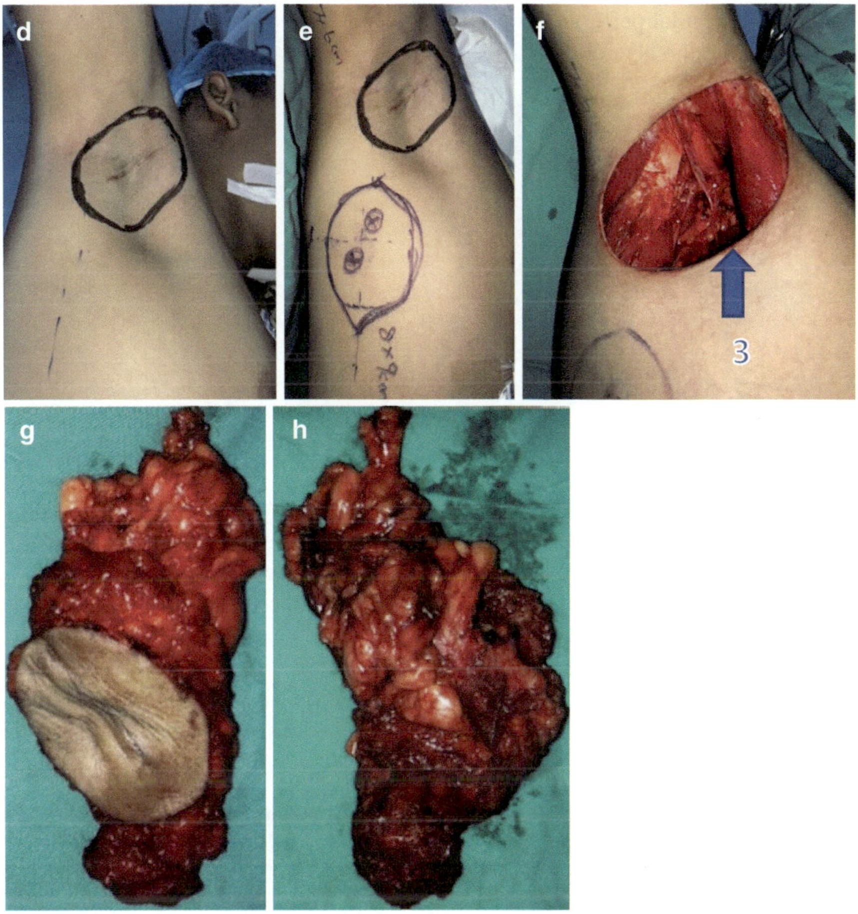

1. Multiple reactive nodes
2. High-intensity surgical scars recurrence
3. Lymph nodes clearance

Thoracoacromial perforator rotational flap was used for closure for early rehabilitation and radiotherapy (Fig. 2i–k)

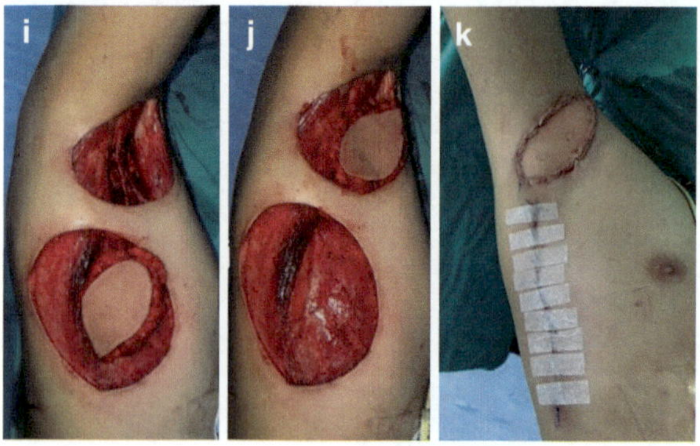

Brachial Plexus Schwannoma

Benign nerve tumour of the brachial plexus can be determined by MRI based on well-defined lesion situated within the plexus with special image characteristic. Schwannoma can be enucleated with preservation of nerve fascicle and minimal motor disability. It must be differentiated from neuroma as surgery for neuroma is complicated with neuropathic pain, and sometimes resection of a segment of nerve is indicated.

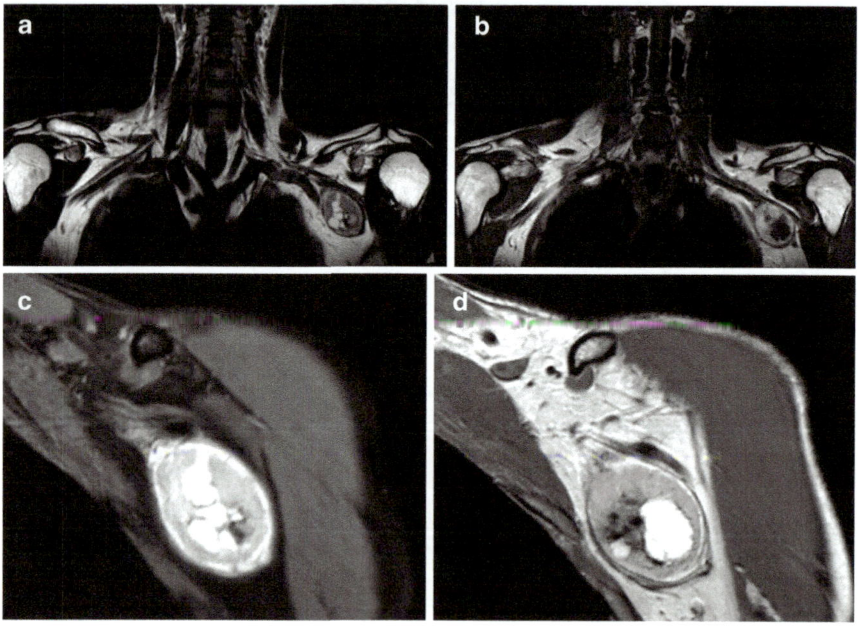

Well-defined ovoid lesion with heterogeneous intensity demonstrating intratumoral cystic lesion with split fat sign. It is inferior to axillary artery tethered to medial cord and ulna nerve most probably a schwannoma (Fig. 3a–d).

Extensile deltopectoral approach and mobilisation of pectoralis minor from coracoid process will expose the brachial plexus and axillary artery for proximal and distal visualisation of the schwannoma and enucleation of capsule with preservation of fasicles (Fig. 3e–i)

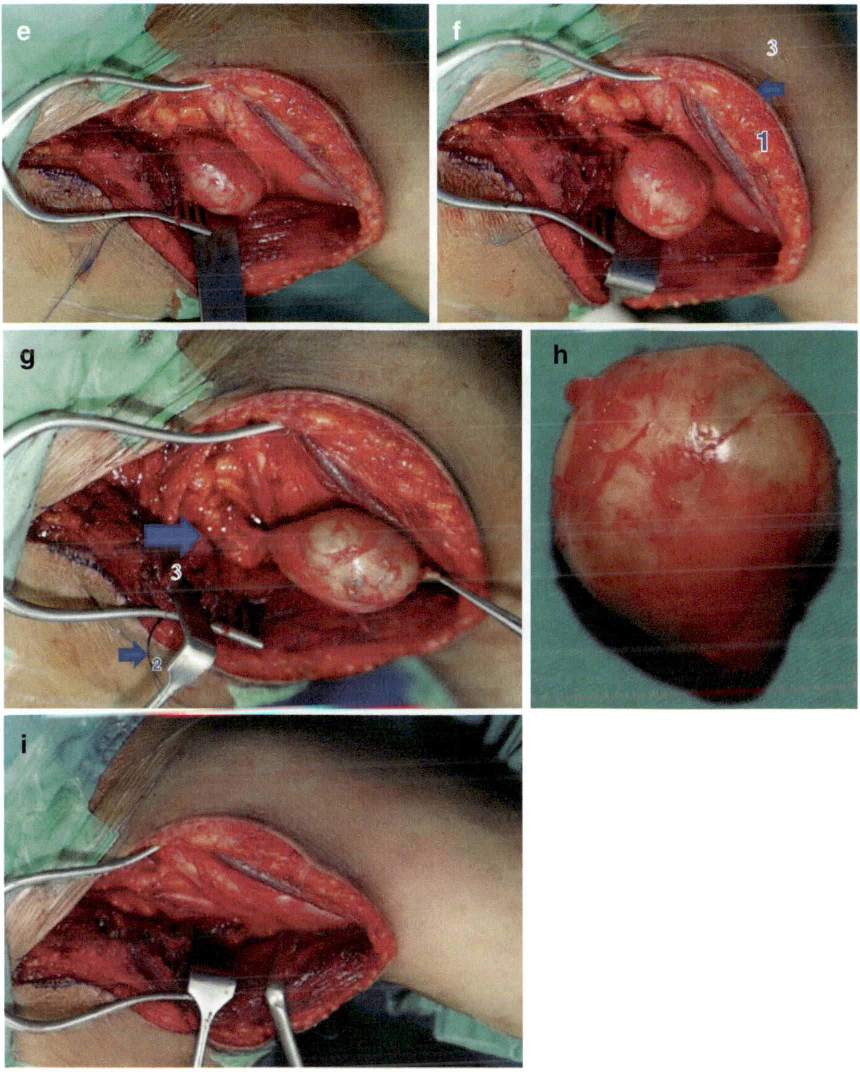

1. Cephalic vein
2. Suture secures pectoralis minor tendon
3. Proximal part ulnar nerve

Pectoralis Major Sarcoma Resection

The pectoralis major is a thick fan-shaped cover of the upper chest composed of the clavicular, sternocostal and abdominal heads and inserts in the lateral lip of the intertubercular groove. It assists in adduction, forward flexion, and medial rotation of the arm. It is innervated by the medial and pectoral nerve from the lateral cord and supplied by the pectoral branch of the thoracoacromial trunk.

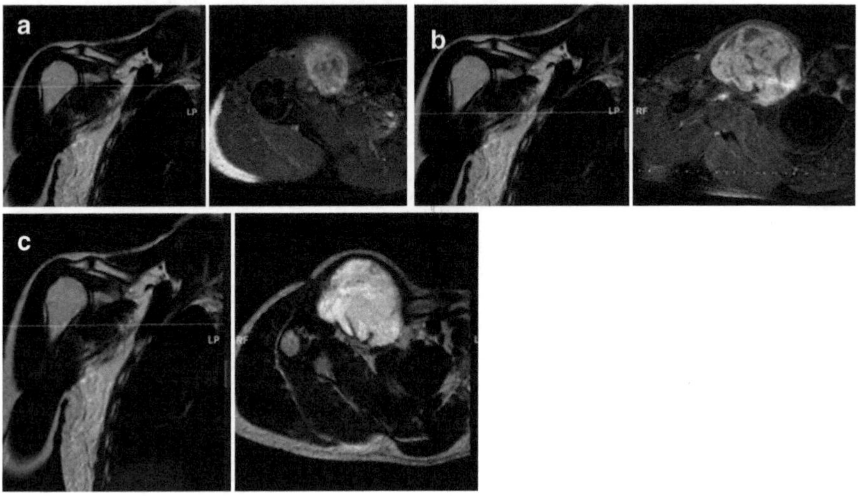

Assessment includes correlation with axillary content and brachial plexus, origin of the pectoralis major and its insertion. This pectoralis major sarcoma was confined to the intra-compartment muscle and protected by the pectoralis minor. There was no direct invasion to the axillary sheath (Fig. 4a–c).

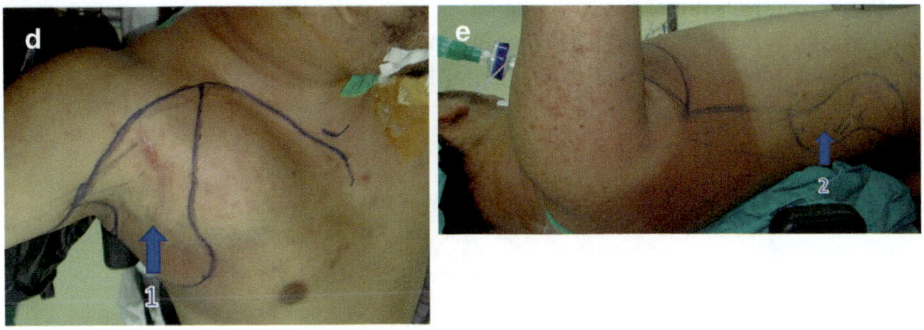

A case of incomplete resection of the pectoralis major sarcoma with axillay scars. There is significant contamination in the axillary fat, which needs to be removed completely. The vascular sheath and neurovascular bundle were not opened in the previous surgery. Limb salvage surgery was possible with minimal surgical contamination and adjuvant radiotherapy was added.

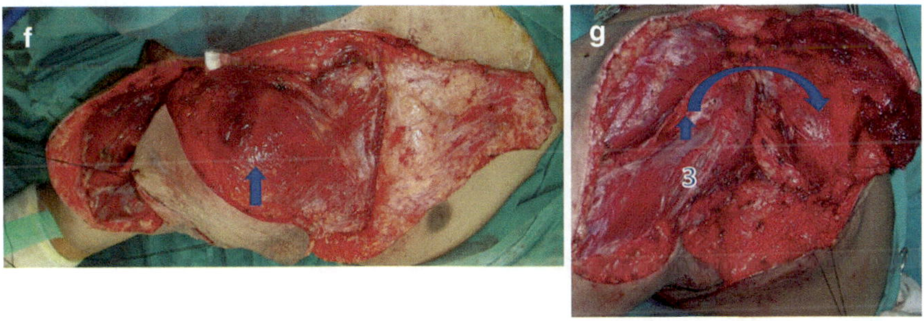

An extensile skin flap is used to expose the entire pectoralis major muscle. A latissimus dorsi flap is planned due to extensive scars and anticipated axillary contamination from the previous surgery. The initial step is identification of the delto-pectoral groove and detachment of the pectoris tendon insertion from proximal humerus (Fig. 4d–g)

1. Previous intralesional surgery surgical scar
2. Latissimus dorsi flap surgical planning incorporating skin resection
3. Pectoralis major detached from medial humerus insertion—mobilisation from axillary vessels and brachial plexus

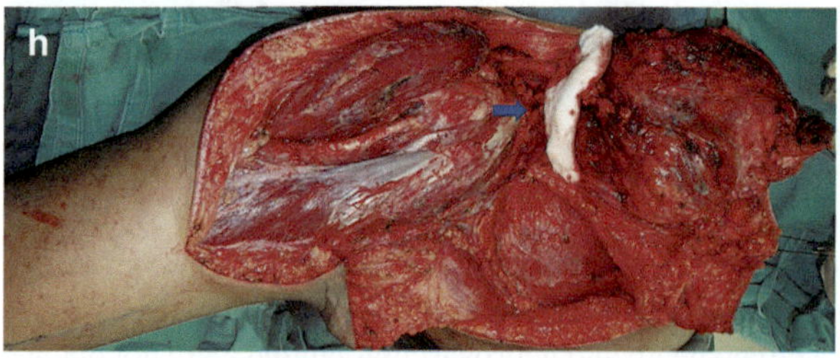

Mobilise the pectoralis major medially together with pectoralis minor and entire axillary fat for adequate margins. The axillary sheath is explored, and the pectoral vessels and nerve are ligated prior to complete resection (Fig. 4h, i)

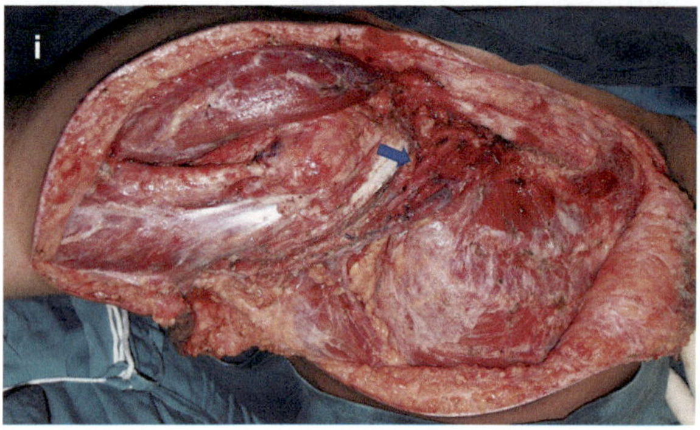

- Brachial plexus and axillary vessels

Surgery completed with a rotational latissimus dorsi flap for closure, early rehabilitation and radiotherapy.

Low-Grade Tumour in the Axillary Space

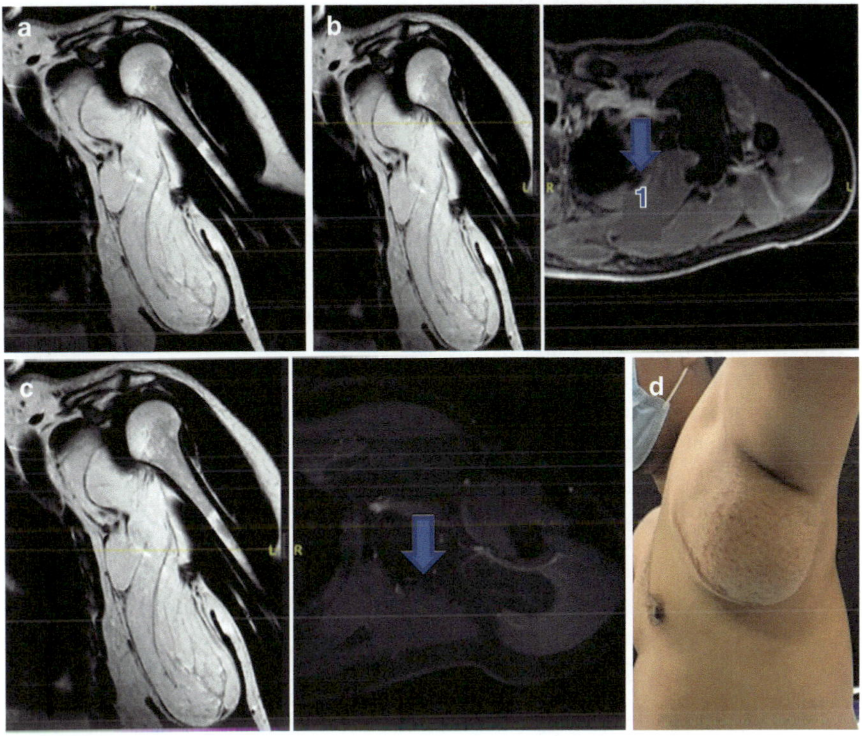

Atypical lipomatous tumour over the axillae with extension to the axillary content. The axillary artery, vein and brachial plexus were within the tumour (Fig. 5a–d). Marginal resection and macroscopic clearance are possible after mobilising the artery and brachial plexus.

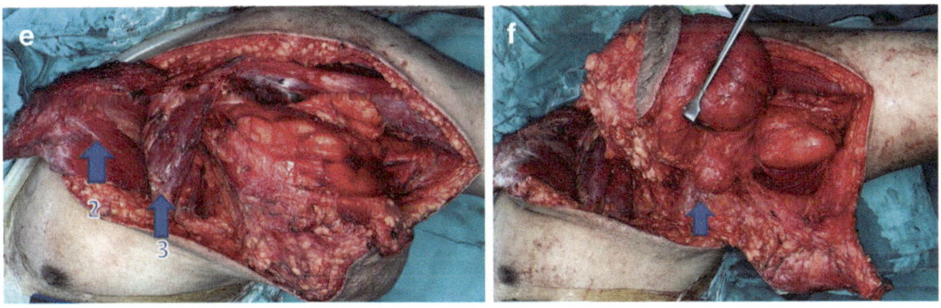

The pectoralis major and minor were mobilised from their attachments to visualise the axillary content. The brachial plexus and artery were mobilised in between the lobule of the lipomatosus lesion. The musculocutaneous nerve must be identified and secured to prevent injury during mobilisation of the entire lesion. Axillary fat was removed in total with the lipomatous lesion to the axillae (Fig. 5e–g)

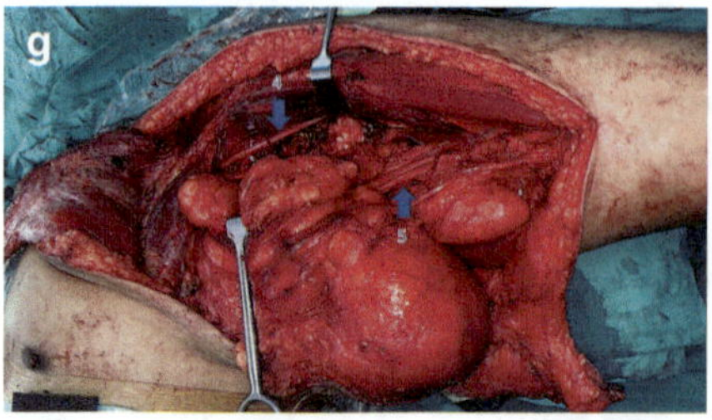

1. Subclavian-axillary artery
2. Pectoralis major mobilisation from humerus insertion
3. Pectoralis minor
4. Musculocutaneous nerve
5. Cord of brachial plexus and axillary artery
6. Reattachment of pectoralis major to humerus insertion for closure (Fig. 5h, i)

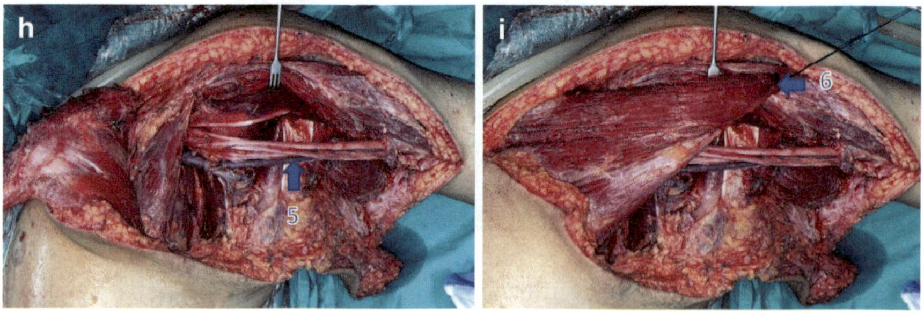

Anatomical reconstruction of the pectoralis major and minor prior to closure (Fig. 5h, i). Due to the benign nature of the lesion, adjuvant local radiotherapy was not given. Surveillance with MRI and CT for recurrence was advised.

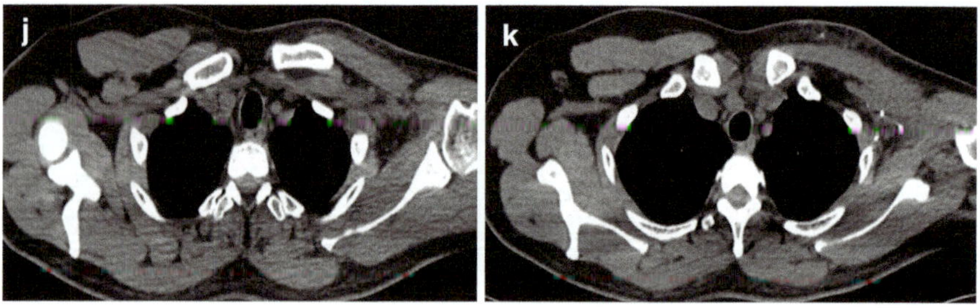

Subsequent contrast CT chest and axilla revealed no evidence of disease (Fig. 5j, k)

Infraspinatus Liposarcoma

A case of recurrent liposarcoma of the scapular area contaminating the subcutaneous tissue and entire infraspinatus and deltoid attachment (Fig. 6a–d)

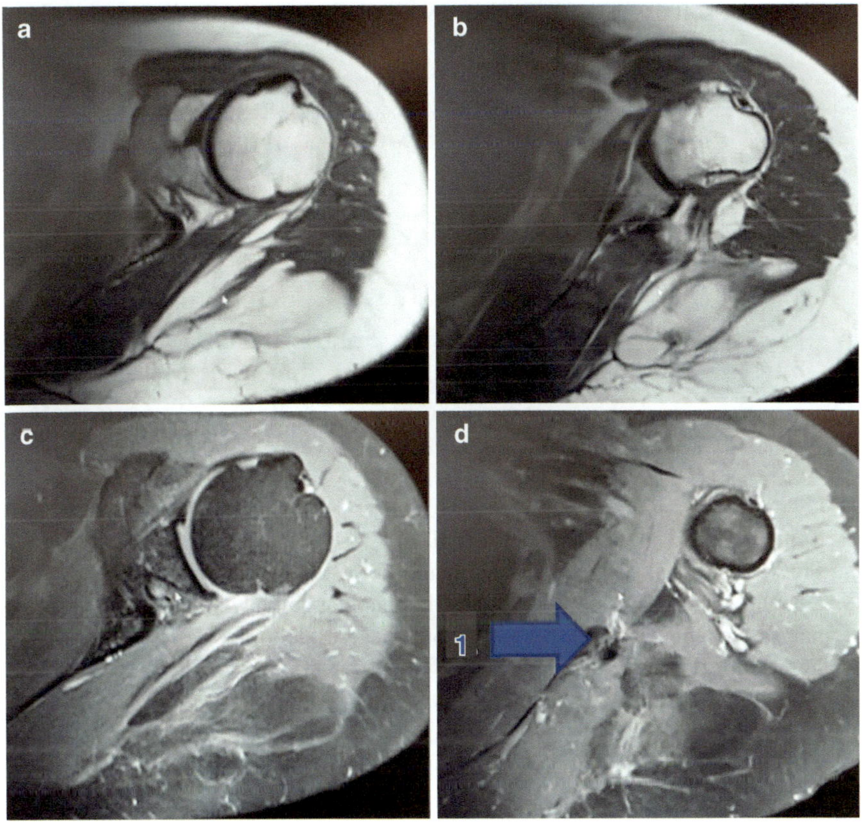

Surgical steps (Fig. 6e–j):

- The contaminated area of the previous resection margin is marked and removed in total with the entire infraspinatus muscle to achieve oncological margin.
- The deltoid attachment to the scapula spine (scapular origin) is removed together with the tumour after elevation of the subcutaneous flap.
- The entire soft tissue defect is closed with a latissimus dorsi advancement flap.

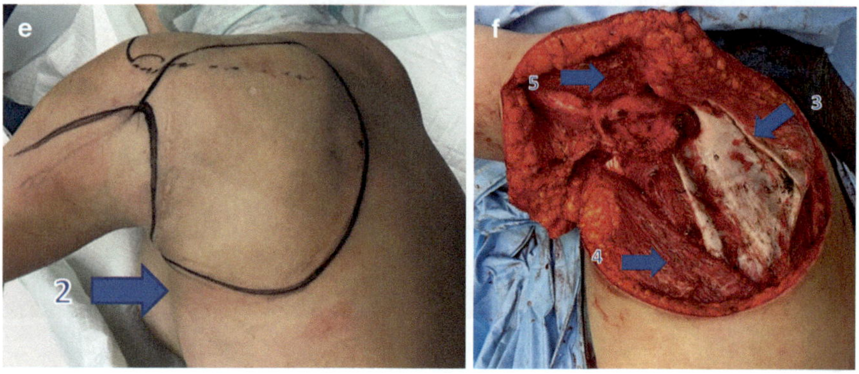

1. Tumour closely attached to the scapula
2. Previous surgical scars and contamination
3. Scapula spine—entire muscle below the scapular spine which includes infraspinatus, teres major and minor and scapula head of deltoid
4. Latissimus dorsi muscle maintained
5. Posterior deltoid

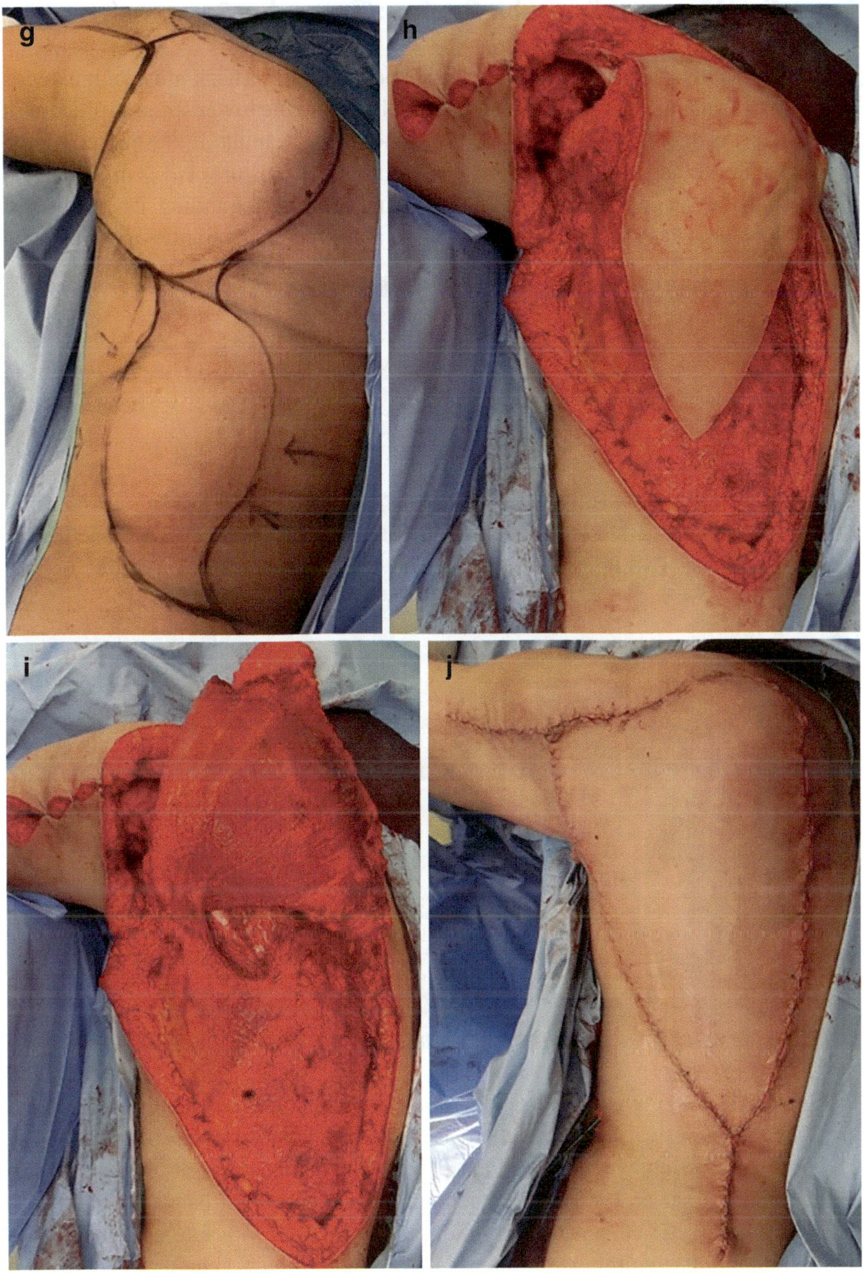
g
h
i
j

Superficial Tumour Scapular Region: 'Trapezius Sarcoma'

The trapezius muscle is a large trapezoid-shaped superficial back muscle. It extends from the external protuberance of the occipital bone to the lower spinous process of the thoracic vertebrae and laterally to the spine of the scapula. It is supplied by the accessory nerve and is an important muscle for back posture and stabilising and mobilising the scapula during shoulder abduction. Understanding its origin and insertion is important for surgical planning to achieve an oncological margin.

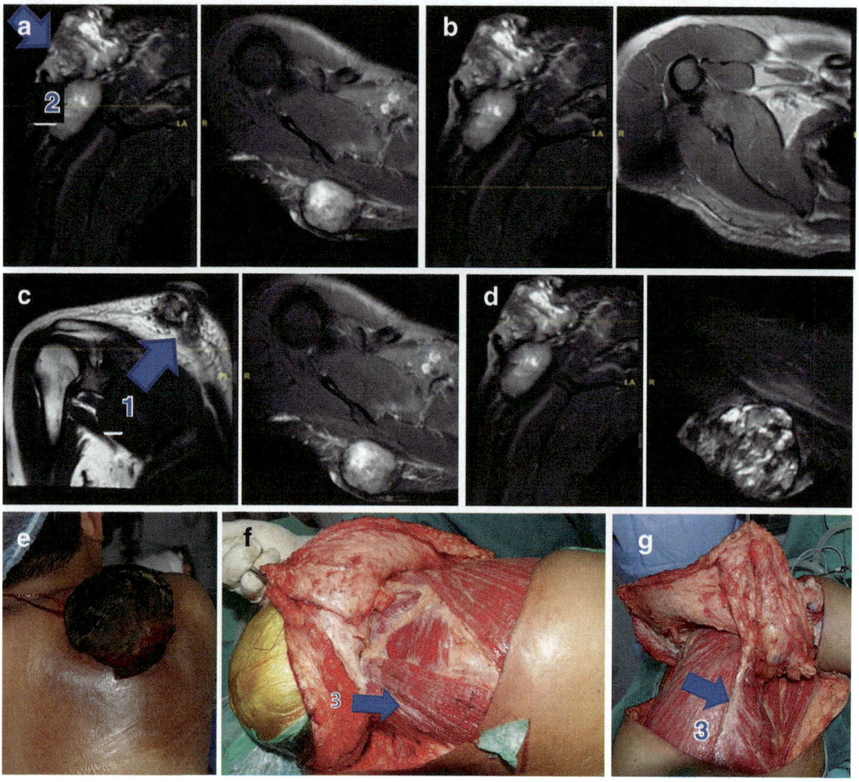

Superficial layer pleomorphic sarcoma of the back with superior fungation involves the trapezius. However, the deep layer muscles were spared (Fig. 7a–e). The trapezius muscle was removed entirely till the spinous process of the thoracic spine, scapula spine and acromion attachment. The fungating area was cleaned with antiseptic, wrapped with gauze, circumferentially secured with sutures, and covered with plastic offsite to minimise contamination. A wide area of skin flap was included in the surgical margin to improve the oncological margin (Fig. 7f–k).

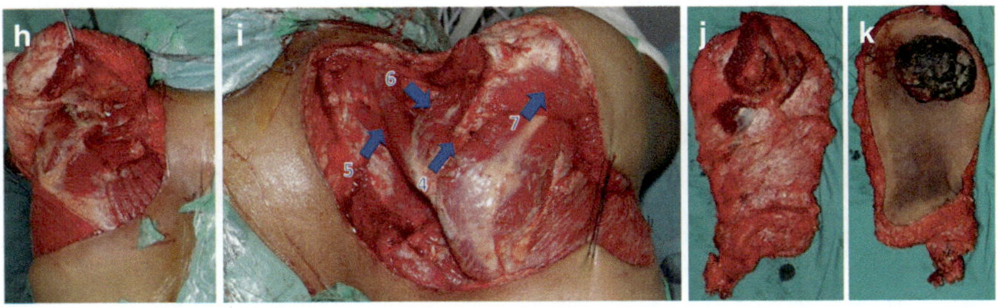

1. Fungating mass trapezius posterior base of neck
2. Inflammation and infiltration to the surrounding skin
3. Medial border of scapula trapezius attachment
4. Scapula spine
5. Levator scapula
6. Supraspinatus
7. Scapula origin of deltoid

The suprascapular and para scapular nodes were removed in total with the sarcoma. The rhomboid muscle, which was adhered to the trapezius muscle, was also included in the margin. The levator scapula muscle was spared. Final closure with rotational latissimus dorsi flap (Fig. 7l, m).

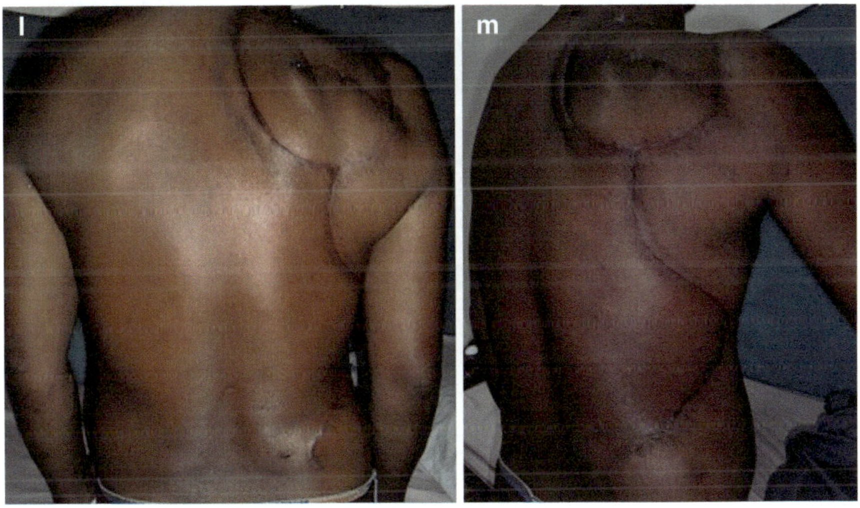

Shoulder Girdle Sarcoma Involving Inferior Scapula

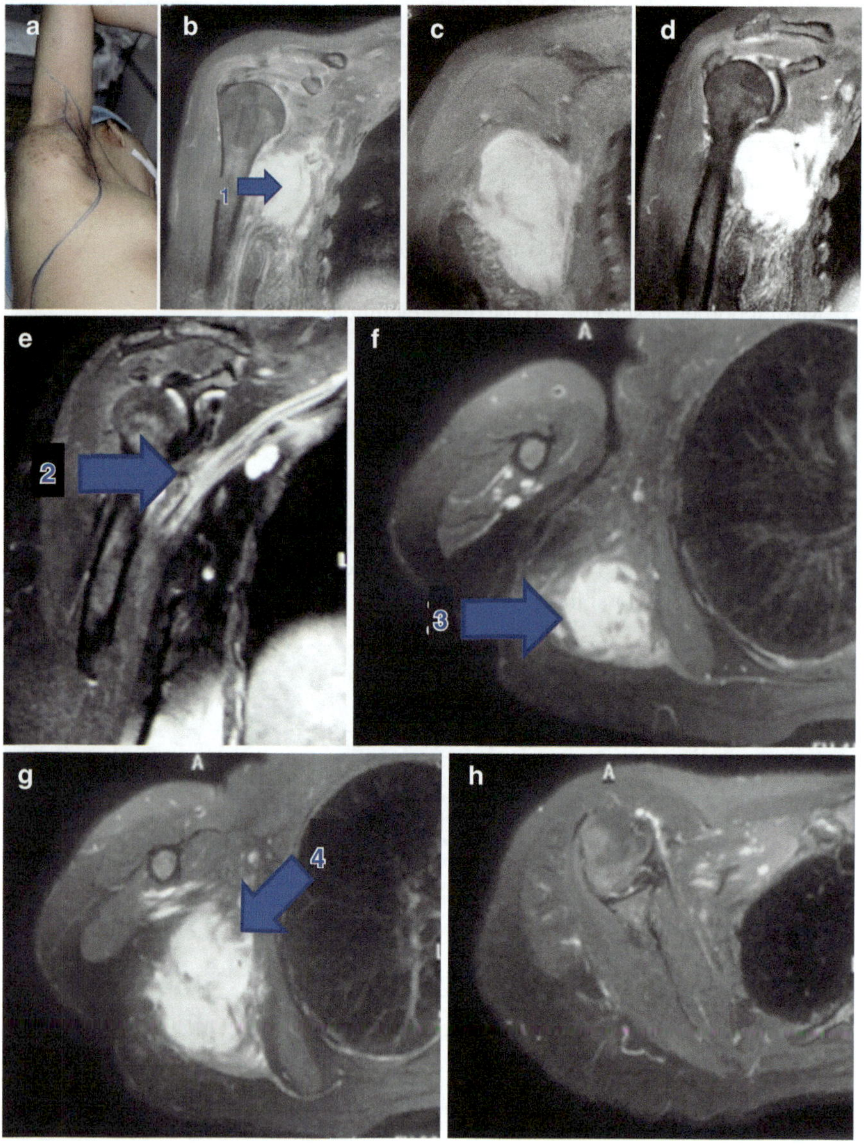

1. Teres major and minor
2. Brachial artery and brachial plexus
3. Infraspinatus
4. Subscapularis

Large sarcoma involving the teres major and minor extending to infraspinatus and subscapularis. The inferior border of the scapula below the scapula spine was involved. The insertion of these shoulder girdle muscles to the humerus was close; however, the bone was not involved. The supraspinatus and shoulder capsules were not involved (Fig. 8a–h)

Surgical steps (Fig. 8i–n):

- Create a fasciocutaneous flap to visualise the entire scapula to its medial border to the level of the scapulae spine. Posterior deltoid must be mobilised from its scapula origin for evaluation of the infraspinatus and teres muscles.
- The flap extends to the infraspinatus and teres origin posterior to the humerus tubercle.
- Mobilisation of the axillary sheath anterior to the subscapularis to the proximal humerus.
- Detachment of the insertion of the infraspinatus, teres major and minor and anteriorly from the inferior part of the subscapularis.
- Tumour is removed in total with the inferior scapula below. The scapula spine and final medial border of the scapula are detached from the trapezius and rhomboids.

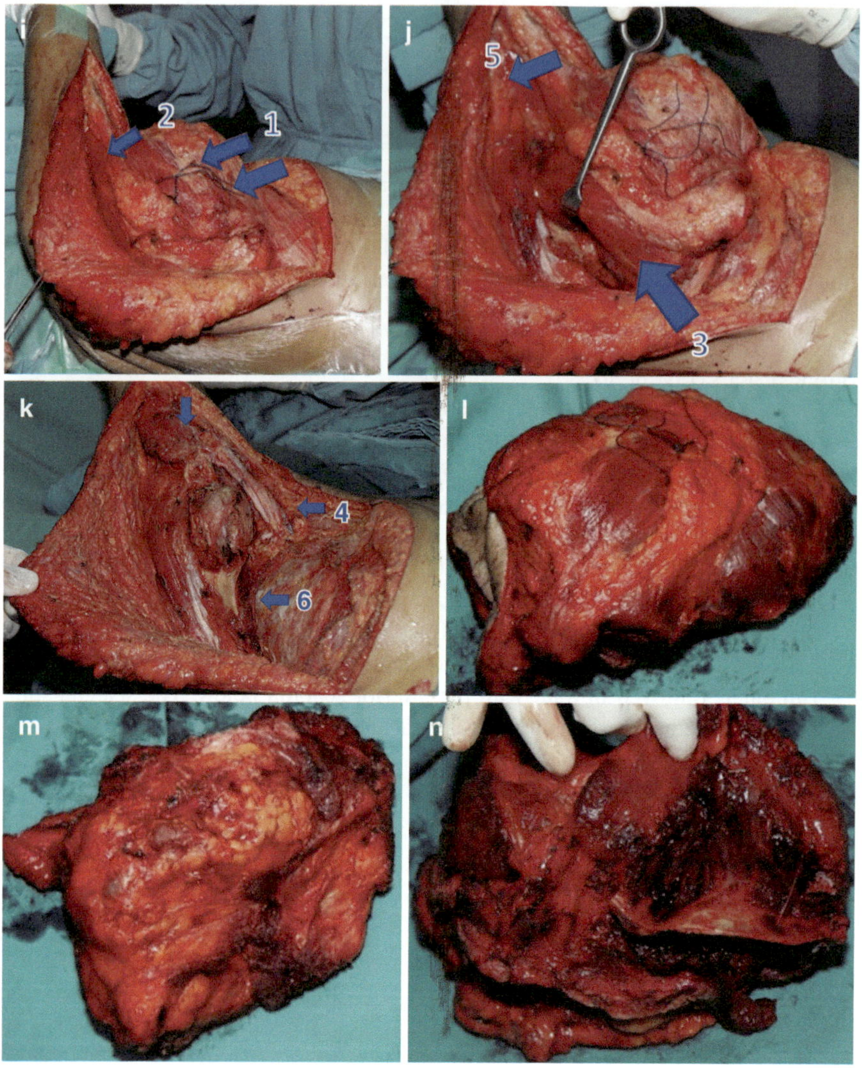
i
2
1
j
5
3
k
4
6
l
m
n

1. Teres major and minor
2. Scapula head of deltoid
3. Infraspinatus
4. Brachial plexus anteriorly
5. Remnant of posterior deltoid
6. Medial border scapula

Adjuvant radiotherapy is necessary due to the narrow surgical margin. Shoulder function expected to be impaired; however, functional abduction is still possible.

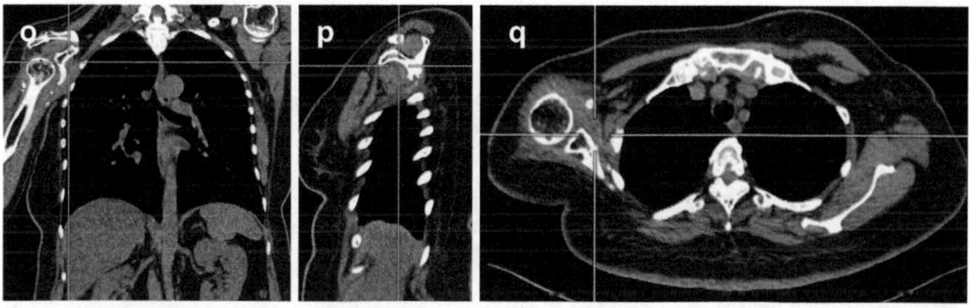

Follow-up CT showed that the humeral head was maintained in the glenoid and part of the superior scapula above the scapulae spine stable was in position (Fig. 8o–q)

Suprascapular Sarcoma

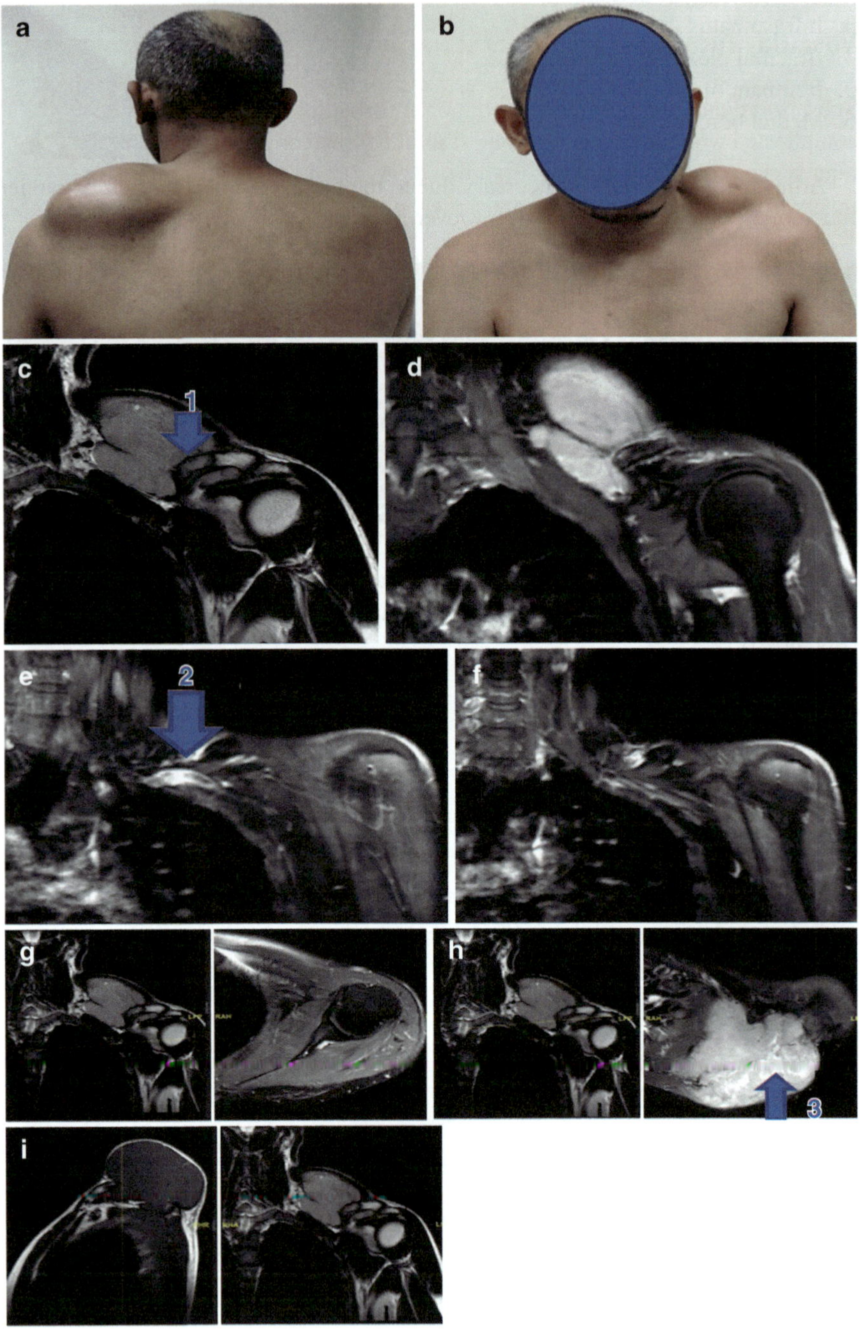

Sarcoma suprascapular region involving the supraspinatus, trapezius and levator scapula. The tumour encircles the lateral half of the clavicle and must be included in the margin. The axillary sheath and brachial plexus were preserved (Fig. 9a–i). Preservation of the deltoid and infraspinatus as shoulder abductor will maintain the function; however, rotation of the scapulae in overhead activities will be restricted due to removal of the scapulae girdle.

1. Supraspinatus and superior part of scapulae
2. Axillary artery and brachial plexus
3. Tumour involving trapezius, levator scapulae and supraspinatus

Surgical steps (Fig. 9j–o):

- Mobilisation of a fasciocutaneous flap from the upper shoulder to the base of the neck.
- Detachment of the superficial muscle for exposure
  - The pectoralis major at the clavicular head from axillary vessels and brachial plexus exploration
  - The trapezius must be included in the oncological margin and sectioned at the medial scapula border
- The clavicle is freed from the plexus medially for osteotomy and the lateral margin is the clavicular acromion joint. Anterior mobilisation of tumour mass will expose the suprascapular nerve.
- Mobilisation of the supraspinatus muscle from the suprascapular fossa. Care must be taken to maintain the suprascapular nerve and vessels for infraspinatus innervation.
- Finally, the levator scapula and rhomboid minor are detached from their insertion at the transverse process spine.

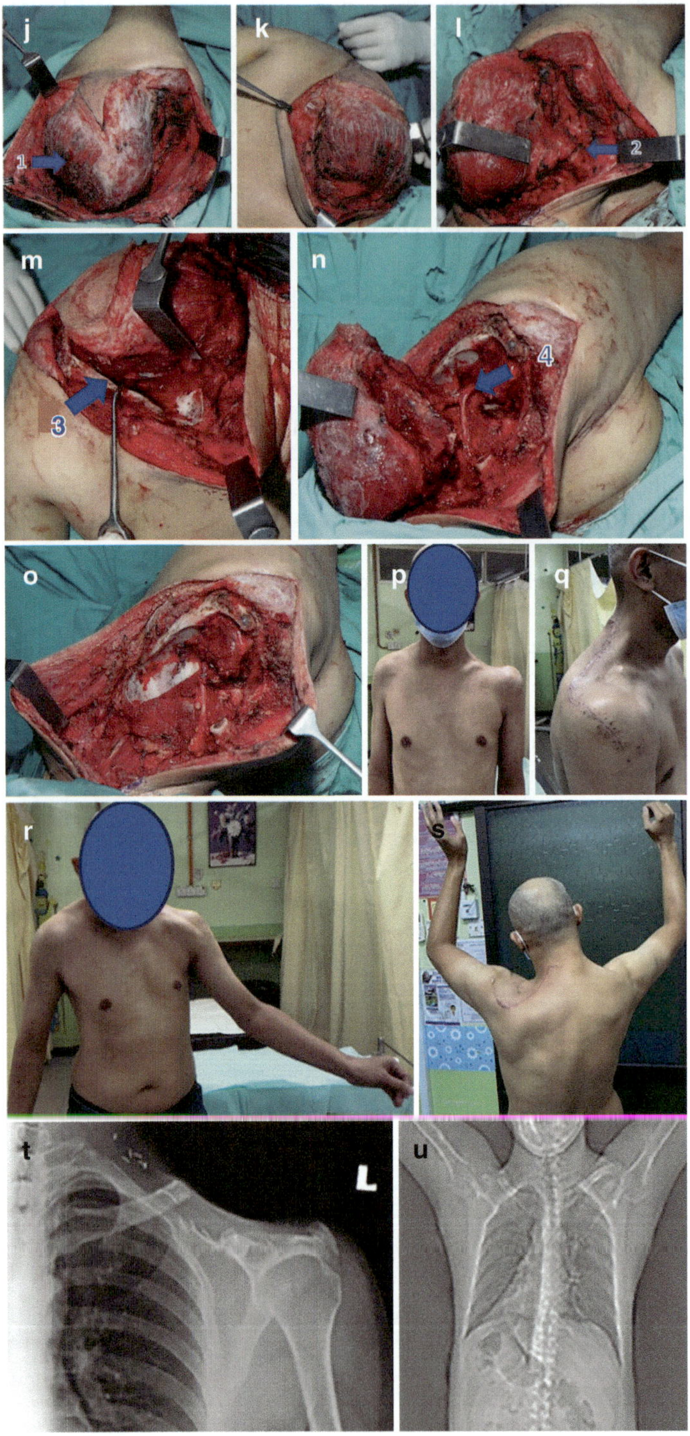
j
k
l
1
2
m
n
3
4
o
p
q
r
s
t
u
L

1. Trapezius muscle
2. Medial clavicle osteotomy
3. Scapula crest elevated and cut for margin
4. Suprascapular nerve

Functional outcome during the postoperative period and after rehabilitation and adjuvant radiotherapy (Fig. 9p–u)

Suggested Reading

1. Behnam AB, Chen CM, Pusic AL, Mehrara BJ, Disa JJ, Athanasian EA, Cordeiro PG. The pedicled latissimus dorsi flap for shoulder reconstruction after sarcoma resection. Ann Surg Oncol. 14(5):1591–5.
2. Cleeman E, Auerbach JD, Springfield DS. Tumors of the shoulder girdle: a review of 194 cases. J Shoulder Elb Surg. 2005;14(5):460–5.
3. Constantine P. Karakousis. Tumor at the shoulder point - atlas of operative procedures in surgical oncology. 83-86 Springer Science 2015
4. Jin JW, Jung SW, Park JY, Jeon JM. Wide resection preserving conjoined tendons of the rotator cuff muscles for undifferentiated pleomorphic sarcoma at the suprascapular fossa–a case report. J Hand Surg (Asian-Pacific Volume). 2023;28(03).
5. Kim JS, Lee JS, Yoon JO, Park JB. Reconstruction of the shoulder region using a pedicled latissimus dorsi flap after resection of soft tissue due to sarcoma. J Plast Reconstr Aesthet Surg. 2009;62:1215e1218.
6. Salemis NS. Intramuscular atypical lipomatous tumour well-differentiated liposarcoma of the pectoralis major masquerading as a breast tumour: management and review of the literature. Int Surg. 2015;100(2):194–8.
7. Stauss R, Graulich T, Pacha O, Omar M. Limb-sparing resection of axillary soft tissue sarcomas. Oper Orthop Traumatol. 2023;35:–377.

Forearm Resection

Wan Faisham Nu'man Bin Wan Ismail,
Mohammad Bin Paiman, Arman Zaharil Mat Saad,
and Wan Azman Wan Sulaiman

Introduction

The forearm comprises unique anatomical structures and is one of the few locations in the body where most muscles run in close vicinity to one another and almost in parallel. Soft tissue sarcomas of the forearm are rare tumours needing special consideration, as their location involves complex anatomy and limited tissue volume. The goal of forearm STS treatment is to perform limb-sparing surgery with wide resection margins, while preserving the function of the distal upper extremity. Surgical margins should never be sacrificed in an attempt to maintain hand function. Wide resection for sarcoma can entail large, deep and complex defects as well as functional deficits. Careful planning is mandatory to achieve functional reconstruction. Immediate reconstruction using free-tissue transfer has advantages of minimising fibrosis and early rehabilitation. Furthermore, motorised functional transfer will improve the functional deficit following resection.

W. F. N. B. W. Ismail (✉)
Prince Court Medical Center, Kuala Lumpur, Malaysia

Orthopaedic Oncology Reconstructive Unit, Universiti Sains Malaysia,
Kubang Kerian, Kelantan, Malaysia

M. B. Paiman
Hand and Microsurgery - Orthopaedic Department, Universiti Sains Malaysia,
Kubang Kerian, Kelantan, Malaysia

A. Z. M. Saad
Plastic Reconstructive & Microsurgery, MSU Medical Centre, Management and Science
University of Malaysia, Shah Alam, Selangor, Malaysia

W. A. W. Sulaiman
Reconstructive Sciences Department, School of Medical Sciences, Universiti Sains Malaysia,
Kubang Kerian, Kelantan, Malaysia

A. Puri, W. F. N. B. W. Ismail (eds.), *Atlas of Orthopedic Oncology Volume 1*,
https://doi.org/10.1007/978-981-95-8958-6_11

Functional Anatomy

The forearm and hand comprise unique anatomical structures and functions classified as extensor muscles and the flexor group which run in close vicinity to one another and almost in parallel. Most muscles originate close to the elbow and extend all the way to the fingertips.

Flexor compartment:
- Includes the pronator teres, flexor carpi radialis, flexor carpi ulnaris, palmaris longus and flexor digitorum superficialis
- Shares a common origin at the medial epicondyle of the humerus
- Is innervated by the median nerve, except for the flexor carpi ulnaris muscle and ulnar border of the flexor digitorum profundus by the ulnar nerve

Extensor compartment:
- Includes the brachioradialis, extensor carpi radialis longus and brevis, extensor digitorum communis, extensor pollicis longus and brevis, extensor digiti minimi, extensor carpi ulnaris and anconaeus
- Crosses the wrist through the anatomical tunnel

Cubital fossa is approached by exposing the antebrachial fascia, and pronator teres is a landmark for radial and ulna artery bifurcation. The supinator is a landmark for posterior interosseous nerve, the main motor extensor of the wrist and finger.

Understanding the forearm's neurovascular structures and their courses is important for assessment of the surgical margin, anticipating functional loss and reconstructive planning. Arteries always accompany major nerves and serve as an indirect guide during contrasted MRI assessment prior surgery. The interosseous branches are unique as they guide the nerve course and are a good recipient for vascularised tissue transfer.

- Median nerve—crosses the cubital fossa medial to the brachial artery and passes between the two heads of the pronator teres and crosses the ulnar artery. It travels between the flexor digitorum superficialis and flexor digitorum profundus and is accompanied by the median artery, a branch of the anterior interosseous artery.
- Ulnar nerve—enters the flexor compartment between the two heads of flexor carpi ulnaris and lies in the lateral border of the flexor carpi ulnaris. It runs between the flexor carpi ulnaris and flexor digitorum profundus and enters the Guyon's canal under the volar carpal ligament near the wrist into the hypothenar eminence.
- Brachial artery bifurcates into the ulnar and radial arteries in the cubital fossa at the level of radial tuberosity.

- Radial artery course deep to the pronator teres, flexor carpi radialis, palmaris longus, and flexor digitorum superficialis and are superficial to the flexor digitorum profundus.
- The ulnar artery courses deep to the flexor digitorum superficialis and lateral to the flexor carpi ulnaris. It continues to the forearm between the flexor carpi ulnaris and flexor digitorum profundus. It gives off palmar and dorsal carpal branches, and courses deep to the palmar carpal ligament through Guyon's canal.
- Both arteries become a superficial palmar branch after giving off a tributary to the deep palmar arch.

Assessment

Recommendations for safe surgical margins in the treatment of forearm and hand sarcomas are still debatable and vary based on tumour size, location and histological grade. Local recurrence in upper limb sarcoma is higher compared to those of the lower limb as an attempt to salvage function can be complicated with narrow surgical margin, even though the mean tumour size is smaller. Surgical margins should never be sacrificed in an attempt to maintain hand function.

Small superficial forearm sarcomas are usually complicated with previous excision biopsy and inadequate margins. Assessment of local contamination and achieving wide oncological margin with simultaneous reconstruction are important for adding adjuvant local radiotherapy. Deep-seated multi-compartment sarcomas need careful evaluation and must involve a multidisciplinary team, especially a reconstructive surgeon, as part of the surgical planning. This includes:

- Assessment of the compartment muscles involved
- Major nerves and vessels—anticipated functional loss and viability and vascular supply to the hand
- Anticipated simultaneous reconstructive procedures
- Local or free flap for closure
- Nerve graft or reverse saphenous graft for vascularity
- Tendon transfer
- Motorised muscle transfer for anticipated functional loss following resection

Benign Tumour Forearm: Marginal Resection

Radiograph and MRI of a 10-year-old boy with slow-growing mass over the forearm. Biopsy revealed lipoblastoma (Fig. 1a–g)

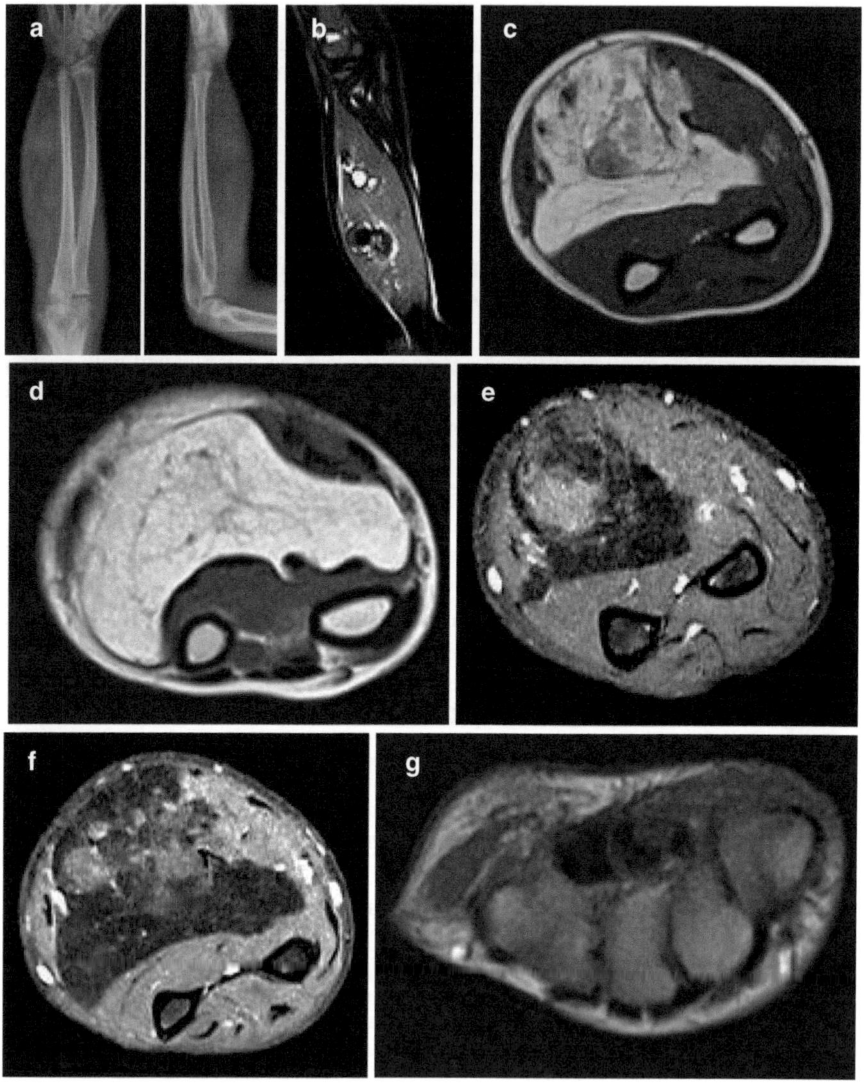

Tumour occupied the space between the flexor digitorum superficialis and profunda. The radial and ulna neurovascular structures were spared.

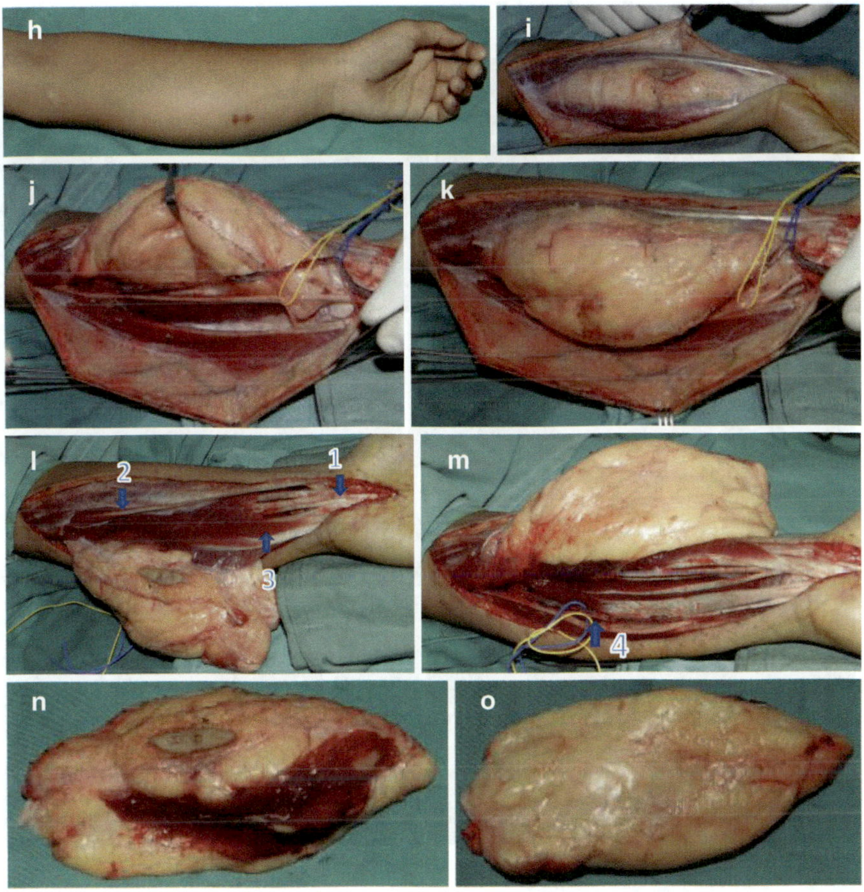

1. Median nerve
2. Flexor digitorum profundus
3. Palmaris longus
4. Ulnar nerve and arteries

Marginal resection with paratenon of the flexor tendon was included as part of the tumour capsule for margin. The ulna neurovascular structures were explored and mobilised from the main tumour. The tumour infiltrated the ulnar border of the flexor digitorum profundus and which was included as margin. The final flexor function was anticipated to be almost normal (Fig. 1h–o).

Atypical Lipoma Proximal Forearm

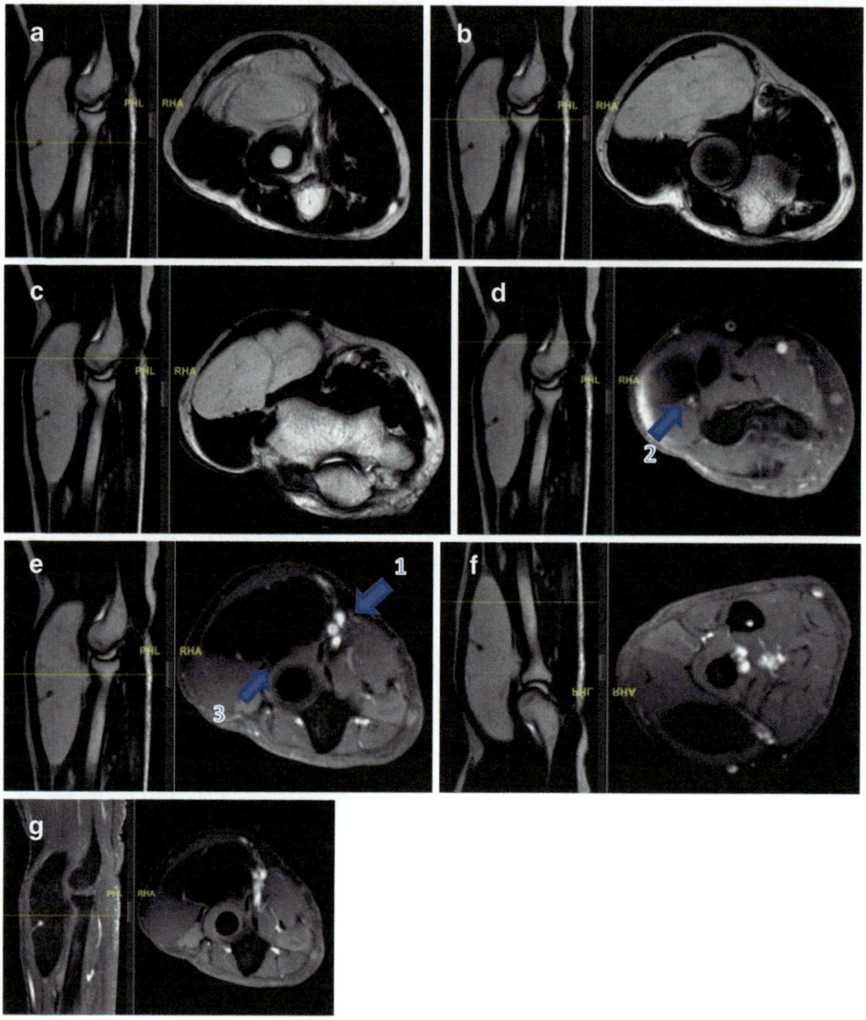

A case of multilobulated intermuscular lipoma, homogenous intensity, well supressed with STIR image and not enhanced with gadolinium. Biopsy confirmed well-differentiated adipose tissue and presence of MDM 2 amplification. CDK 4 did not suggest any malignancy. The lesion was within the course of the radial nerve and very close to brachial artery and median nerve (Fig. 2a–g)

1. Brachial artery and median nerve
2. Radial nerve with posterior interosseous artery
3. Supinator muscle

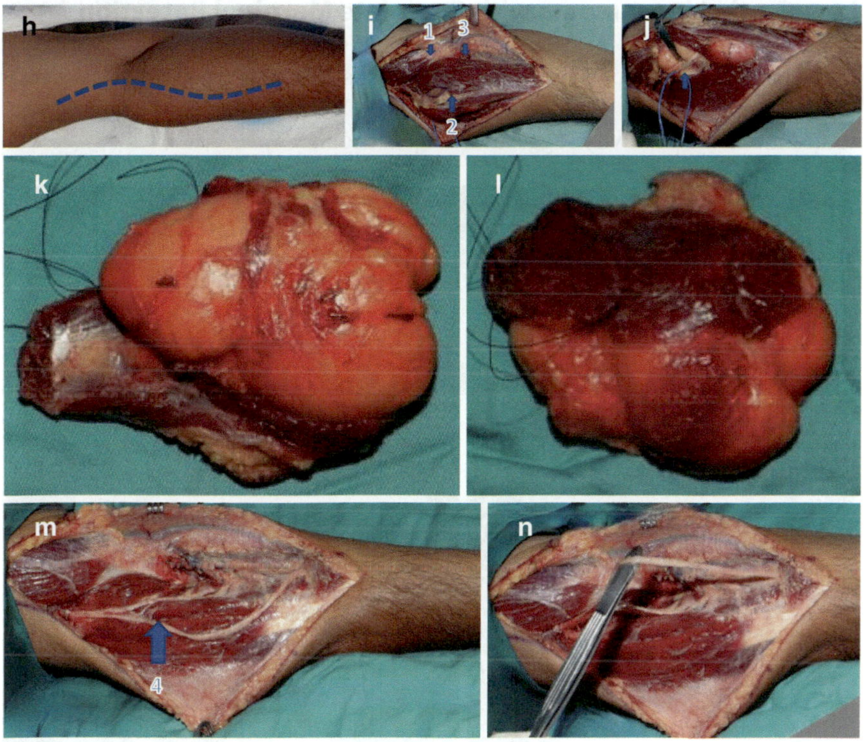

1. Biceps tendon
2. Brachioradialis
3. Brachial artery and median nerve
4 Radial nerve—posterior interosseous nerve and superficial radial nerve

Elevation of a fasciocutaneous flap exposed the entire antecubital area up to the lateral border of the brachioradialis. Proximal exploration of the radial nerve between the brachialis and brachioradialis plane for mobilisation of tumour mass after detaching the brachioradialis origin. The entire course of the radial nerve and its motor and sensory branch was preserved, and the interosseous lipoma was removed with an intact capsule to minimise possibility of recurrence. (Fig. 2h–n)

Low-Grade Liposarcoma with Complete Marginal Resection

Low-grade atypical lipoma presented after 3 years with tumour occupying the volar compartment of entire forearm. MDM-2 and CDK-4 molecular testing demonstrated moderate positivity suggestive of liposarcoma.

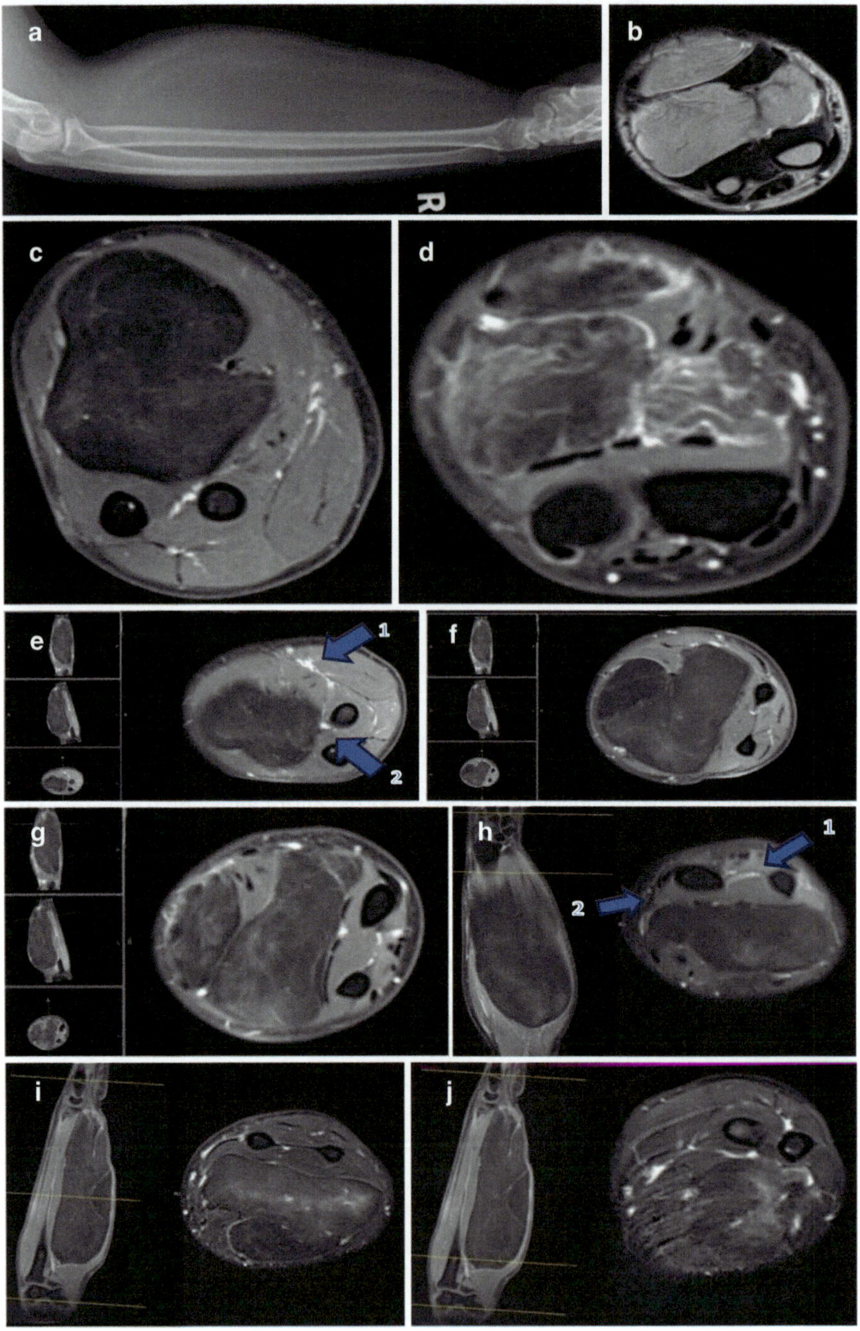

1. Radial neurovascular
2. Ulna neurovascular

Well-circumscribed fatty lesion occupied the entire volar compartment from cubital fossa to the wrist joint. The proximal lesion displaced radial and ulnar vessels but remained intact throughout its course. The carpal tunnel area was not involved but had to be exposed for proper mobilisation of entire tumour. The lesion described as fat intensity in T1 sequence was supressed on T2 but demonstrated heterogeneity and uptake of gadolinium suggestive of liposarcoma (Fig. 3a–j)

Surgical steps (Fig. 3k–r)

- Extensile exposure from elbow and carpal tunnel release for mobilisation of proximal extension and exploration of brachial vessels and branch of radial and ulnar vessels.
- Mobilisation of brachioradialis muscle and exploration of radial vessels and median nerve which is closely attached to the tumour capsule
- The tumour situated between flexor digitotur superficialis and profundus is mobilised ulnarly together with muscle attached and synovial lining to improve surgical margin.
- Mobilisation of tumour from proximal border of flexor carpi ulnaris and ulnar neurovascular structures.

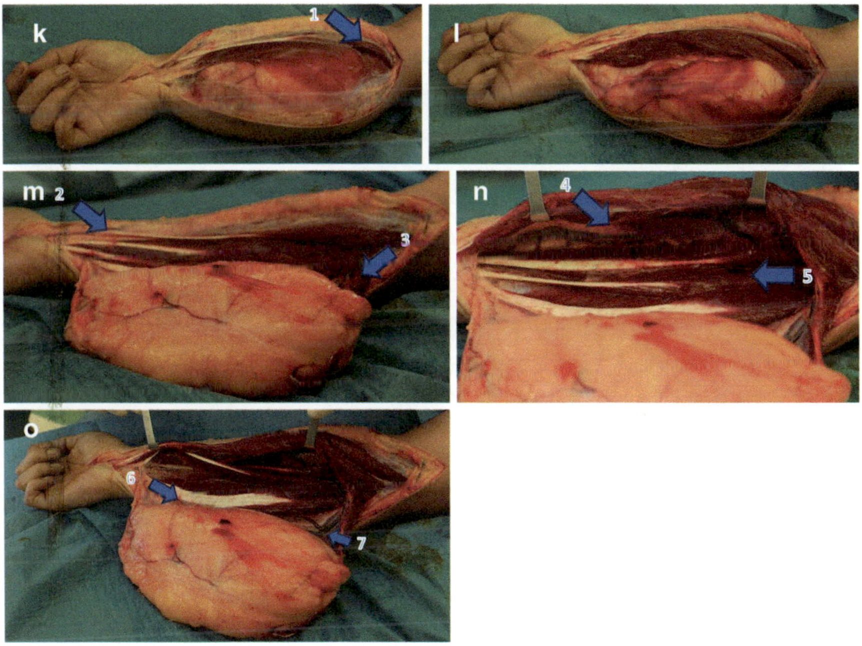

1. Brachioradialis
2. Median nerve
3. Flexor carpi ulnaris
4. Radial vessels
5. Flexor digitorum superficialis
6. Flexor digitorum profundus
7. Ulnar vessels and nerve

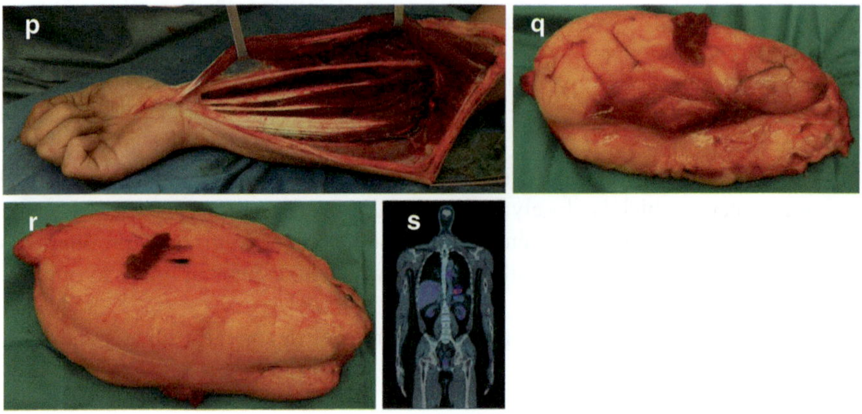

Patient received radiotherapy to the entire forearm and had good hand wrist function. PET scan after 5 year showed no local recurrence (Fig. 3s).

'Whoops' Surgery Forearm

Recurrence of sarcoma presented after excision biopsy with involved margins on final histopathology evaluation.

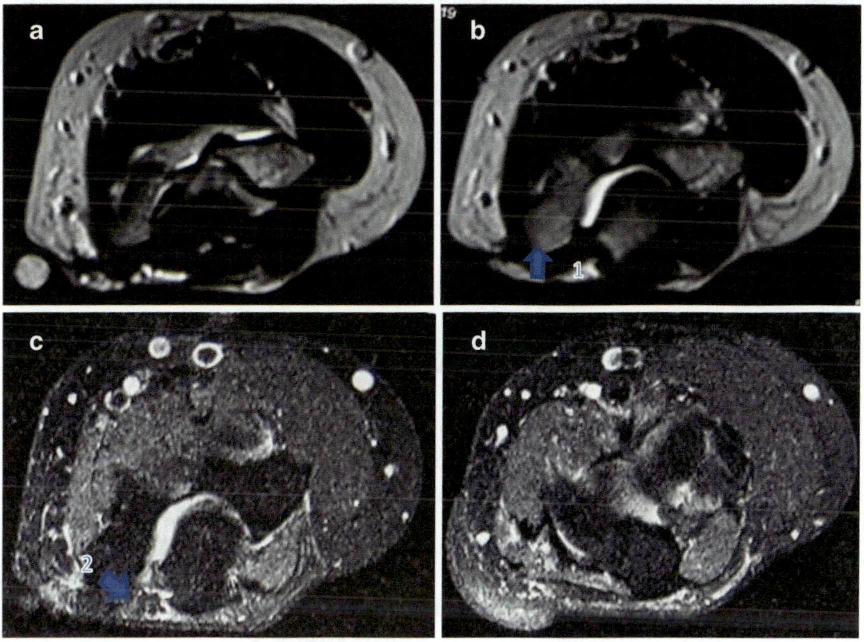

Inflamed scars at the medial epicondyle of posterior humerus with presence of high-intensity lesion within the subcutaneous and flexor origin. Ulnar nerve crossed the surgical area and was at risk for local contamination and required epineural resection. Large skin and subcutaneous tissue needed to be removed to achieve oncological margins and a flap was needed for closure of the exposed bone and nerve (Fig. 4a–d)

1. Ulnar nerve
2. Common flexor origin

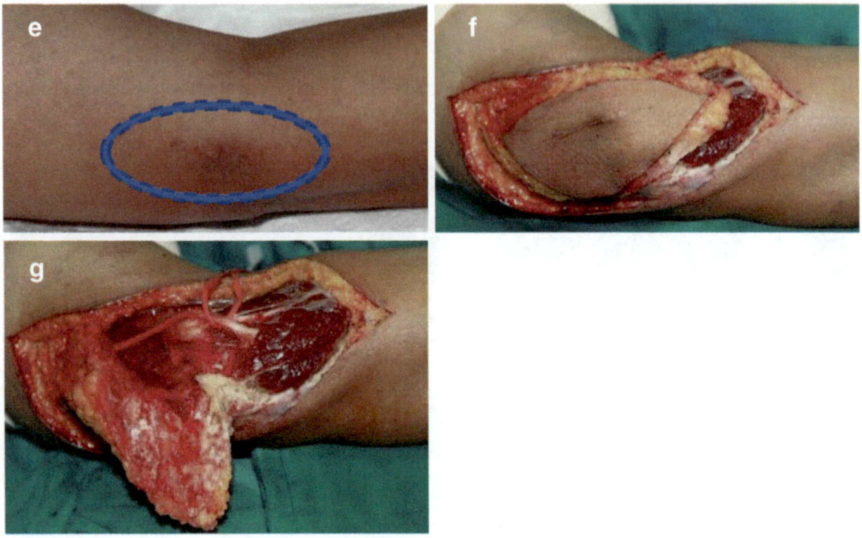

Wide margin surgery including 3 cm border of skin with the subcutaneous and fascia with cuff of flexor origin. The ulna nerve was mobilised and epineural dissection was performed for better oncological margin (Fig. 4e–h)

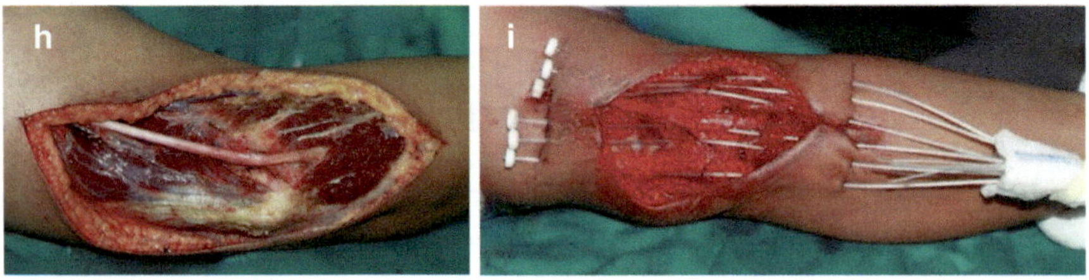

Local brachytherapy followed by external beam radiation to improve local control. Rotational flap from the posterior interosseous artery is an option for elbow coverage to improve soft tissue cover and is resilient to local radiotherapy (Fig. 4i, j)

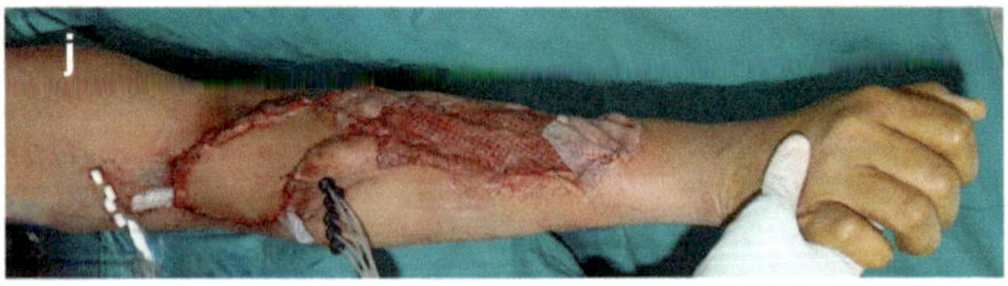

Brachioradialis Sarcoma

Surgical Step for Forearm Sarcoma

Wide fasciocutaneous flaps elevated for evaluation of the superficial layer of the muscle for definitive planning of resection:

- Exploration of the major neurovascular structures related to the border of the sarcoma
- Excision of tumour medially and laterally with cuff of compartment tissue
- Proximal and distal excision of muscles compartment for at least 3 cm
- Assessment of tissue loss and functional deficits
- Soft tissue covers included primary reconstruction with tissue transfer

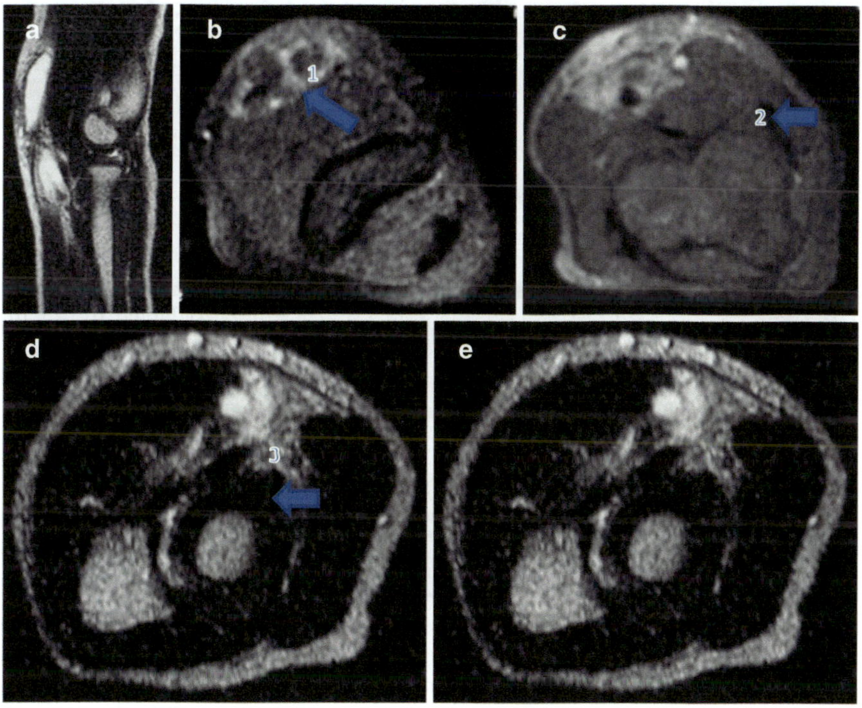

Sarcoma arising from the brachioradialis muscle in close proximity to the brachial artery, median nerve, supinator muscle and radial nerve. Resection of the entire mass with wide margin surgery causes significant disability and poor hand function (Fig. 5a–e)

1. Brachioradialis muscle
2. Brachial artery and median nerve
3. Supinator muscle—indirect structures for assessment of posterior interosseous nerve

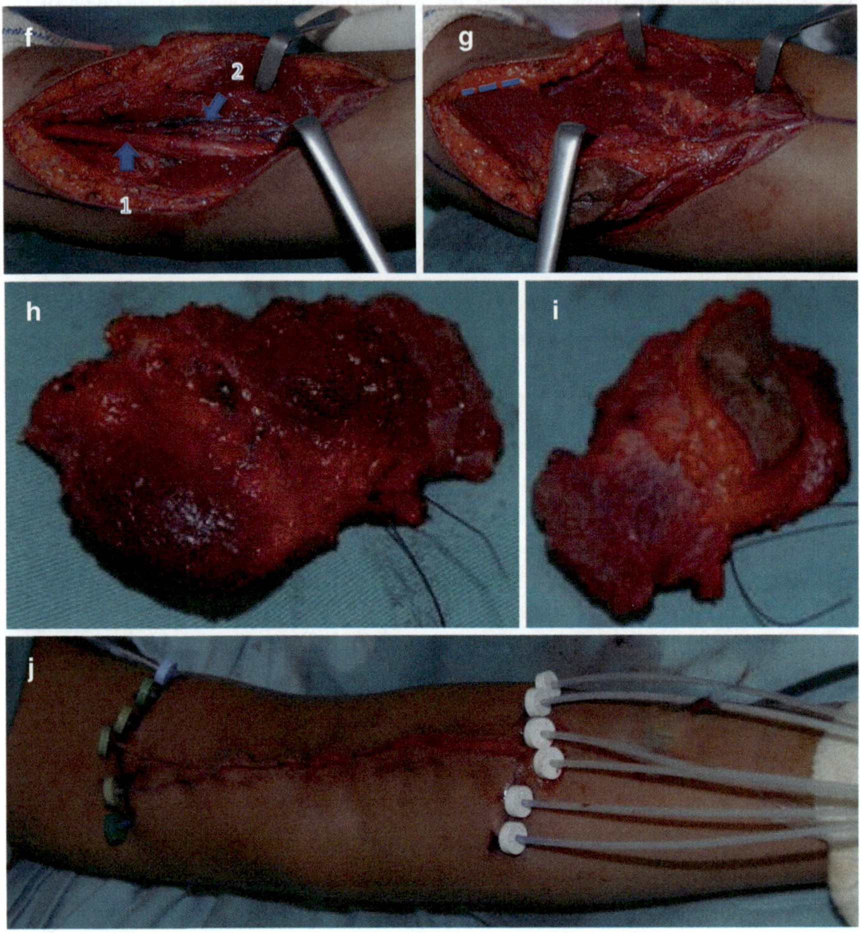

Mobilisation of the brachioradialis from the brachial artery and median nerve, plane of the brachioradialis from the extensor carpi radialis created with cuff of normal tissue. The brachial artery and median nerve are approached by incising the fascia at the level of the antecubital fossa. The brachial artery bifurcates into the radial branch and ulnar artery in front of the pronator teres. The proximal brachioradialis is detached from the origin and elevated from the supinator muscle with proper care and protection of the radial nerve (Fig. 5f–j)

Brachytherapy was utilised for early radiation treatment as surgical margin was narrow.

1. Median nerve
2. Brachial artery
3. Lever of proximal resection of the brachioradialis from its origin

Forearm and Wrist Sarcoma with Median Nerve Resection

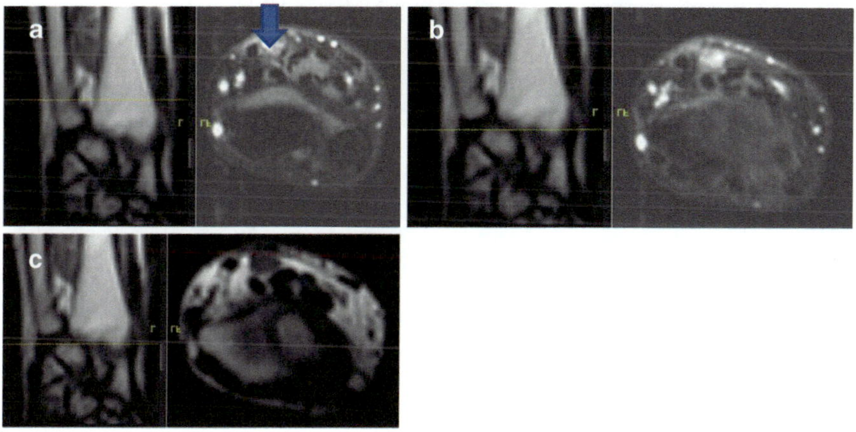

A case MPNST of peripheral median nerve, initially explored and found attached to the median nerve (Fig. 6a–c)

- Median nerve lesion and inflamed subcutaneous tissue

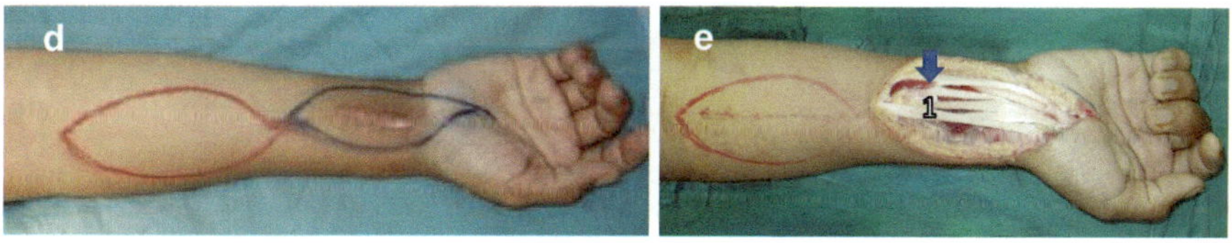

The contaminated surgical scar was resected with exposure of the carpal tunnel area. A segment of the median nerve with 3 cm proximal and distal margin was resected together with the synovial lining of the flexor tendon to improve local clearance. The segment loss of the median nerve was grafted with the sural nerve (Fig. 6d, e)

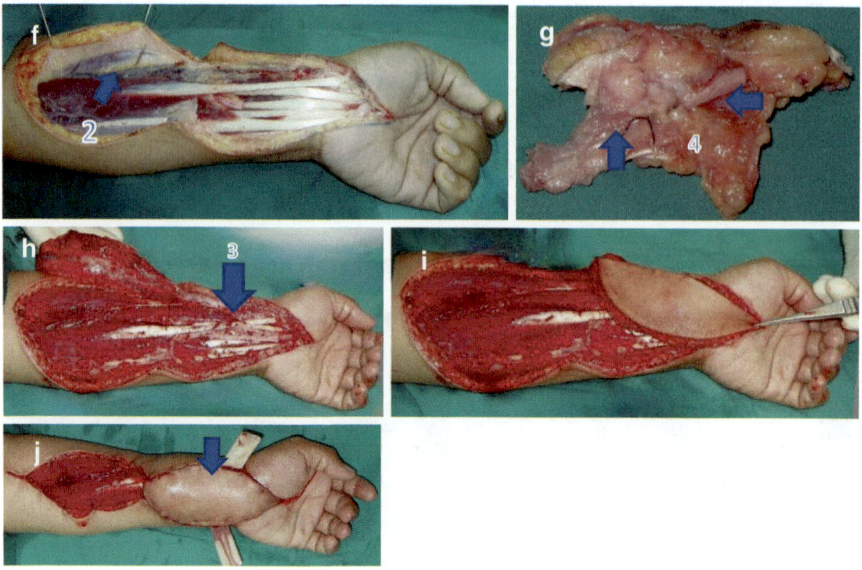

1. Median nerve—proximal and distal stump
2. Radial artery—radial forearm flap
3. Sural nerve graft
4. Median nerve resected—synovial lining flexor tendon

Distally based radial forearm fasciocutaneous flap based on the radial artery was raised to cover the potentially contaminated area for flexibility of the joint and radiotherapy (Fig. 6f–k). Three years after treatment, there is no evidence of local recurrence; however, median nerve has only partially recovered in terms of distal motor function of the hand (Fig. 6l, m)

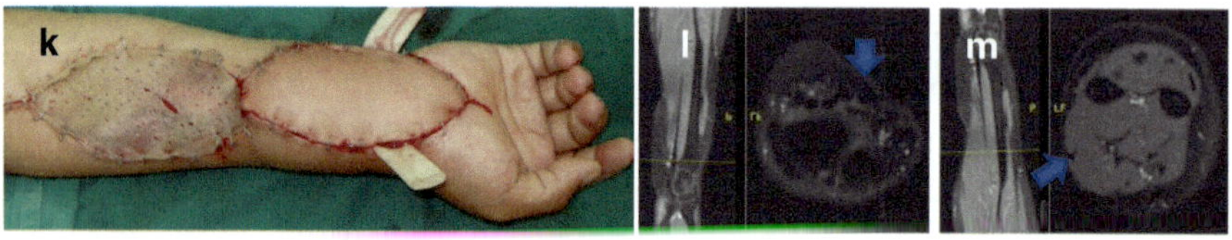

- Flap
- Skin grafting

Common Extensor Origin Sarcoma: Motorised Flap Transfer

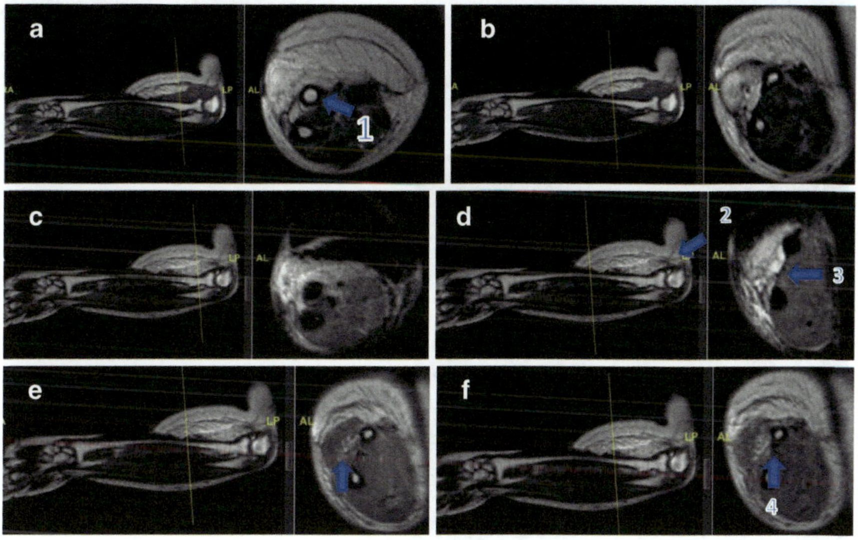

A case of pleomorphic sarcoma with the entire extensor muscles, extensor carpi radialis longus and brevis, brachioradialis and supinator muscle infiltrated by the tumour. The lateral elbow capsule and radial head were involved and excised together for margin (Fig. 7a–f)

1. Supinator muscle closely attached to the mass
2. Common extensor origin
3. Interosseous membrane
4. Brachial artery divides into the radial and ulnar artery

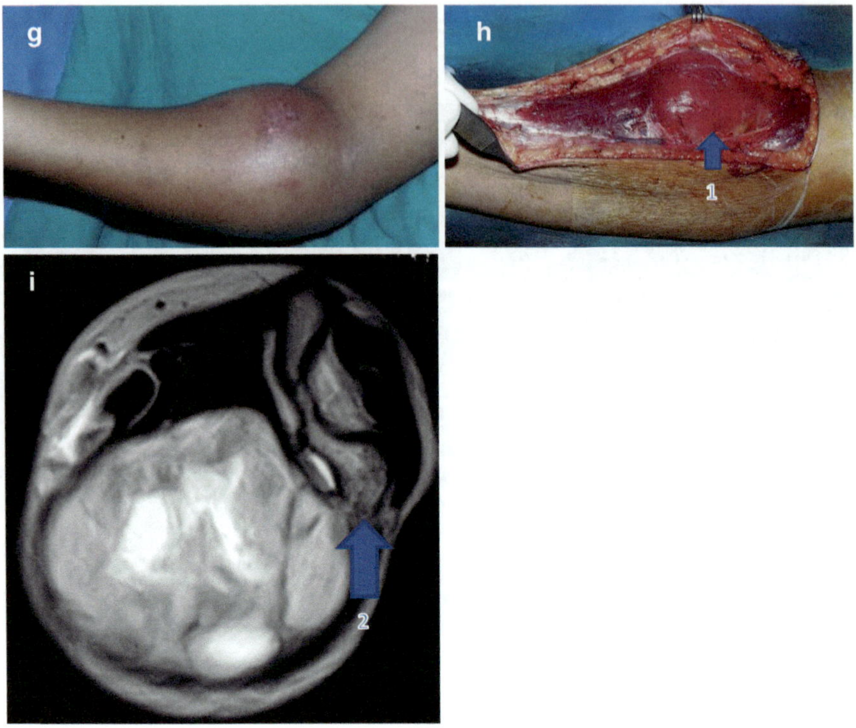

The brachioradialis muscle and extensor carpi radialis longus and brevis were exposed at their origin from the lateral supracondylar ridge and lateral epicondyle of the humerus (Fig. 7g–i)

1. Brachioradialis muscle as a landmark for tumour resection
2. Lateral ridge humerus—common extensor origin

Mobilisation of the brachial artery and median nerve from the main tumour. The entire lateral compartment of the extensor group and supinator was elevated from the periosteum of the distal humerus and radial head. Capsule and annular ligament were included as tumour margin (Fig. 7j, k)

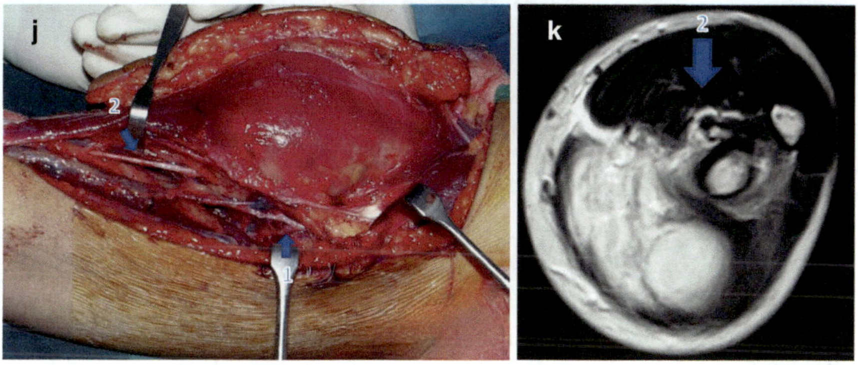

Exploration of the brachial artery by incising the antebrachial fascia. The radial and ulnar artery branch above the pronator teres was explored at the medial tumour border. The brachioradialis is a landmark for mobilisation of the entire extensor tumour. Care must be taken to include the supinator muscle as tumour border as it is attached and close to tumour.

1. Brachial artery and its division
2. Superficial radial nerve

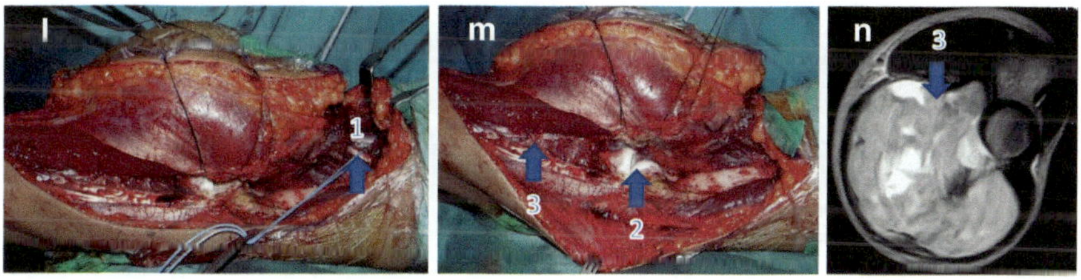

Radial nerve emerges between the brachioradialis and brachialis muscles, and bifurcates into the superficial branch of the radial nerve and deep branch posterior interosseous nerve. The posterior interosseous branch pierces the supinator muscle and enters the back of the forearm. The entire extensor compartment from the lateral extensor ridge was mobilised, and the entire capsule and supinator muscle were included as margin (Fig. 7l–o)

1. Radial nerve
2. Radial head—capitulum exposed after elevation of lateral capsule
3. Supinator muscle

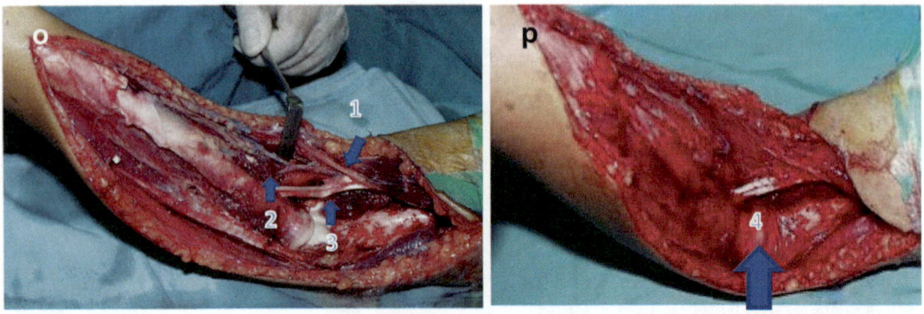

Lateral capsule and annular ligament of the radial head were reconstructed by allograft fascia. A latissimus dorsi flap was used as motorised extensor muscle and tagged to the remnant tendon using the remnant of the radial nerve (Fig. 7p–u)

1. Median nerve
2. Radial artery
3. Biceps insertion at the radial tuberosity
4. Capsular and annular ligament reconstruction with fascia latae

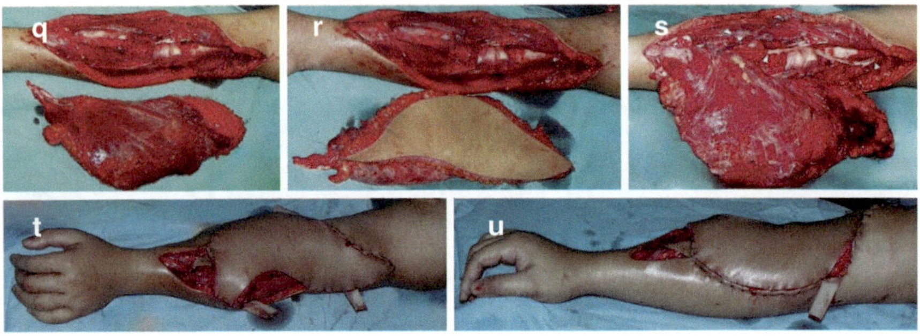

Partial Flexor Compartment: Motorised Flap

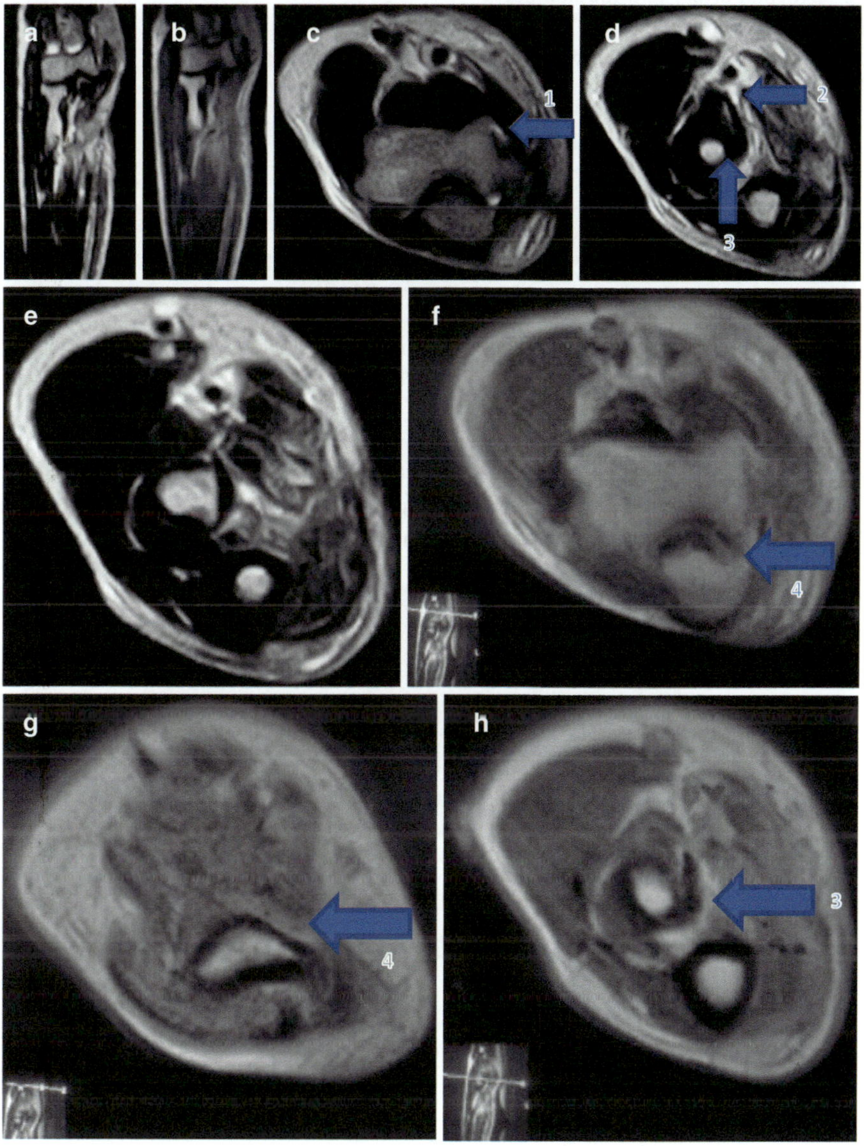

A case of ‘whoops’ pleomorphic sarcoma medial compartment elbow involving the entire flexor compartment to the origin at the medial epicondyle ridge humerus. The proximal pronator teres muscle was infiltrated to the periosteum of the ulna and abutting the interosseous membrane and supinator muscle. The ulna nerve was involved; however, the brachial artery and median nerve above the pronator muscle were clear of direct infiltration (Fig. 8a–h).

1. Medial ridge epicondyle humerus—common flexor origin
2. Brachial artery and median nerve
3. Supinator muscle
4. Periosteum of the ulna was intact with no bony infiltration

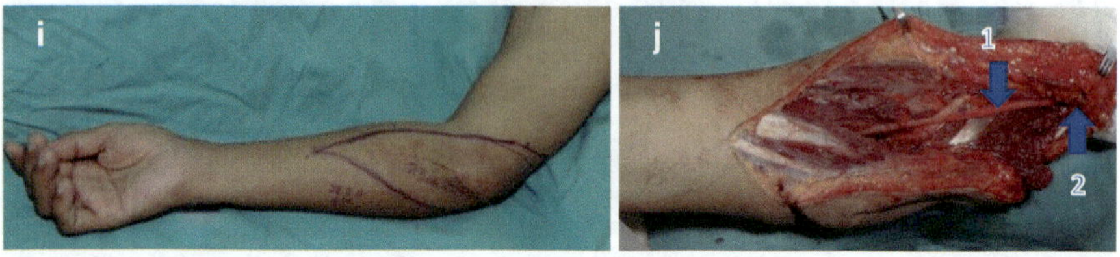

Fasciocutaneous flap created to expose antebrachial fascia for mobilisation of the brachial artery and median nerve to the distal forearm. The entire flexor compartment of the forearm, except the lateral flexor digitorum and pollicis, was maintained and spared. The origin of the flexor group and pronator teres was detached from the medial ridge of humerus. The medial periosteum of the ulna was elevated for better oncological margin. Ulnar nerve was explored and transacted as the pronator teres muscle was involved entirely and trapped the nerve within (Fig. 8i–k).

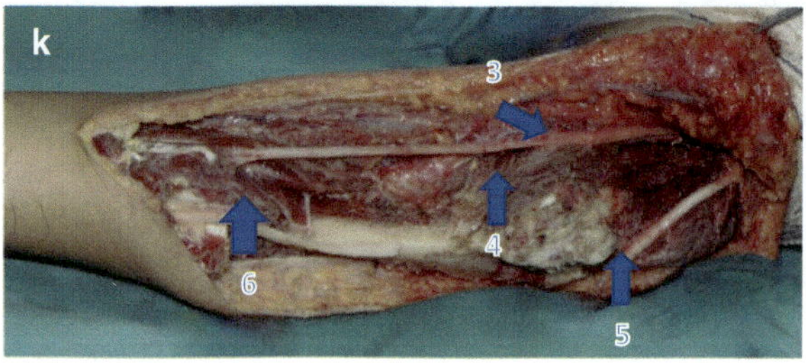

1. Median nerve
2. Ulna nerve
3. Radial artery
4. Brachialis muscle insertion
5. Proximal and distal stump ulnar nerve
6. Distal ulnar artery stump

Flexor wrist and finger reconstruction with motorised latissimus dorsi flap and defect closure. Thoracodorsal nerve anastomosed to the proximal stump ulnar nerve for motorised latissimus dorsi. (Fig. 8l, m)

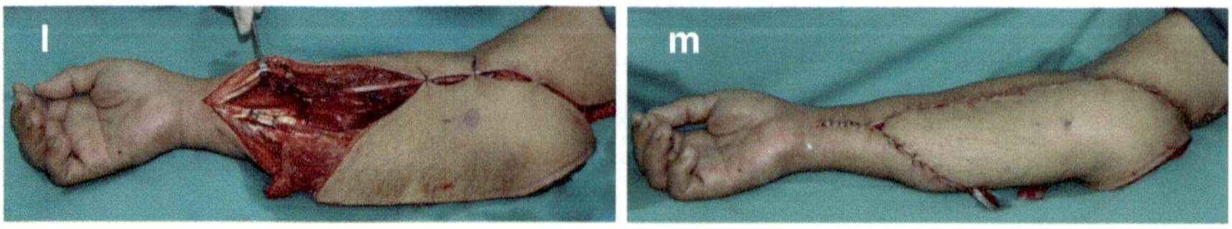

Flexor Compartment with Involvement of Radius

Large sarcoma over the forearm occupying multiple compartments is best managed by amputation as resection of multiple tendons and nerves in an attempt to salvage the hand will lead to poor function. Advancement of microsurgery and motorised flaps allow for more wider resection, flexibility closure and restoration of function with a motorised flap.

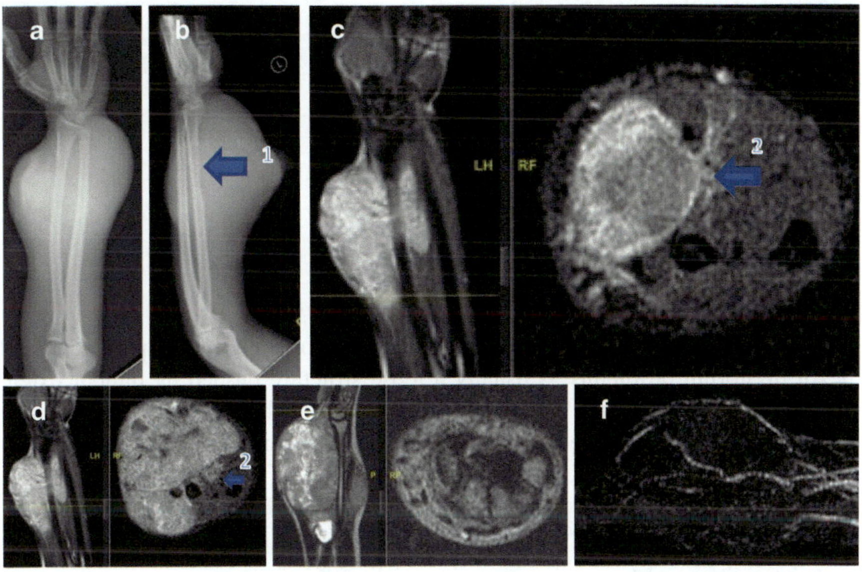

Large tumour occupying the radial ventral forearm, involving the radial flexor structures and infiltrating the anterior cortex of the radius. The carpal tunnel of the wrist joint was free from tumour infiltration. MRI showed the radial artery was pushed medially by the mass; however, it remained intact (Fig. 9a–f)

1. Anterior radial cortex erosion
2. Radial artery and median nerve

Large sarcomas of the ventral forearm often require skeletonisation of important neurovascular structures. Resection of tumour in multiple loose tendon structures is accomplished en bloc with grossly involved adjacent structures. Additional margin may be obtained by removing structures or tissues whenever there is a 'clear' plane between the tumour mass and adjacent structures. This should be entered so that the adjacent grossly uninvolved structures may be preserved (Fig. 9g, h).

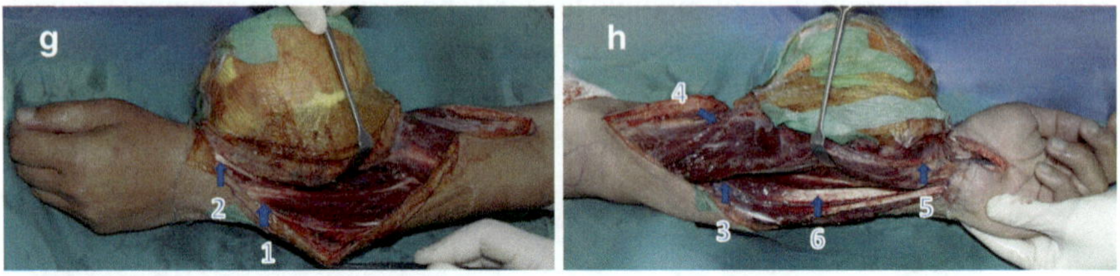

1. Extensor digitorum communis
2. Extensor pollicis longus
3. Radial artery
4. Flexor digitorum superficialis muscle
5. Median nerve
6. Flexor digitorum profundus tendon

The median nerve, which lies between the flexor digitorum superficialis and flexor digitorum profundus, is usually a loose structure pushed by tumour extension. It is not involved and can be dissected. In cases where it is circumferentially involved, the median nerve may be sacrificed with minimal motor disability provided the long flexor is functioning well.

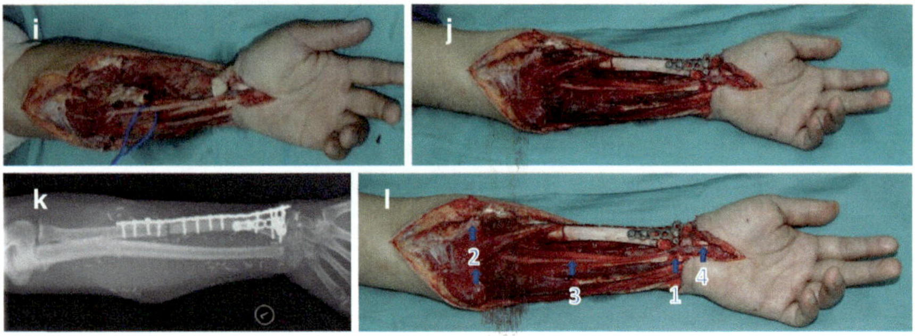

Flexor digitorum superficialis, radial border of the flexor digitorum longus and radial artery were resected with the tumour. Segment of bony defect was reconstructed with an intercalary distal radius allograft and stabilised with two plate constructs (Fig. 9i–l)

1. Flexor digitorum superficialis remnant
2. Radial artery stump
3. Median nerve
4. Stump of the flexor pollicis longus and radial border of both the flexors digitorum

The index and middle fingers lose their cascade without an intact long flexor and need to be reconstructed for function. Motorised gracilis with large fasciocutaneous nerve and a motor to the gracilis were anastomosed to anterior interosseous nerve for motor function (Fig. 9m)

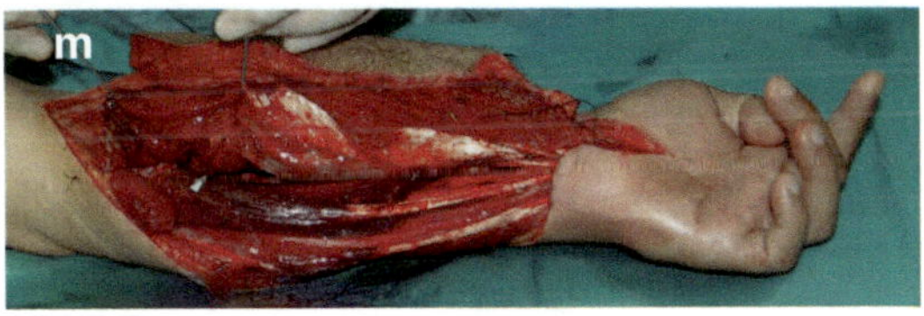

Suggested Reading

1. Lazerges C. Soft tissue sarcomas of the forearm, wrist and hand. Hand Surg Rehabil. 2017;36:233–43.
2. Lucattelli E, Lusetti IL, Cipriani F, Innocenti A, De Santis G, et al. Reconstruction of upper limb soft-tissue defects after sarcoma resection with free flaps: a systematic review. J Plast Reconstr Aesthet Surg. 2020;74:755–67.
3. Baroudi MR, Ferguson PC, Wunder JS, Isler MH, Mottard S, Werier JA, Turcotte RE. Forearm soft tissue sarcoma: tumors characteristics and oncologic outcomes following limb salvage surgery. J Surg Oncol. 2014;110:676–81.
4. Muramatsu K, Ihara K, Doi K, Hashimoto T, Taguchi T. Sarcoma in the forearm and hand: clinical outcomes and microsurgical reconstruction for limb salvage. Ann Plast Surg. 2009;62:28–33.
5. Muramatsu K, et al. Musculoskeletal sarcomas in the forearm and hand: standard treatment and microsurgical reconstruction for limb salvage. Anticancer Res. 2013;33:4175–82.
6. Vetter M, Germann G, Bickert B, Sauerbier M. Current strategies for sarcoma reconstruction at the forearm and hand. J Reconstr Microsurg. 2010;26:455–60.

Major Amputation for Sarcoma

External Hemipelvectomy

Wan Faisham Nu'man Bin Wan Ismail,
Arman Zaharil Mat Saad, Wan Azman Wan Sulaiman,
Zulmi Wan, and Ahmad Sukari Halim

External hemipelvectomy 'hindquarter amputation' is a major surgical procedure whereby the hemipelvis at the level of sacro-iliac joint and symphysis pubis is removed together with the limb. It is indicated where oncological margin cannot be achieved with preservation of a viable limb. Pelvic or proximal femur sarcomas that requires hemipelvectomy usually present late, have a poor response to chemotherapy or are recurrent after primary internal hemipelvectomy. Critical structures for functions preservation in pelvic resections are the hip joint, femoral neurovascular structures and sciatic nerve. If more than two are involved, an external hemipelvectomy is justified. The decision to perform a hemipelvectomy is made when partial pelvic resection does not allow for safe surgical margin or results in a functionless limb. Even though hemipelvectomy has devastating results, it provides the possibility of surgical cure or palliation for pelvic malignancies that could otherwise not be excised with preservation of the limb.

W. F. N. B. W. Ismail (✉)
Prince Court Medical Center, Kuala Lumpur, Malaysia

Orthopaedic Oncology Reconstructive Unit, Universiti Sains Malaysia,
Kubang Kerian, Kelantan, Malaysia

A. Z. M. Saad
Plastic Reconstructive & Microsurgery, MSU Medical Centre, Management and Science University of Malaysia, Shah Alam, Selangor, Malaysia

W. A. W. Sulaiman · A. S. Halim
Reconstructive Sciences Department, School of Medical Sciences, Universiti Sains Malaysia, Kubang Kerian, Kelantan, Malaysia

Z. Wan
Prince Court Medical Center, Kuala Lumpur, Malaysia

A. Puri, W. F. N. B. W. Ismail (eds.), *Atlas of Orthopedic Oncology Volume 1*,
https://doi.org/10.1007/978-981-95-8958-6_12

Hemipelvectomy is commonly indicated as a large size and massive extension tumour to surrounding structures whereby anatomically the local barrier and compartmentalisation are breeched. Understanding the anatomical barrier and careful MRI evaluation is critical to achieve negative oncological margin with external hemipelvectomy.

Surgical Anatomy

Understanding the 3D skeletal anatomy of pelvic organs, abdominal wall muscles, pelvic floor and major vessels and nerves is important for surgical planning to achieve oncological clearance and minimise surgical morbidity.

Important skeletal anatomy for evaluation of the osseous margin:

- Sacroiliac joint—tumour crossing the joint requires resection of the alar of the sacrum or part of the sacrum with good osseous margin.
- Symphysis pubis being a fibrocartilaginous structures serves as a good tumour barrier. This is important for tumour margin for hemipelvectomy.
- The hemipelvectomy osseous margin can be modified based of marrow extension and soft tissue involvement (diagram below).

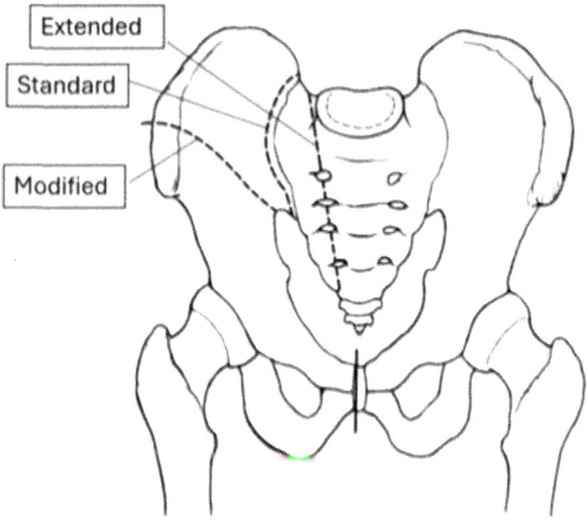

Vessel Anatomy

- Abdominal aorta bifurcates at the level L4 to form the common iliac, travels laterally over the sacrum alar and branches to the internal iliac artery at the sacroiliac joint.

- The internal iliac descends to the greater sciatic notch and branches into several arteries that supply the gluteal muscle. These are important for viability of the posterior flap and classic posterior flap hemipelvectomy.
- External iliac vessels are directly related to the medial brim of ilium; however, it is protected by the thick iliopectineal fascia.
- In cases with gluteus muscle involvement, the external iliac vessels is explored and maintained for anterior flap hemipelvectomy.
- Sarcomas with anterior pelvic extension may either push or infiltrate the external iliac vessels, involvement of the vessel need a posterior flap hemipelvectomy or fillet from the distal femoral or popliteal vessels.
- Obturator artery runs at the medial acetabulum together with the obturator nerve to the obturator fossa and must be ligated for hemipelvectomy.

Abdominal Wall and Pelvic Floor

- Ilium is covered by the iliacus muscle that provides a good anatomical boundary against anterior tumour extension. Posteriorly, the gluteus maximus and medius origin are attached to the ilium and can be infiltrated by posterior extension of tumour.
- Iliopectineal fascia that covers the medial brim provides a good barrier against tumour extension to the pelvic organ.
- Obturator internus covers the medial wall of the acetabulum. Posteriorly the sacrospinous ligament is attached to the spinous process and pelvic floor muscle iliococcygeus and ischiococcygeus.
- Sartorius and inguinal ligament is attached to the ASIS and must be evaluated prior to resection.

Pelvic Visceral

- Urinary bladder can be pushed or infiltrated by medial extension of tumour.
- Ureter, an intraperitoneal structure, lies on the peritoneal surface and crosses medially at the common iliac bifurcation to the sciatic notch and inserts into the trigone of the bladder. Large tumour with medial extension needs a ureteric stent for easy palpation during surgery to minimise risk of injury.
- Colon and rectum must also be identified and protected before completing the amputation.
- In female patients, the ovaries, fallopian tubes, uterus, cervix, and vagina require identification and protection.

Major nerve: the sciatic and femoral nerves are sacrificed in hemipelvectomy. Care must be taken to prevent phantom pain, particularly in patient with chronic pain prior to hemipelvectomy.

- Adequate analgesics and early treatment with good analgesic, neuropathic pain medication and tricyclic anti-depressant
- Nerve procedures, such as epineural ligature flat, cauterisation nerve stump and sometimes in chronic pain patient with neuropathic pain; centro-central union using femoral sciatic nerve apposition and concomitant nerve coaptation

Assessment

Hemipelvectomy is done in the following cases:

- Pelvic tumour with extensive involvement of the major vessels and nerve, hip joint and massive soft tissue involvement with anticipated poor function
- Recurrent pelvic or proximal femur sarcoma
- Primary lesion of the pelvis or hip joint with progressive disease on chemotherapy
- Disabling infection following primary pelvic resection
- Failure of multiple revision pelvis prosthesis

Assessments include:

- Osseous involvement for definitive osteotomy:- classically is hemipelvectomy osteotomy is done through the symphysis pubis and sacroiliac joint as these are natural barrier to tumour extension
- Main vessels: external iliac or internal iliac involvement will determine the type of flap coverage
- Pelvic organ involvement: bladder, ureter and colorectal area
- Pelvic floor and anterior abdominal wall

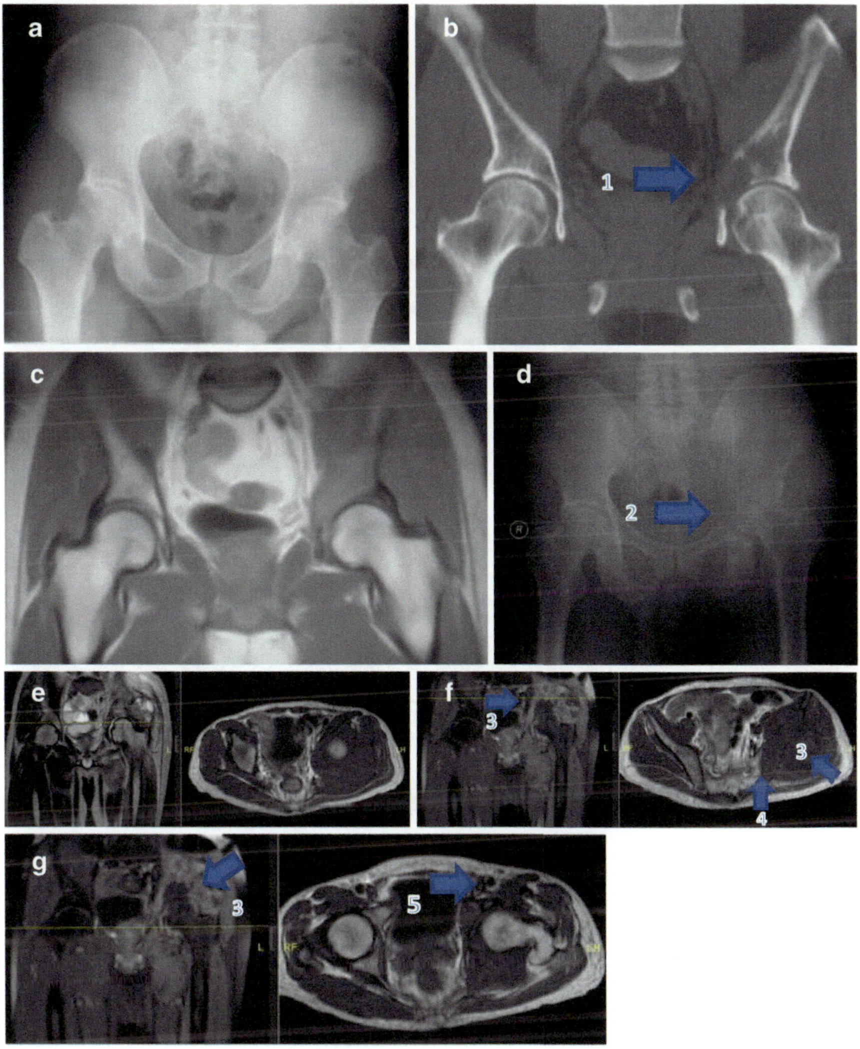

A 56-year-old man presented with periacetabular osteosarcoma, poor response to chemotherapy with extension to the entire ilium and acetabulum. Massive soft tissue extension to the iliopsoas and gluteus muscle (Fig. 1a–g)

- 1.Peri acetabulum osteosarcoma
- 2. Extensive acetabulum destruction

- 3. Infiltration entire hemipelvis
- 4. Sacro iliac joint
- 5. External iliac vessels

Assessment for recurrence tumour is sometimes complicated with implant interference in either a CT scan or MRI. Currently, there is a software available to minimise interference and get better images for evaluation of margin (Fig. 1h–p).

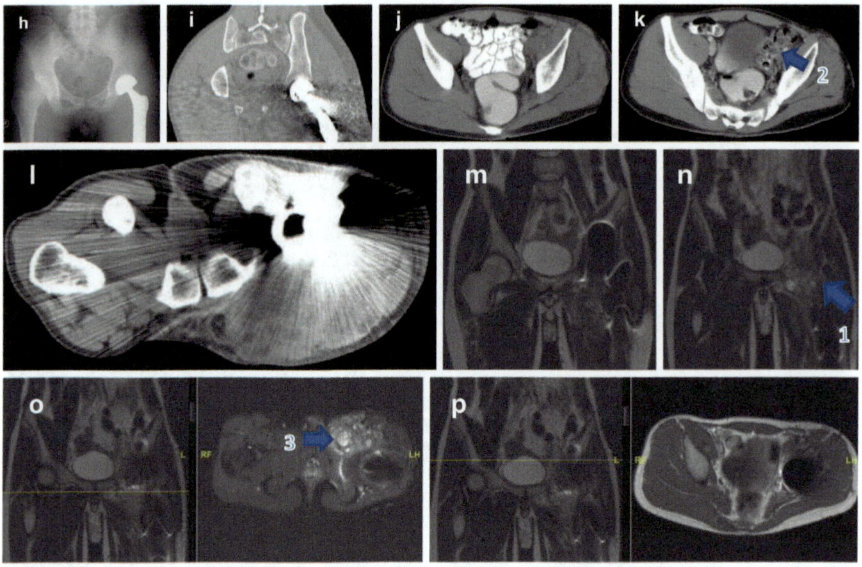

Evaluation of structures and infiltration above the implant are possible for safer surgical margin for hemipelvectomy.

1. Hip joint contamination
2. External iliac vessels—multiple nodes
3. Soft tissue recurrence around hip capsule and adductor

Internal hemipelvectomy of entire hemipelvis (type I-III) was complicated with chronic pain and poor function. Reconstruction to the remnant Lumbar 5 to provide stability is always complicated with higher hip joint centre, disability and chronic pain. Both patients ended up with external hemipelvectomy (Fig. 1q–y).

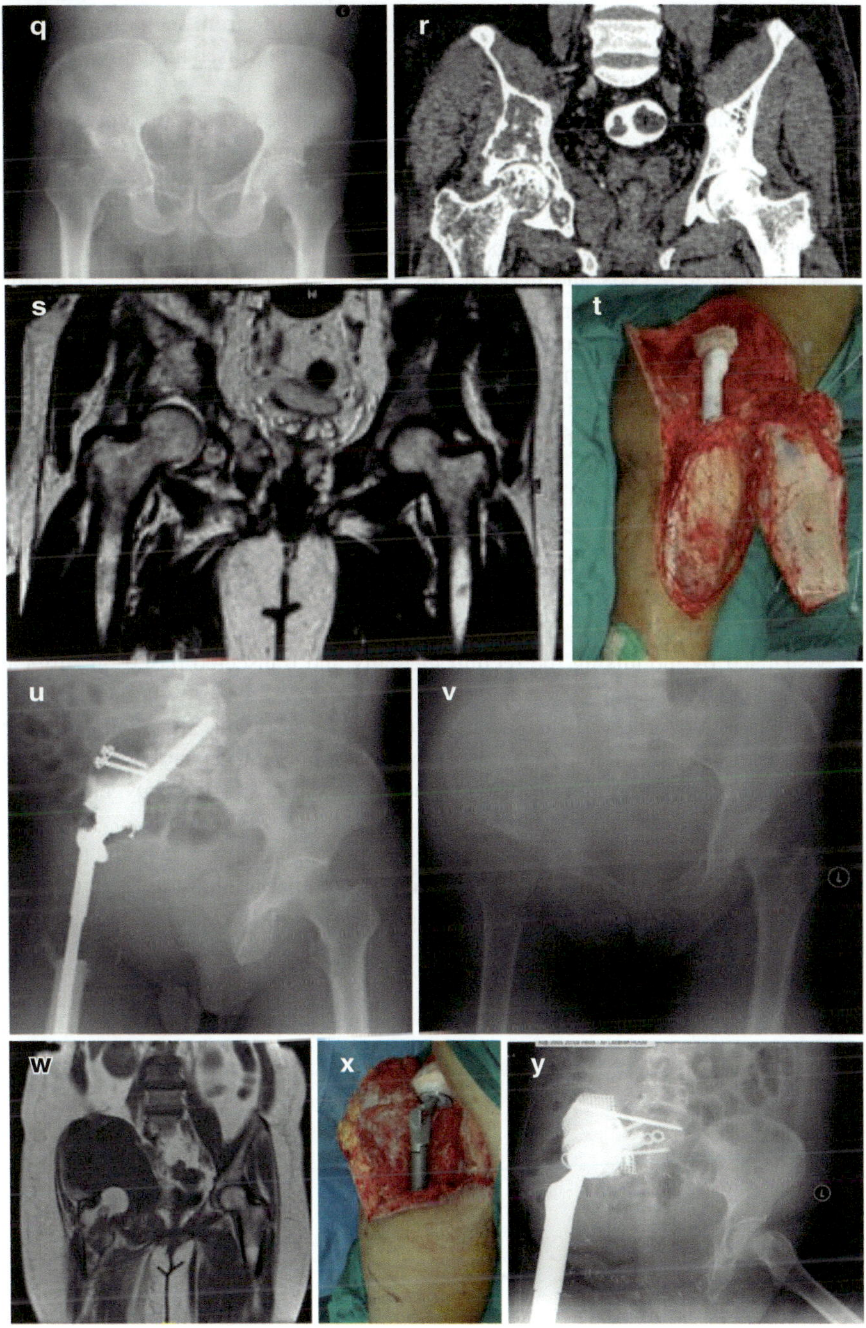

Surgical Steps of Hemipelvectomy (Fig. 2a–j)

- Flexible lateral position is important for exploration and evaluation of the entire pelvis up to sacroiliac joint.
- The inner pelvis is approached through the retroperitoneal space by elevating the inguinal ligament and detaching the abdominal muscle from the pelvic brim to the quadratus lumborum muscle. The peritoneum is mobilised medially exposing the iliopsoas muscle and iliac vessels medially.
- The common iliac vessels are visualised. Care must be taken to protect the internal iliac vessels through the entire sciatic foreman anteriorly.
- The iliacus muscle provides a good anterior anatomical boundary and must be removed in total as surgical margin.
- Anterior sacroiliac joint must be identified for osteotomy, mobilisation of the common iliac vessels and internal iliac vessels before entering greater sciatic foreman. It is an important step to minimise vessels injury prior to osteotomy.
- The urinary bladder and urethra are protected for symphysis pubis osteotomy.
- The gluteus maximus is mobilised from the femoral insertion exposing the short rotators and sacroiliac joint posteriorly. The inferior gluteal vessels must be protected, mobilising them from the greater sciatic foreman posteriorly by detaching piriformis tendon.
- The gluteus medius, minimums and tensor fascia latae muscle are good anatomical boundaries against for posterior extension of tumour and are usually removed in total for oncological clearance (Fig. 2d).
- Osteotomy of each structure allows the pelvic to be displaced laterally and opened for visualisation of the pelvic floor. Levator ani, obturator internus are visualised by mobilising the rectum medially and transected based on surgical margin (Fig. 2a, b, i, j).
- Complete transection of the sacrotuberus and sacrospinous ligament will help mobilisation of the hemipelvis for completion of amputation, and final resection of pelvic floor diaphragm with good margin: levator ani, Iliococcygeus, pubococcygeus, piriformis and obturator internus (Fig. 2a, b).
- Finally, the internal iliac vessels are freed from the greater sciatic notch to posterior in continuity with the gluteus maximus and skin flap. Failure to do this can cause flap necrosis and wound dehiscence.

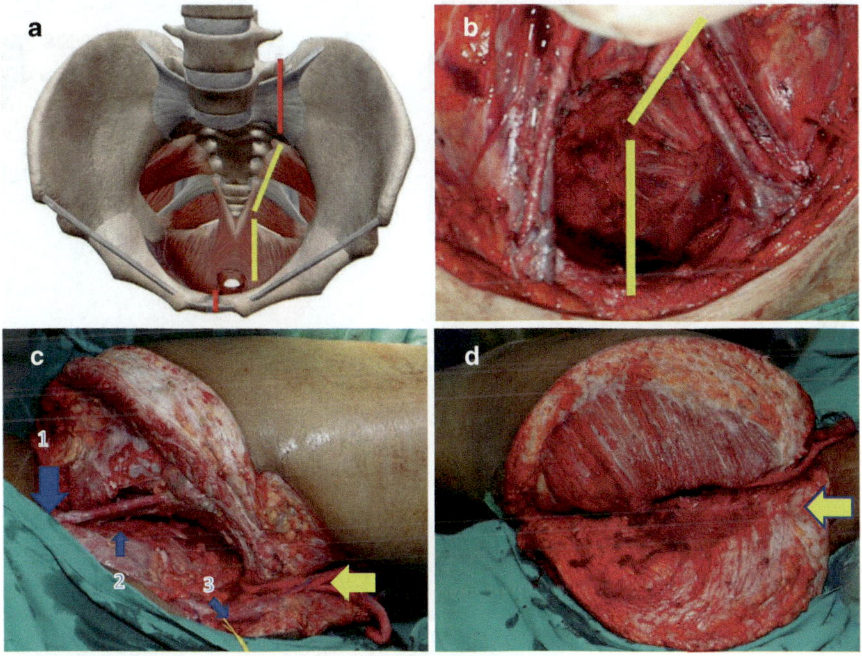

Osteotomy over the symphysis pubis and sacroiliac joint: (Fig. 2c, d, f, g)

- Direct control using osteotome
- Gigli saw

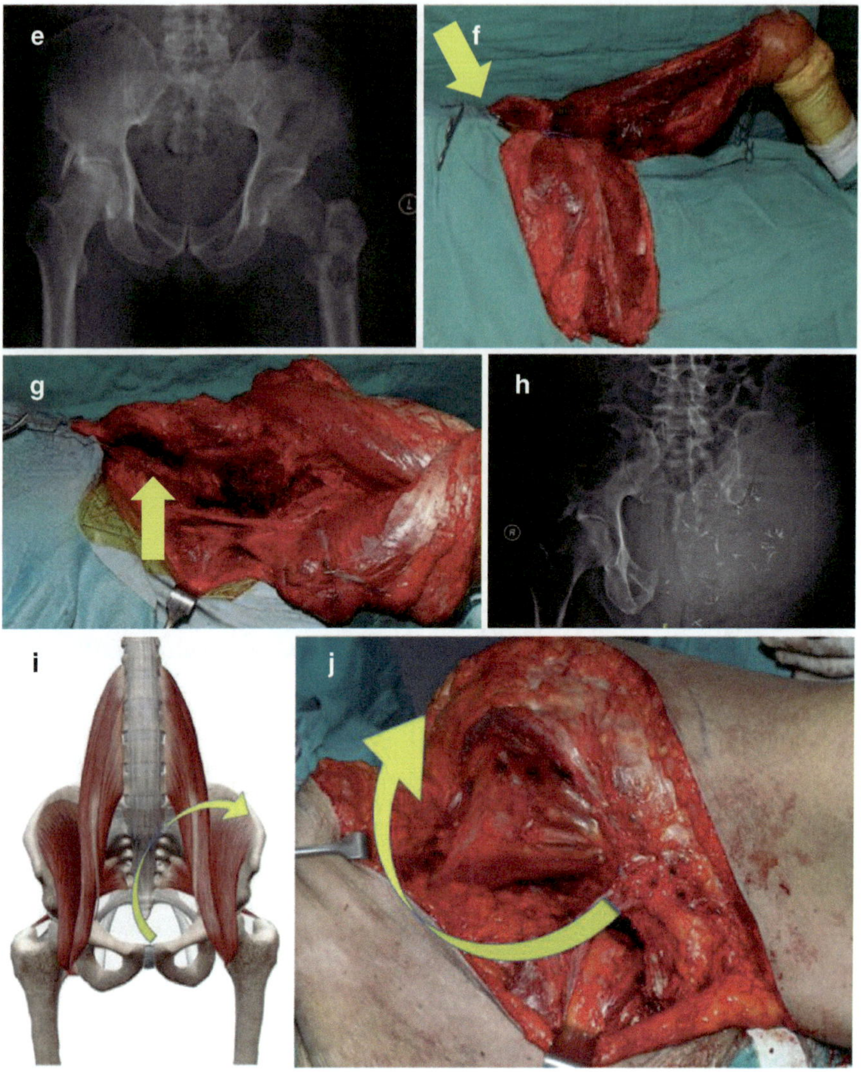

1. External iliac artery
2. Spermatic cord
3. Internal iliac vessels

Posterior Flap Hemipelvectomy

The entire gluteus maximus muscle is preserved for myo-cutaneous flap closure. The inferior gluteal vessels branching from the internal iliac branch must be preserved for viability of the flap for posterior flap hemipelvectomy.

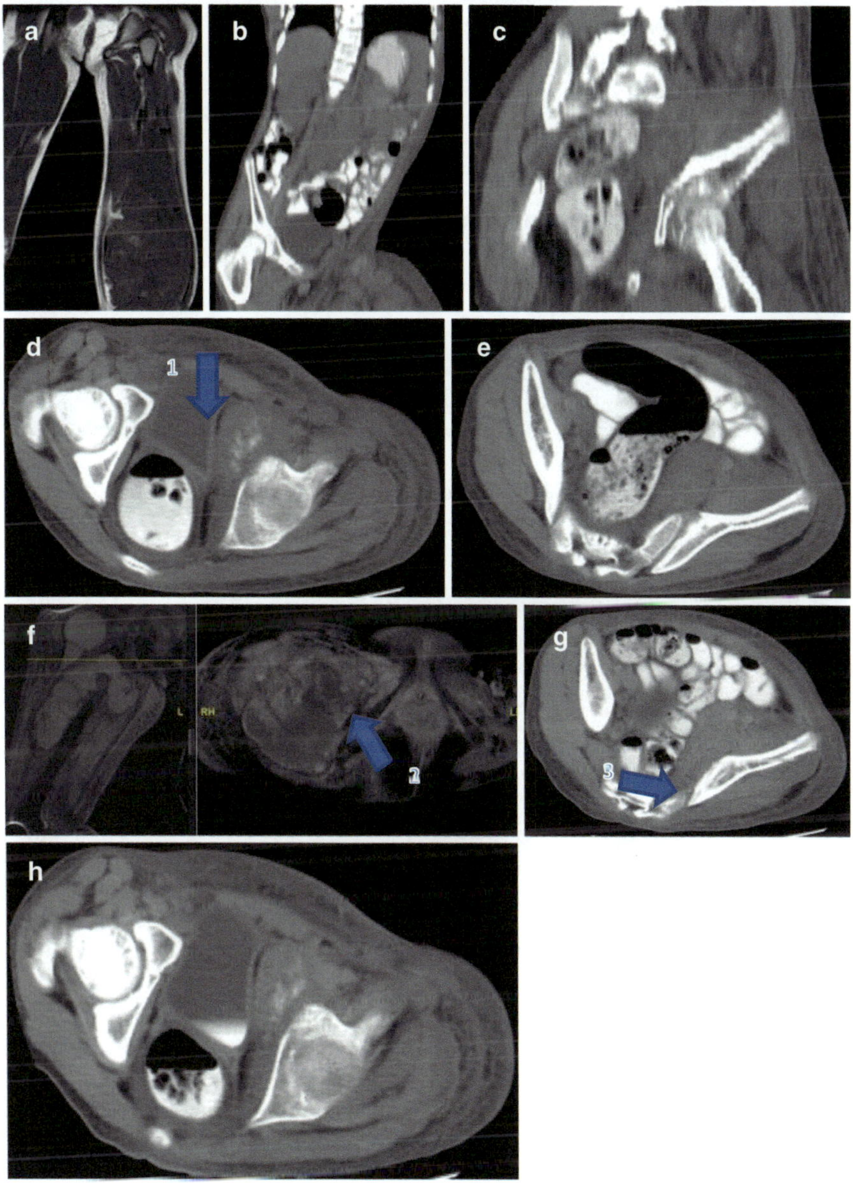

Osteosarcoma of the entire femur responded poorly to chemotherapy. CT and MRI evaluations revealed intrapelvic extension to the iliopsoas muscle. The posterior structures were spared and the internal iliac vessels over the sciatic foramen were not involved (Fig. 3a–h).

1. Direct infiltration iliopsoas muscle
2. Adductor compartment involvement
3. Tumour at the anterior sacroiliac joint
4. External iliac artery
5. Spermatic cord
6. Internal iliac vessels

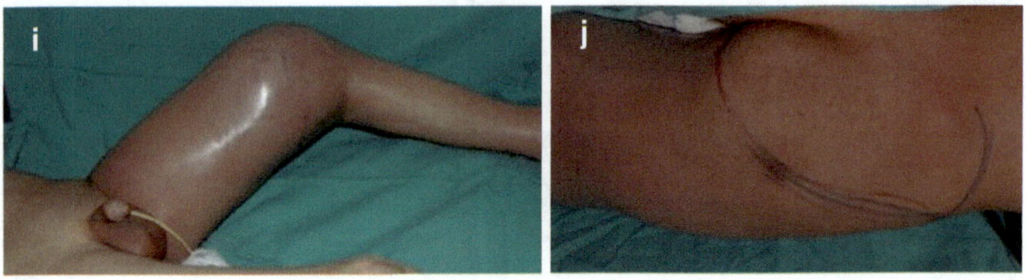

Clinical photo of extensive osteosarcoma over thigh with preservation of gluteal muscle (Fig. 3i, j)

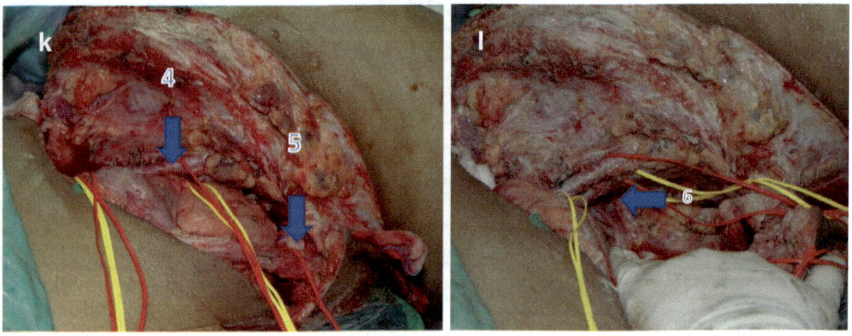

Pelvic structures are approached through the retroperitoneal space by reflecting three layers of the abdominal muscle and inguinal ligament. This structure is rarely invaded by the tumour. However, resection of the abdominal muscle is possible for exploration of the pelvic structures. External iliac vessels and vas deferens are identified and protected. The iliacus and psoas muscle are good anatomical boundaries against tumour extension. The internal iliac vessels is explored and must be secured and released from the greater sciatica notch for posterior flap hemipelvectomy (Fig. 3k–n).

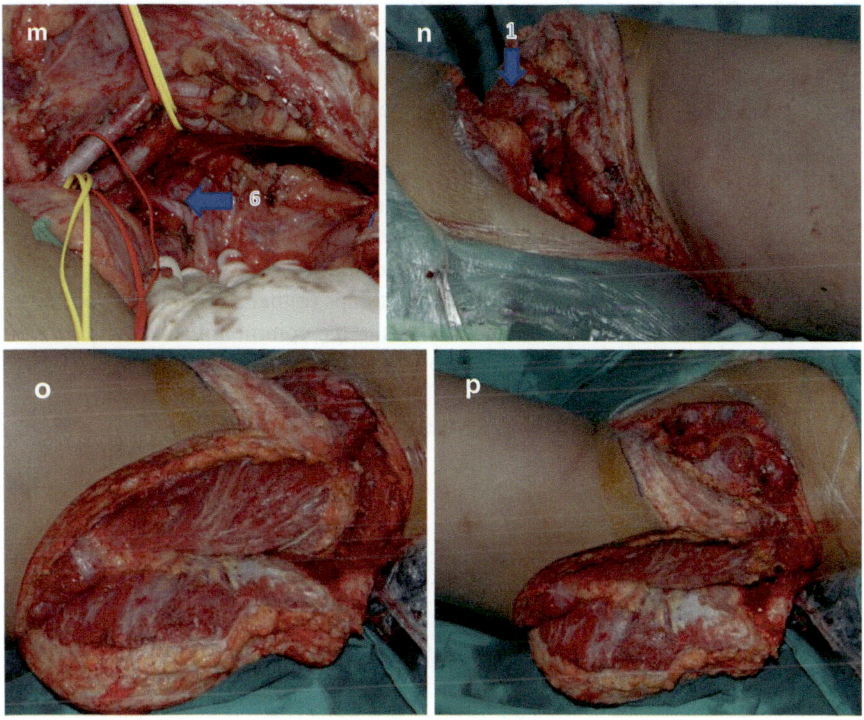

The internal iliac vessels and posterior branch of the superior and inferior gluteal vessels are carefully protected during sacroiliac osteotomy. It is important for posterior gluteal flap viability (Fig. 3m–r).

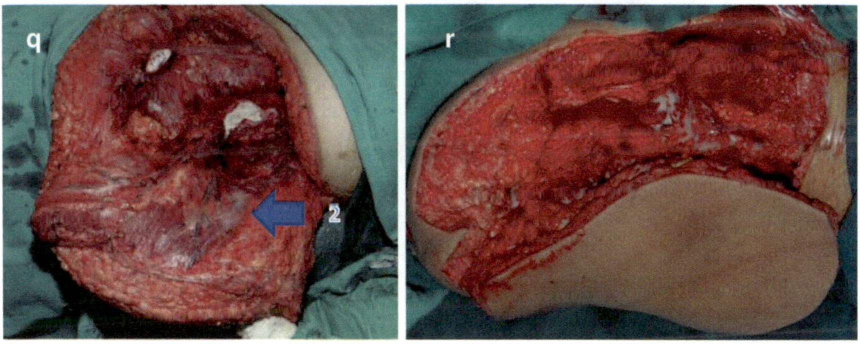

1. Tumour contained within fascia covering iliopsoas.
2. Gluteal vessels.

Anterior Flap Hemipelvectomy

Anterior flap hemipelvectomy is done for pelvic tumour with posterior infiltration to the gluteus maximus muscle. Sarcoma involving the inferior sacroiliac joint and greater sciatic notch where mobilisation of the internal iliac and gluteal branch vessels poses a risk of contamination and vessels injuries are indications for anterior flap hemipelvectomy. The anterior myocutaneous flap utilises the femoral vessels and its branch for supplying the entire quadriceps compartment of the thigh. In such cases, where mobilisation of the external iliac and femoral vessels poses a risk of contamination, a free tissue transfer from fillet flaps (either from thigh or leg) of the amputated limb can be used with anastomosis to the common iliac vessels.

Options for anterior flap hemipelvectomy are:

- Local fasciocutaneous flap with femoral vessels
- Anterior myofascial cutaneous flap
- Free fillet flap from the amputated limb
- Distant free flap

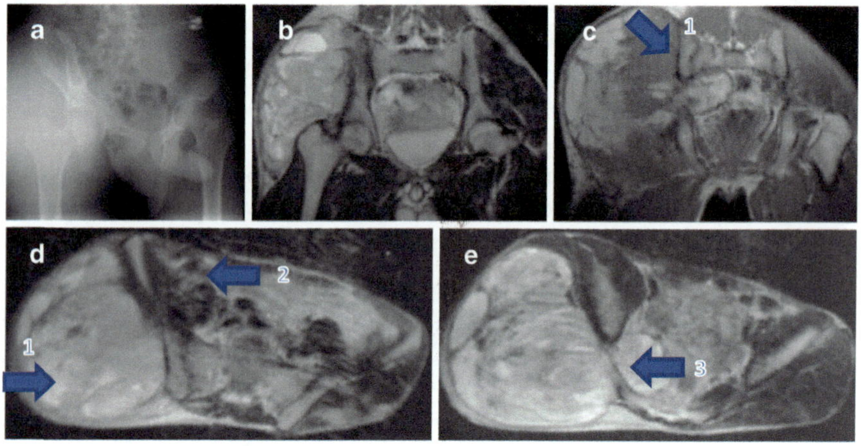

A case of MPNST sciatic nerve with the entire gluteus muscle involved with iliac wing infiltration. The tumour follows the course of the sciatic nerve and enters the inner pelvis through the greater sciatic foreman and infiltrates the gluteal and internal iliac vessels (Fig. 4a–e).

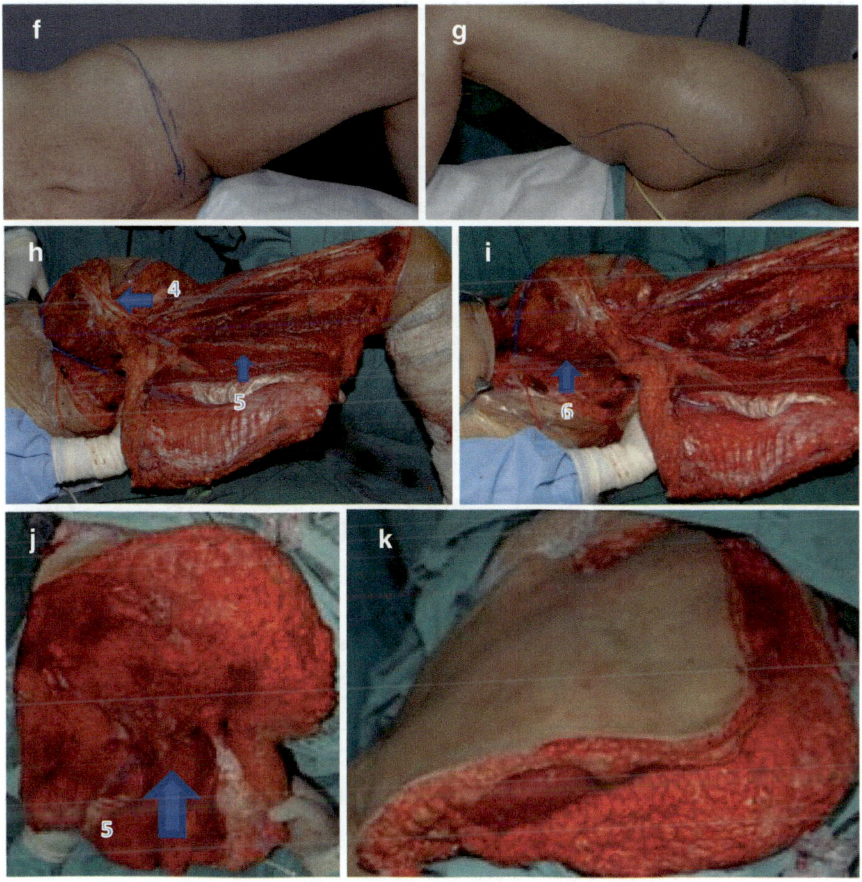

The femoral vessels were mobilised with the entire quadriceps muscle leaving the vastus medialis. Care must be taken to mobilise the medial row perforator and descending branch of the femoral circumflex for vascularity to the entire lateral thigh. The profunda femoral vessels were ligated, the adductor and posterior compartment were not taken as flap for closure (Fig. 4f–k)

1. Extensive gluteal involvement
2. External iliac vessels
3. Sciatic nerve and L5 S1 S2 root extension
4. Inguinal ligament
5. Femoral artery with sartorius muscle
6. Common iliac vessels

Modification of Anterior Flap Hemipelvectomy

A case of dedifferentiated chondrosarcoma of proximal femur with pathological fracture of proximal femur. The gluteus maximus attachment showed infiltration and the adductor muscle showed infiltration to the level of the inferior pubic rami and ischium. The vastus intermedius and lateralis were involved (Fig. 5a–f). The anterior flap was designed to include the sartorius and vastus medialis as part of the cover as the gluteus maximus was partially resected. The ilium was partially resected for peri acetabulum margin (Fig. 5g–j).

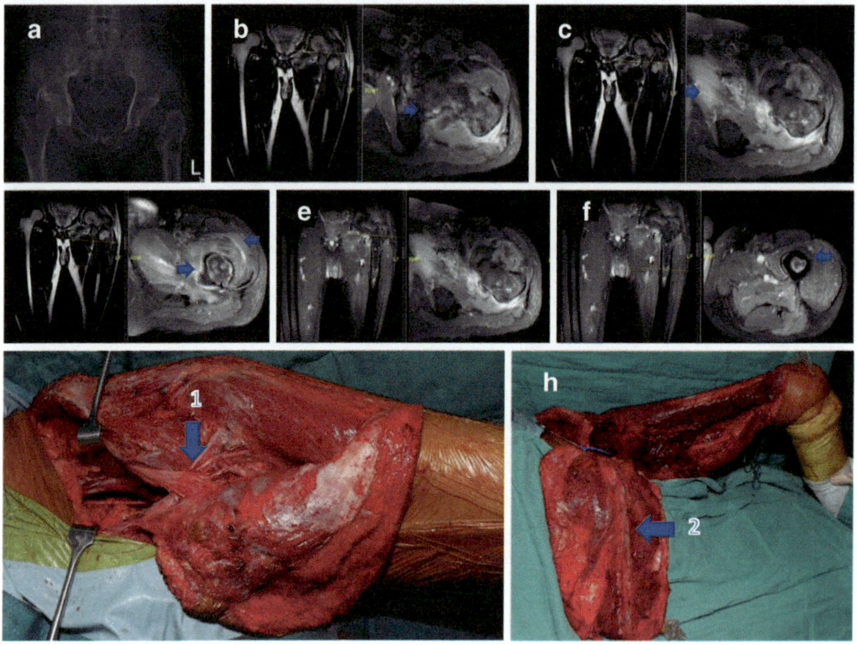

1. Femoral nerve was transacted for mobilisation of the flap
2. Femoral vessels with sartorius and vastus medialis
3. Remnant gluteus medius

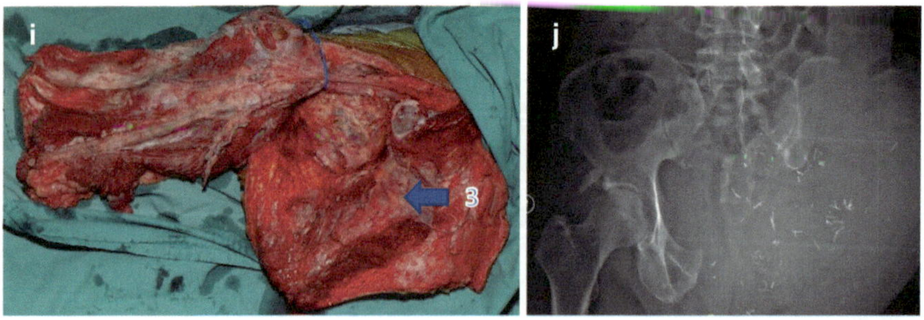

Fillet Flap from Entire Thigh

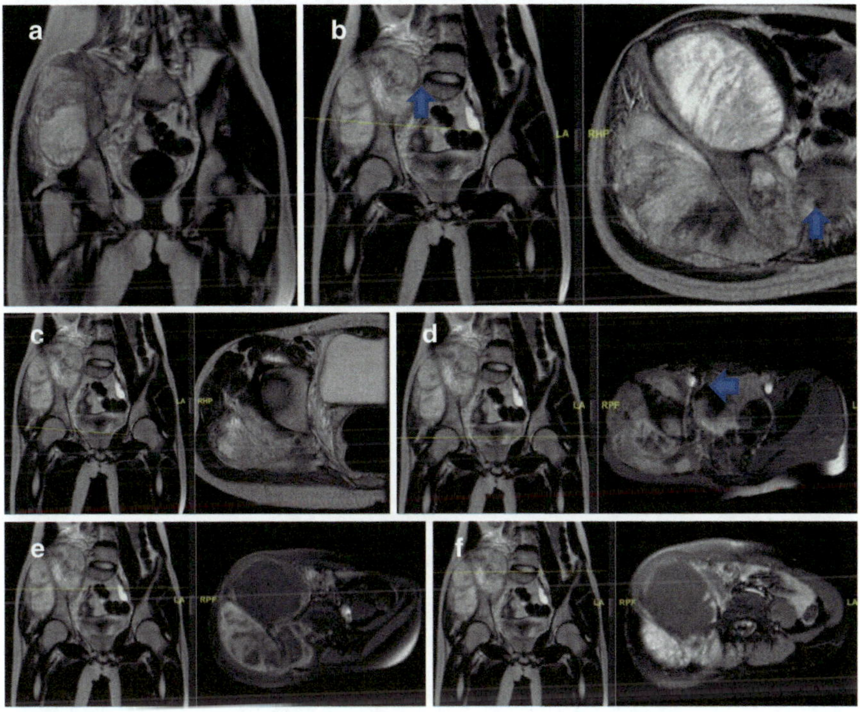

A case of poorly differentiated chondrosarcoma with entire hemipelvis involvement and extension to the alar of the sacrum (Fig. 6a–f). Rotation of entire anterior thigh flap is possible as the external iliac and femoral vessels were not involved (Fig. 6g–i).

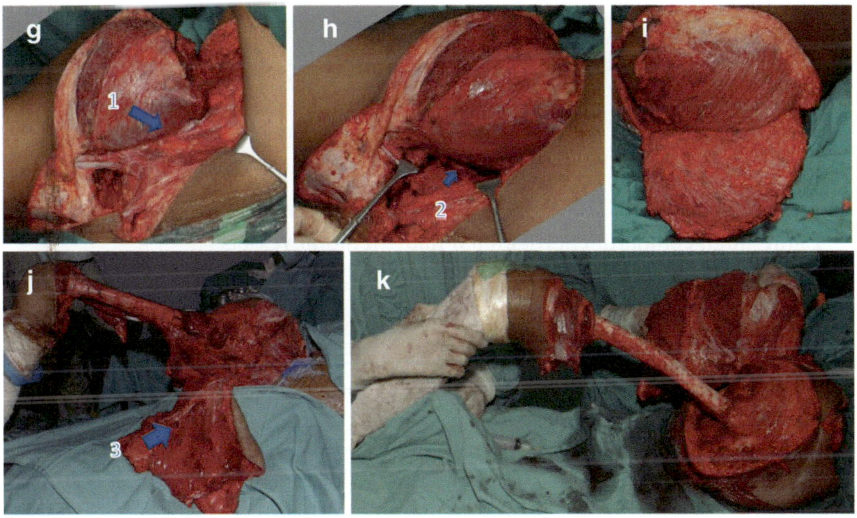

Both superficial and profunda femoral vessels were mobilised together with the entire thigh muscle flap. Lateral approach through the septum and mobilising the entire muscle sub-periosteally had maintained the perforator of the profunda artery to the posterior compartment (Fig. 6j–n).

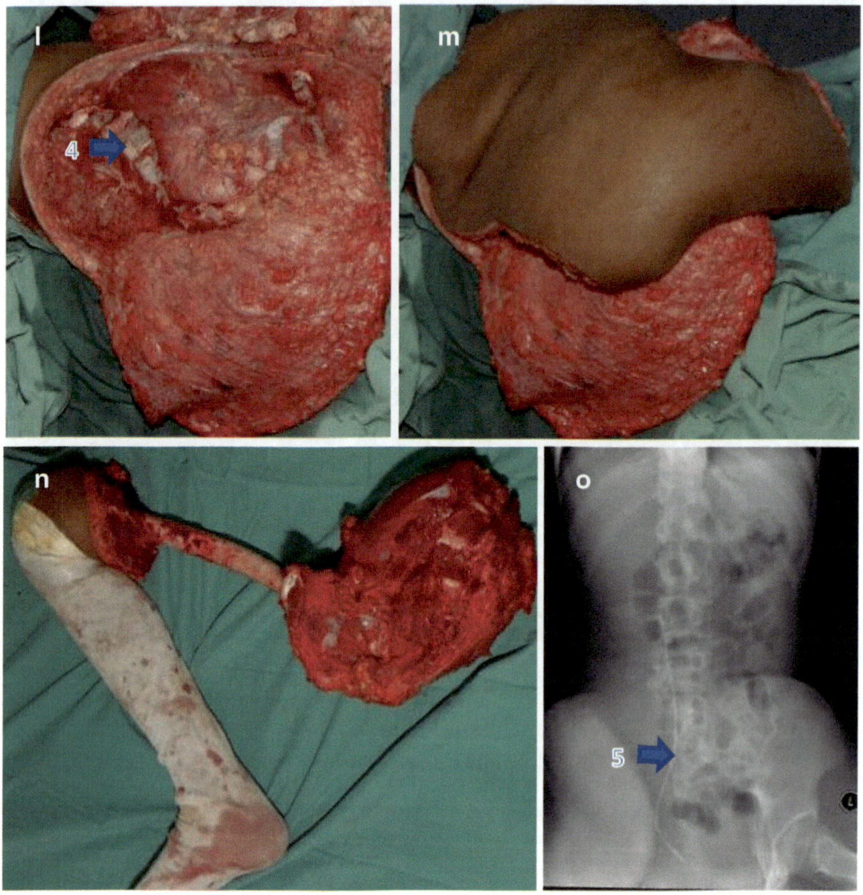

1. External iliac artery
2. Internal iliac vessels
3. Entire thigh compartment rotational flap—femoral vessels
4. Alar of sacrum involvement
5. Remnant half sacrum (Fig. 6o)

Free Vascularised Fillet Flap from Leg Muscle

Extensive sarcoma with pelvic extension and infiltration of the anterior thigh muscle is not suitable for rotational thigh flap (Fig. 7a–d). The fillet tissue from the remaining distal amputated segment either from the lower thigh or leg can be used for vascular bulk transfer. Remnant of common or external iliac can be used as recipient free fillet flap for anastomosis.

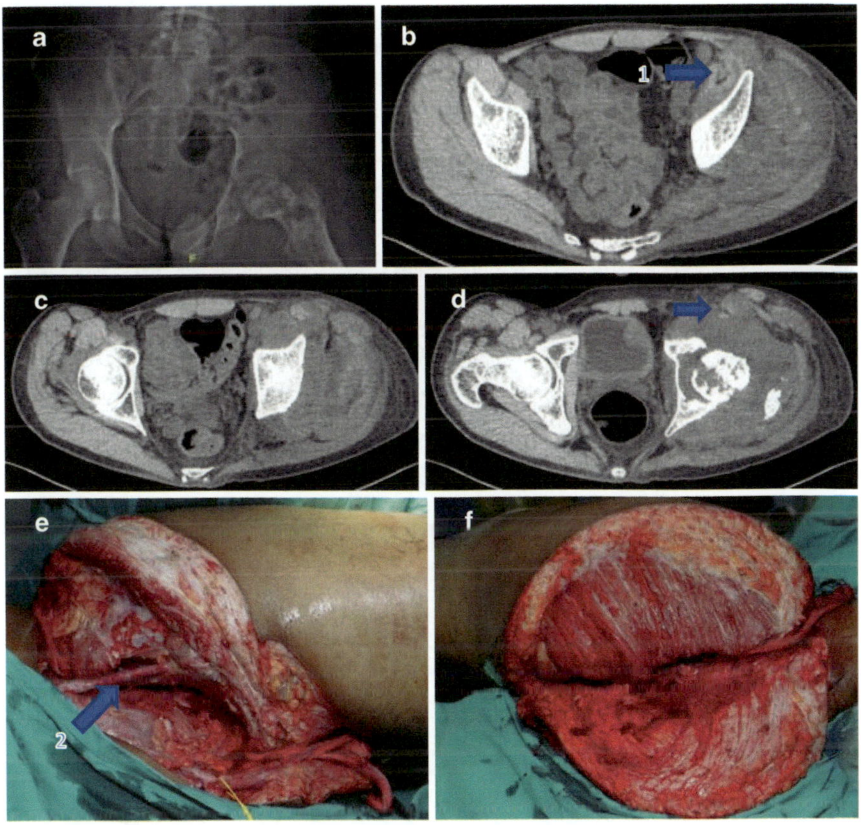

Proximal femur osteosarcoma with soft tissue extension to the gluteus maximus and anterior pelvis. The femoral vessels were within the tumour mass that precluded the thigh flap. Option was limited to free the fillet leg flap from the popliteal vessels (Fig. 7e, f).

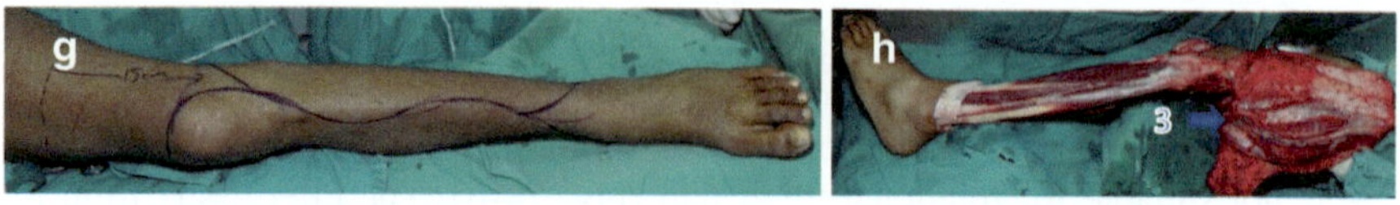

1. External iliac artery involved
2. Common iliac vessels
3. Popliteal vessels

The flap using the popliteal vessels with deep and superficial posterior compartment as bulk muscle. The entire leg skin and fascia were mobilised together with the muscle to allow the pedicle perforator to be maintained (Fig. 7g–i).

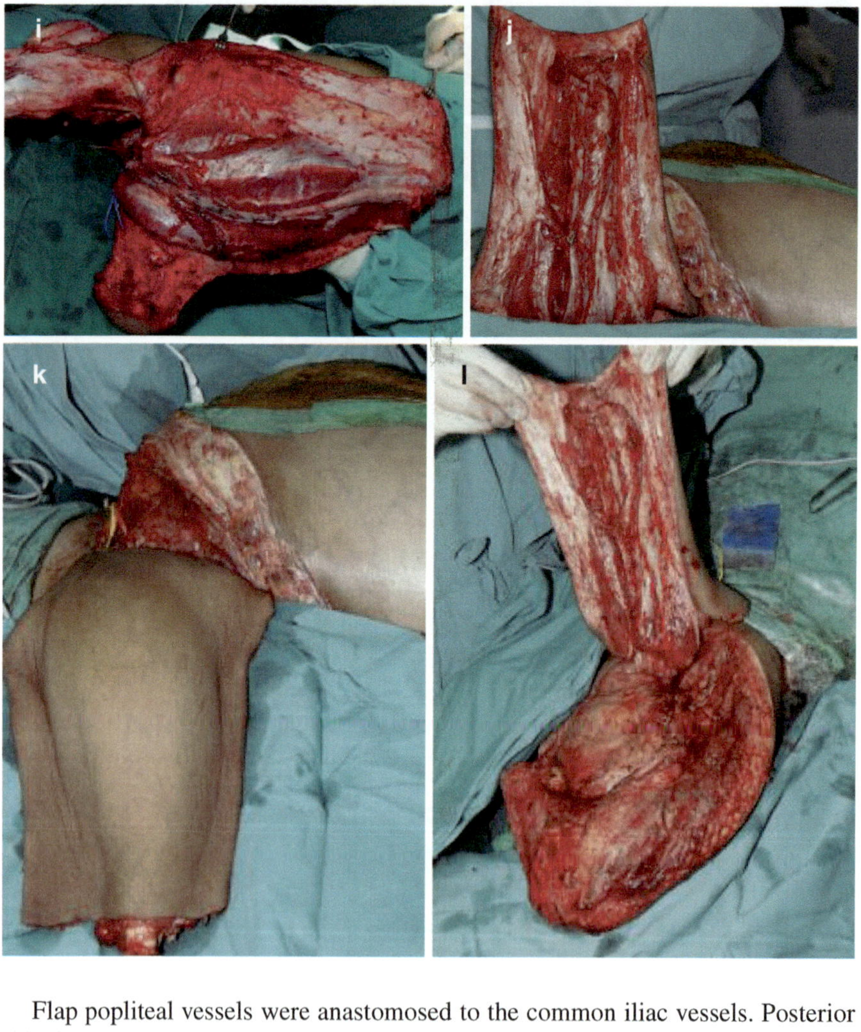

Flap popliteal vessels were anastomosed to the common iliac vessels. Posterior skin flap through random pattern supply was created prior to flap procedures as a reserve procedure if complication of the flap failure occurred (Fig. 7j–l).

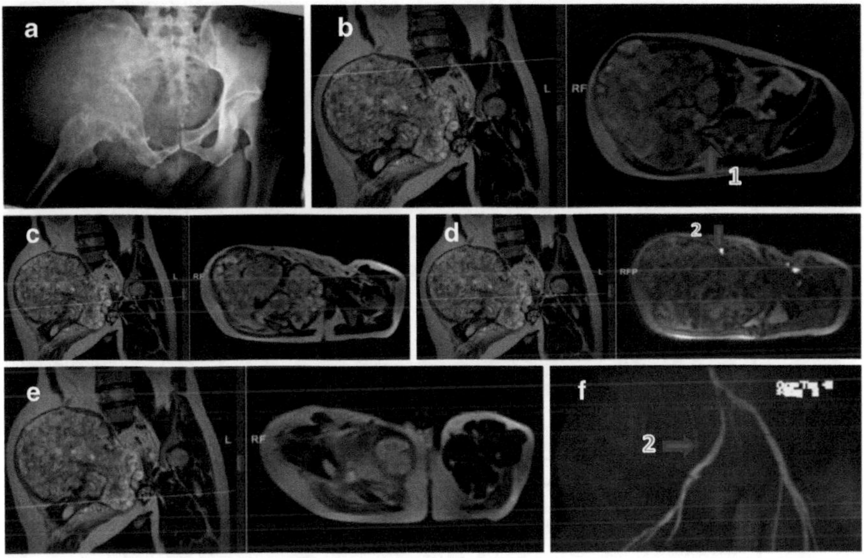

Extensive chondrosarcoma involving the anterior and posterior pelvis with direct involvement of the external and internal iliac vessels (Fig. 8a–f). The flap was taken from the lower thigh as main superficial femoral supply with the proximal tibia and entire knee fasciocutaneous flap (Fig. 8g–m).

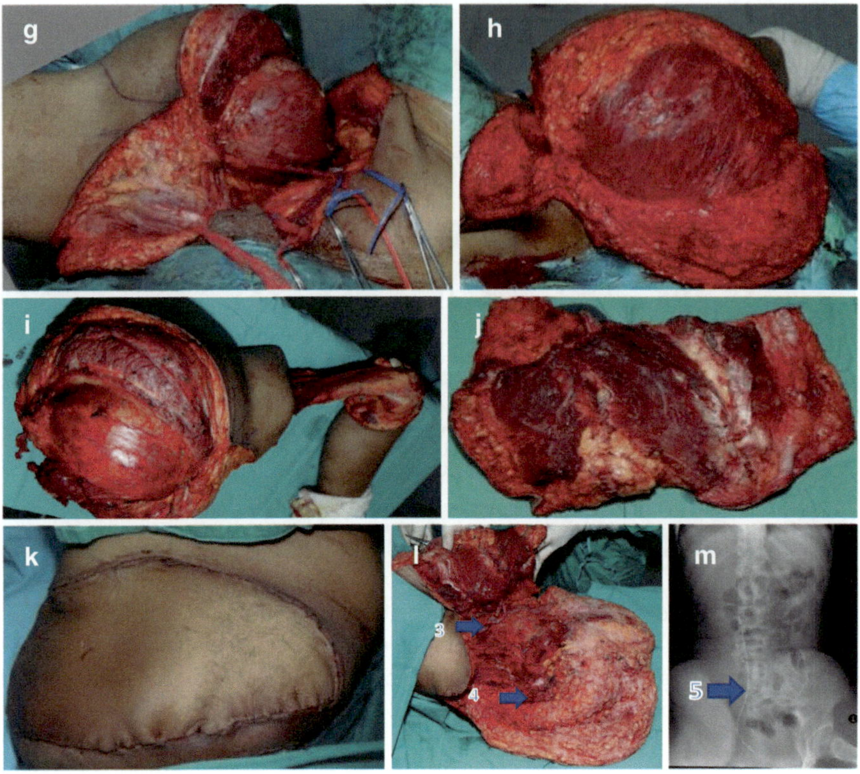

1. Ala of the sacrum involved
2. Common iliac artery pushed by the tumour
3. Femoral vessels anastomosed to common iliac vessels
4. Osteotomy at the sacral foramina
5. Ureteric stent in situ

Suggested Reading

1. Senchenkov A, Moran SL, Petty PM, Knoetgen J III, Tran NV, Clay RP, Bite U, Johnson CH, Barnes SA, Sim FH. Soft-tissue reconstruction of external hemipelvectomy defects. Plast Reconstr Surg. 2009;124:144–55.
2. Mat Saad AZ, Halim AS, Faisham WI, Azman WS, Zulmi W. Soft tissue reconstruction following hemipelvectomy. Eight years' experience and literature review. Sci World J. 2012;2012:702904.
3. Constantine P. K. Hemipelvectomy (Hindquarter amputation) & variants of hemipelvectomy. In: Atlas of operative procedures in surgical oncology. Springer Science; 2015. p. 361–75.
4. Knox K, Bitzos I, Granick M, Datiashvili R, Benevenia J, Patterson F. Immediate reconstruction of oncologic hemipelvectomy defects. Ann Plast Surg. 2006;57(2):184–9.

5. Kulaylat MN, Froix A, Karakousis CP. Blood supply of hemipelvectomy flaps: The anterior flap hemipelvectomy. Arch Surg. 2001;136:828–31.
6. Malawer MM, Wittig JC. Anterior Flap Hemipelvectomy 208–216 operative technique in orthopaedic surgical oncology. Lippincott Williams & Wilkins, A Wolters Kluwer; 2012.
7. Malawer MM, Wittig JC. Posterior Flap Hemipelvectomy 197–207 operative technique in orthopaedic surgical oncology. Lippincott Williams & Wilkins, A Wolters Kluwer; 2012.
8. Sugarbaker PH, Chretien PA. Hemipelvectomy for buttock tumors utilizing an anterior myocutaneous flap of quadriceps femoris muscle. Ann Surg. 1983;197:106–15.
9. Yamamoto Y, Minakawa H, Takeda N. Pelvic reconstruction with a free fillet lower leg flap. Plast Reconstr Surg. 1997;99:1439–41.

Forequarter Amputation

Wan Faisham Nu'man Bin Wan Ismail

Introduction

Forequarter amputation is a surgical procedure for removal of the upper extremity together with the scapula en bloc. It is an amputation for malignant tumours around the shoulder not suitable for limb salvage surgery. Indications mainly include large sarcoma with poor response to chemotherapy, recurrent disease or sarcoma displacing or infiltrating the subclavian vessels and brachial plexus in which achieving oncological margin with limb salvage surgery is not possible.

Surgical Anatomy

The subclavian and axillary vessels exit above the first ribs from the brachiocephalic trunk and lies posterior to the pectoralis major and minor below the coracoid process:

- They lie directly above the subscapularis muscle—direct approach for brachial plexus and artery through anterior approach by detaching pectoralis major and mirror attachment is best. However, exploration from posterior between the thoracic cage and subscapularis after elevating the entire scapula is possible especially for tumours with anterior chest extension.
- The suprascapular anastomosis, a system connecting the subclavian and axillary artery and forming circulatory vessels around the scapula, can be very vascular in large tumour.

W. F. N. B. W. Ismail (✉)
Prince Court Medical Center, Kuala Lumpur, Malaysia

Orthopaedic Oncology Reconstructive Unit, Universiti Sains Malaysia, Kubang Kerian, Kelantan, Malaysia

A. Puri, W. F. N. B. W. Ismail (eds.), *Atlas of Orthopedic Oncology Volume 1*,
https://doi.org/10.1007/978-981-95-8958-6_13

Scapular Muscle Attachment

- The supraspinatus and infraspinatus cover the posterior aspect of the scapula and must be removed in total as oncological margin.
- The subscapularis muscle provides anterior anatomical boundaries and protects the rib cage from tumour infiltration. Elevation of the scapula from the posterior border will reveal the subclavian and axillary vessels at the apex of the axillary space
- The muscle attached to the medial border scapula, rhomboid major and minor, levator scapula and trapezius must be transacted for lateral mobilisation of the scapulae
- Muscle attached to the lateral border of scapula, teres major and minor are elevated together with the scapula from the thoracic cage and removed in total with the entire limb. The latissimus dorsi muscle is transacted at the tip of the scapula and the superior remnant is included as margin. Care must be taken to ligate the thoracodorsal artery during this manoeuvre.

Clavicle Muscle Attachment

- The clavicular head of the pectoralis major must be evaluated for tumour extension and oncological margin.
- The pectoralis minor is attached to the coracoid process and originates from the second to fourth ribs. Mobilisation from the ribs below the pectoralis major provides a good margin.

Assessment

Assessment for surgical margin for forequarter amputation includes:

- Infiltration or extension to the chest wall
- Scapula tumour with anterior extension
- Involvement of the pectoralis major and minor
- Extension to the axillary space
- Medial margin of the scapulae
- Superior infiltration to the brachial plexus in malignant nerve sarcoma
- Contamination of the axillary space and involvement of the nodes

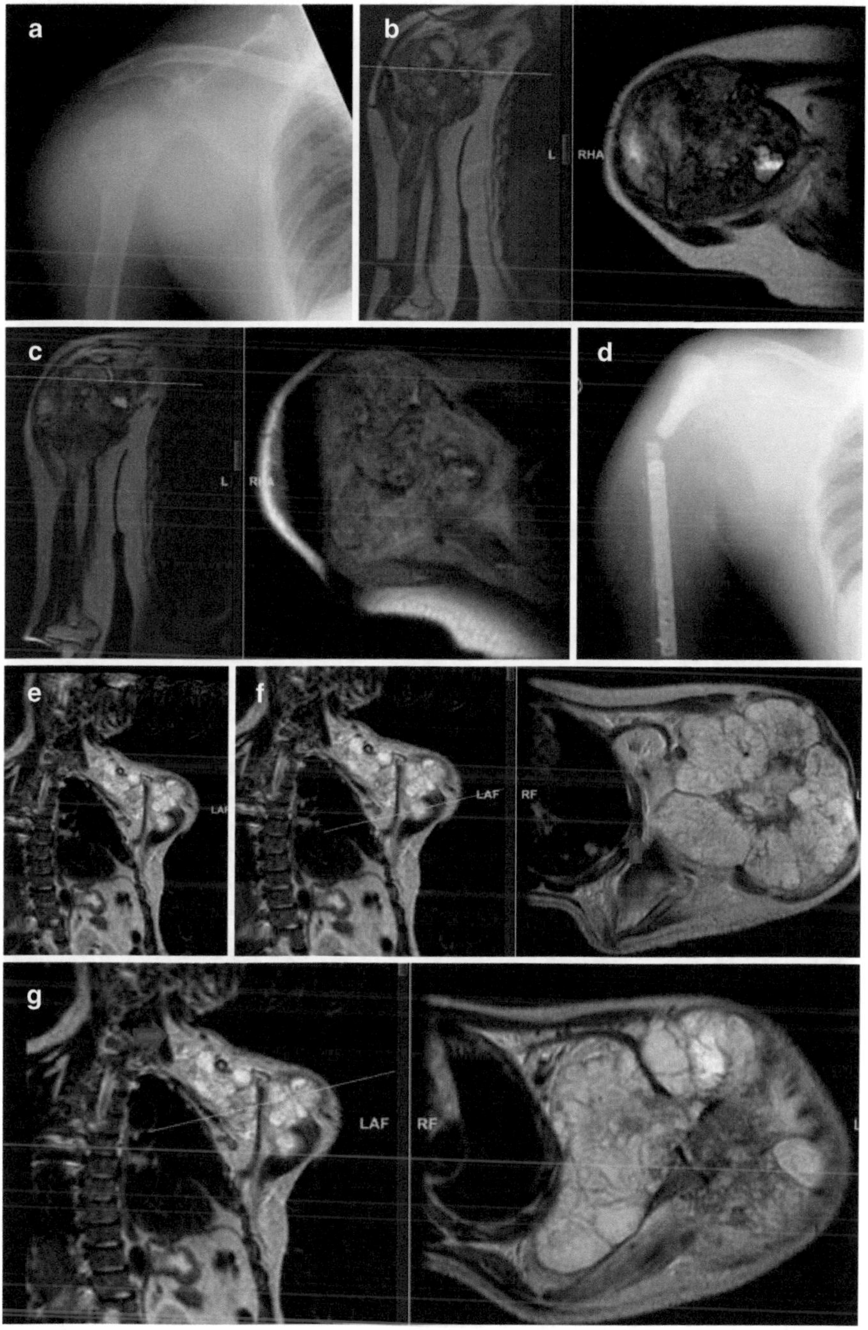

Proximal humerus tumour with glenoid extension proximal humerus tumour treated with resection and allograft reconstruction. The surgical margin was free with 20% necrosis index. The patient had early recurrence at 12 months and local MRI showed axillary contamination and that the entire scapulae was involved.

There was extension to the base of neck; however, the chest wall was not involved. This necessitated a forequarter amputation (Fig. 1a–g).

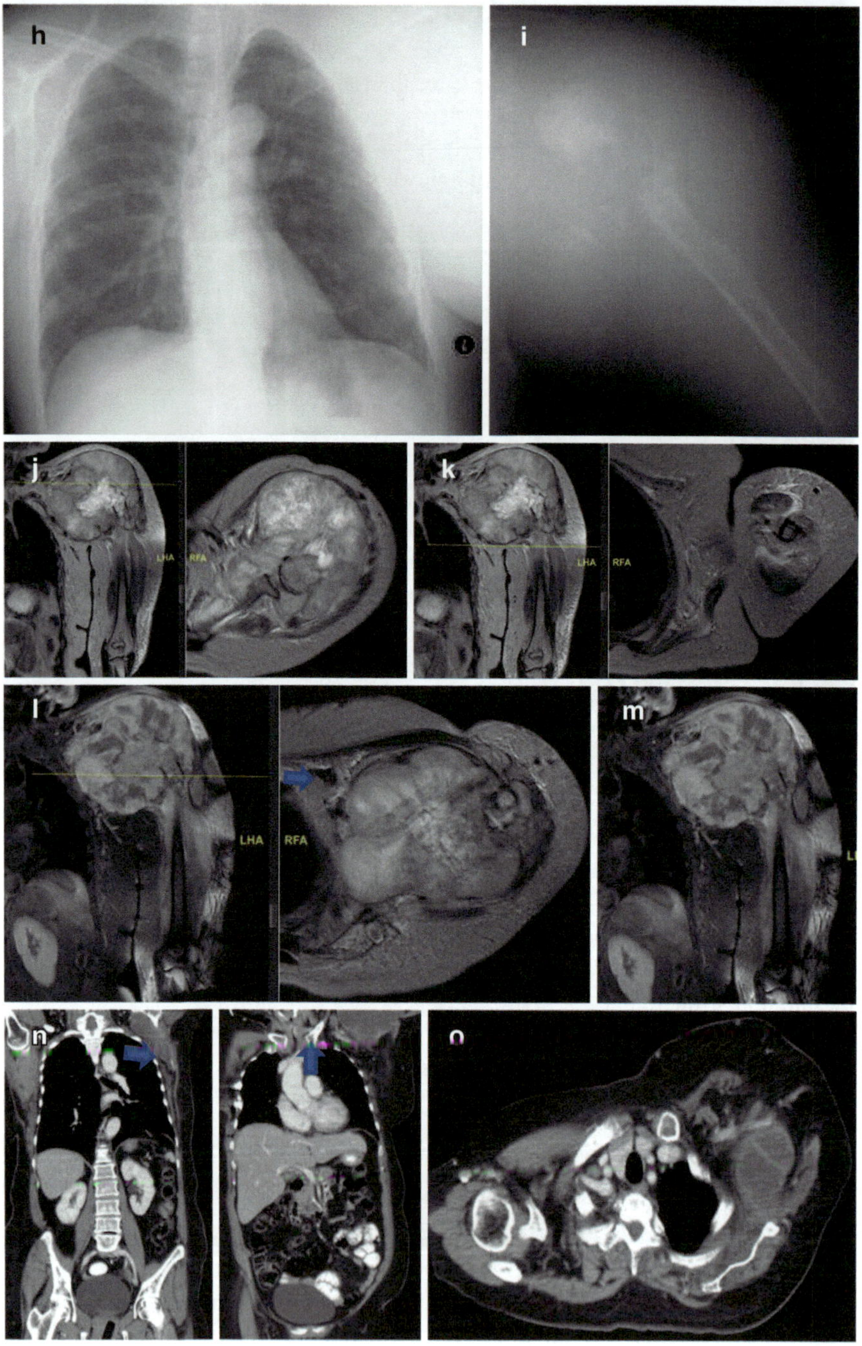

A case of proximal humerus osteosarcoma aggressive behaviours with pathological fracture and poor response to two chemotherapy cycles. The tumour mass involved the entire proximal humerus and scapula and was closely attached to thoracic cage on the MRI. Spiral CT in limb abduction showed that the thoracic cage was free thus enabling a forequarter amputation (Fig. 1h–o).

Surgical Steps: Posterior Approach for Forequarter Amputation (Fig. 2)

- The patient is placed in a direct lateral position as majority of the surgery is performed mainly through a posterior approach (Fig. 2a–c).
- The upper extremity is covered with a sterile stocking so that it can be manipulated as the procedure evolves.
- The posterior approach is started by creating a posterior skin flap medially. The exposure was utilised by detaching the scapula from the rhomboids, trapezius, levator scapulae and latissimus dorsi muscle (Fig. 2d).
- The scapula is lifted from the chest wall with the subscapular muscle by detaching the latissimus dorsi at its lowest points (Fig. 2e–g).
- The limb is moved anteriorly to improve posterior exposure to the axillary fossa. The brachial plexus and clavicle acted as pivotal points to protect the vessels from being avulsed.
- Complete the dissection anteriorly by creating the flap to the exposed pectoralis major and transection of both the pectoralis major and minor for margins (Fig. 2h).
- Both the subclavian and axillary artery and vein are ligated 1 cm from the chest wall before all the plexus is sectioned and the clavicle is osteotomised. The subclavian-brachial vessels and axillary content are included in the surgical margins (Fig. 2i).

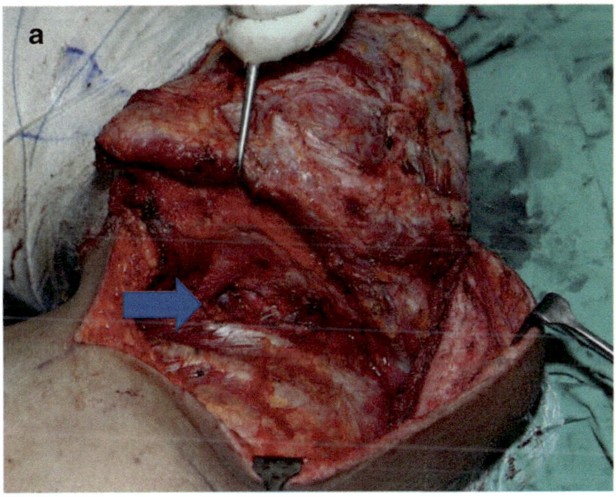

- Axillary artery and brachial plexus below the mid clavicle from a posterior approach

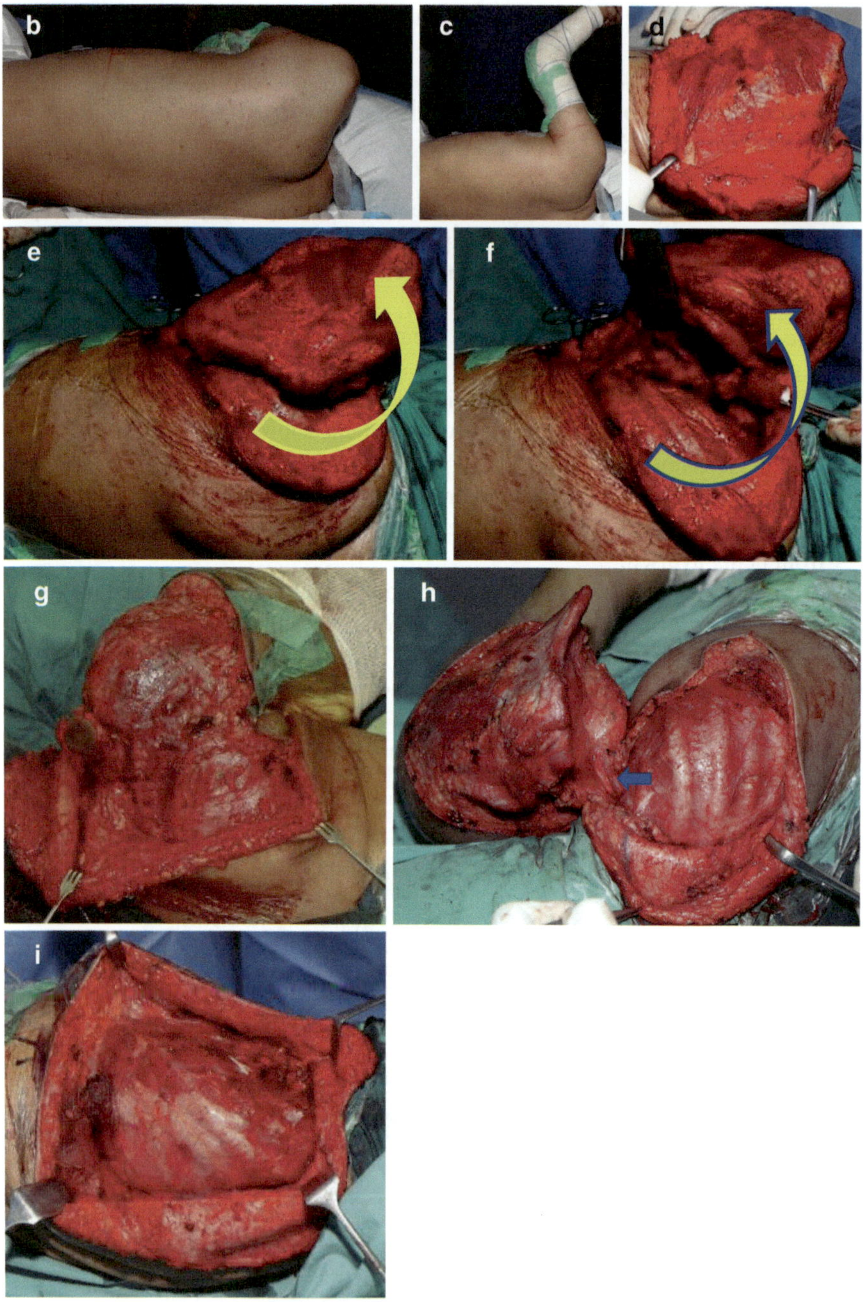

Forequarter Amputaion with Entire Root Brachial Plexus Margin

A case of neurofibrosarcoma with involvement of the entire brachial plexus to the cervical root region that required exploration and resection for better oncological margin.

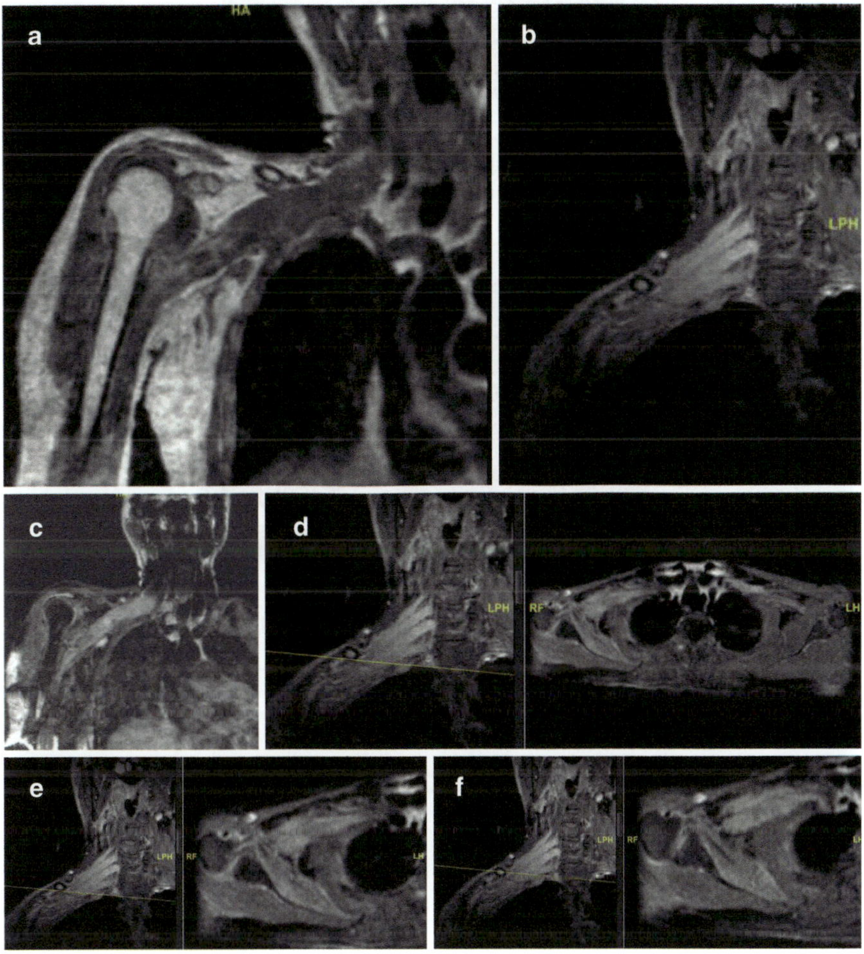

The entire brachial plexus showed significant enhancement on the gadolinium scan that suggested direct local infiltration to the root. No evidence of extension to the spinal cord (Fig. 3a–f).

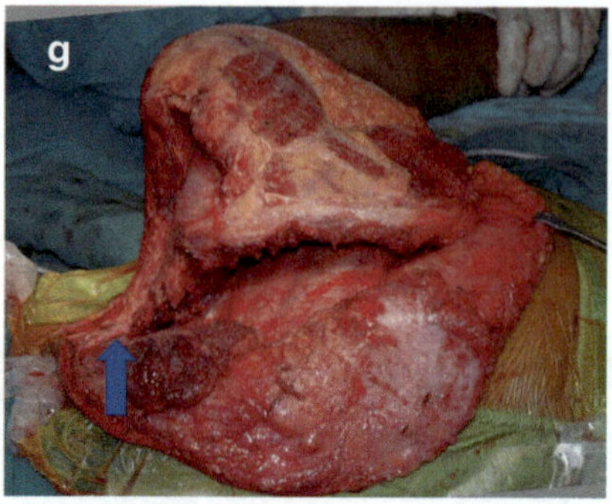

Mobilisation of the posterior flap and exploration of the plexus between the scalenus muscle for complete resection of the plexus.

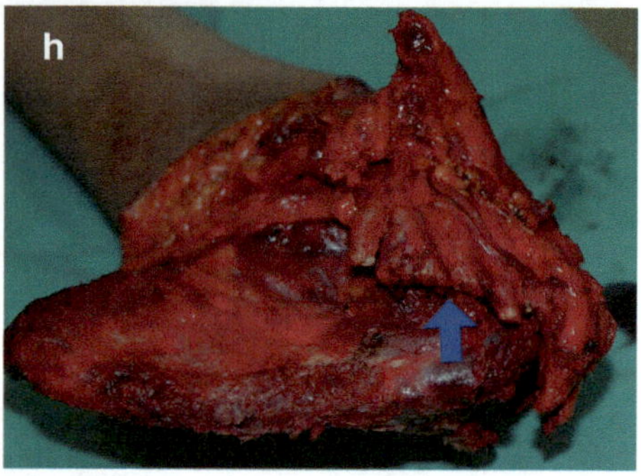

The entire upper limb with the scapula was removed in total with the entire brachial plexus to the root (Fig. 3g, h).

Defect Closure After Forequarter Amputation

Large sarcoma arising from proximal humerus with extraarticular glenoid extension infiltrates the anterior periscapular muscle and rarely involves skin and subcutaneous tissue. In forequarter amputation, the periscapular and chest wall structures was removed leaving a small area for coverage. Ample random pattern fasciocutaneous tissue around periscapular region can be utilised for reliable closure of amputated stump. In cases with anterior skin involved, posterior fasciocutaneous flap can be used to cover the anterior defect Tumour extending to the axillary region with wide skin involvement requires lateral shoulder fasciocutaneous tissues over the deltoid for coverage and minimise tension.

In cases with massive skin infiltration, particularly scapula tumour whereby local fasciocutaneous tissue is not adequate, split skin grafted can be harvested from amputated forearm limb for skin coverage. Exposed ribs with intact soft tissue and periosteum are adequate for the success of grafting. Fillet flap from the amputated limbs is used for restoration of the shoulder silhouette and provides additional stability and better body contour. In cases the thoracic cage is involved, distal forearm is used for coverage of osseous defect. Free tissue transfer is an option but most of forequarter amputation is done with palliative intent, short surgical intervention with minimal reconstruction is a priority to minimised major complication of surgery and anaesthesia.

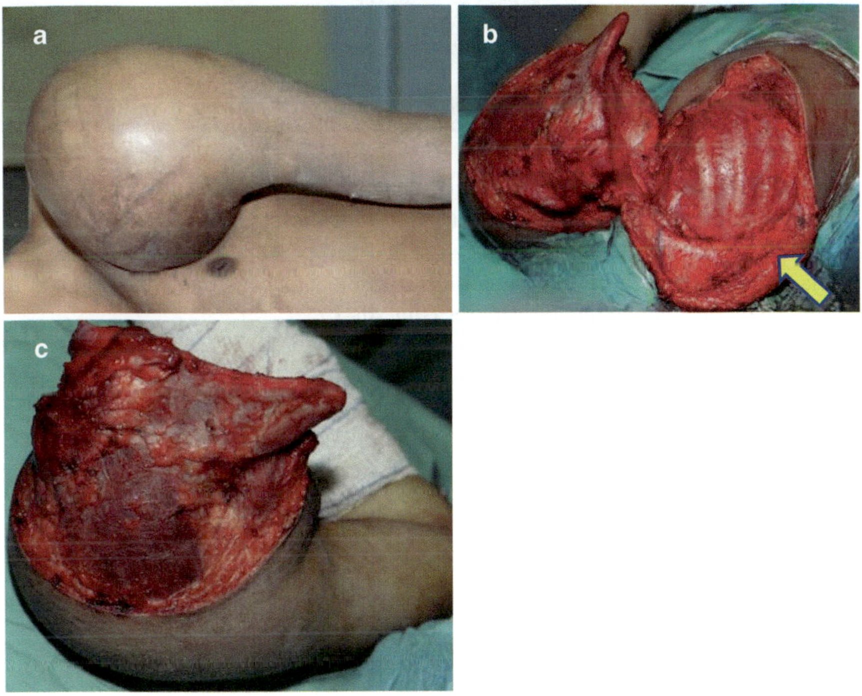

Proximal humerus osteosarcoma with anterior soft tissue extension—utilised posterior fascio cutaneous flap over scapula for closure of forequarter amputation stump (Fig. 4a–c).

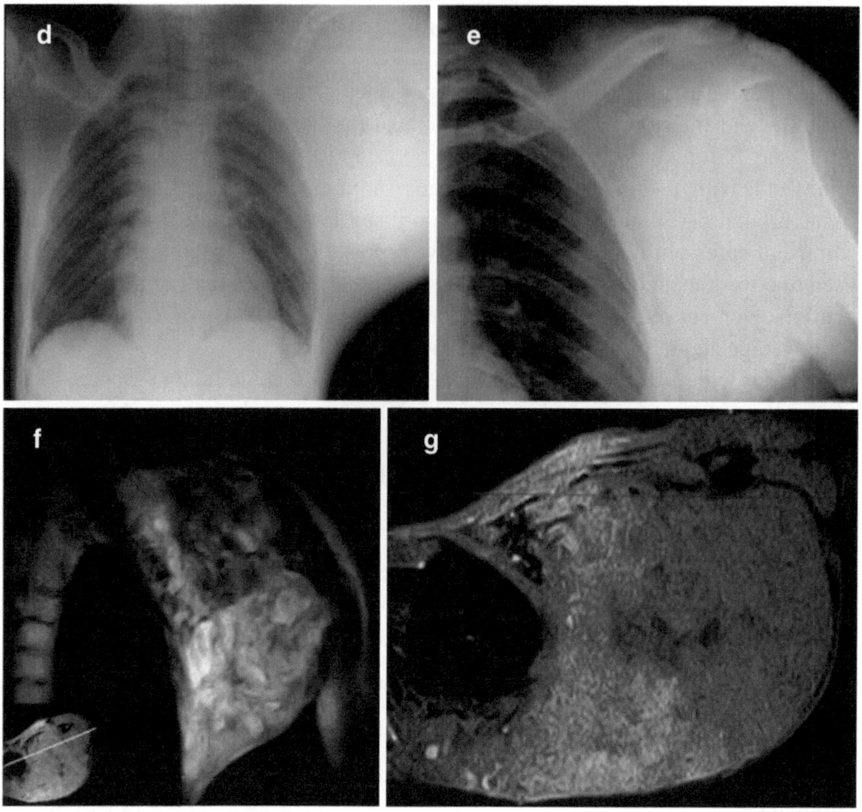

De-differentiated chondrosarcoma of scapula with massive extension to the periscapular area, axillary structures and pectoralis muscle (Fig. 4d–g). The fasciocutaneous tissue around scapula was stretched and possible infiltrated by the sarcoma. Random pattern of anterior posterior fasciocutaneous flap was designed to minimise reconstructive flap procedures (Fig. 4h–k).

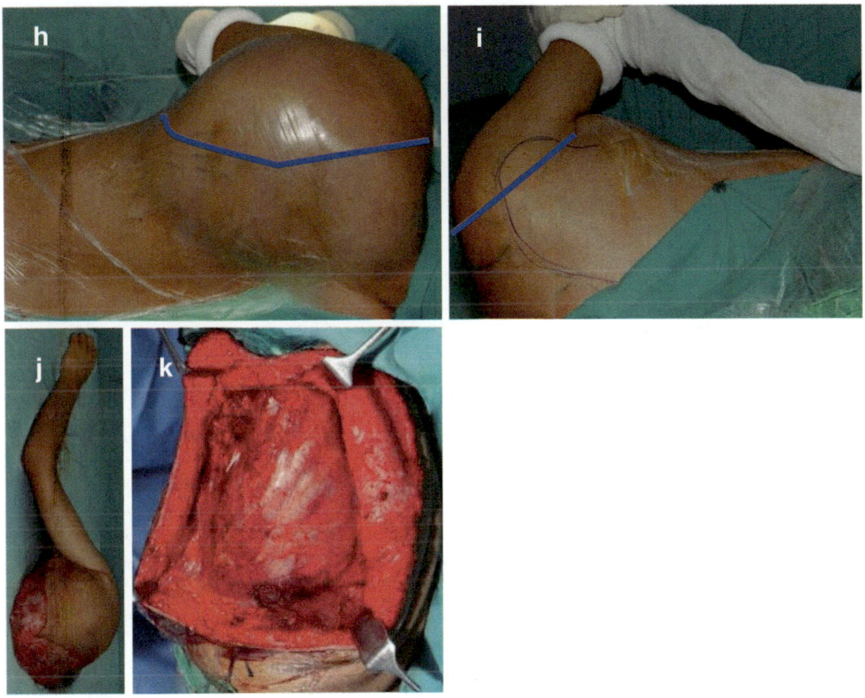

A case of soft tissue sarcoma with local recurrence. Medial forearm and axillary region presented with multiple skin nodule indicating local skin infiltration. The fasciocutaneous flap was designed to include lateral arm and deltoid region for better closure due to large skin involvement around the axillary region (Fig. 4l–n).

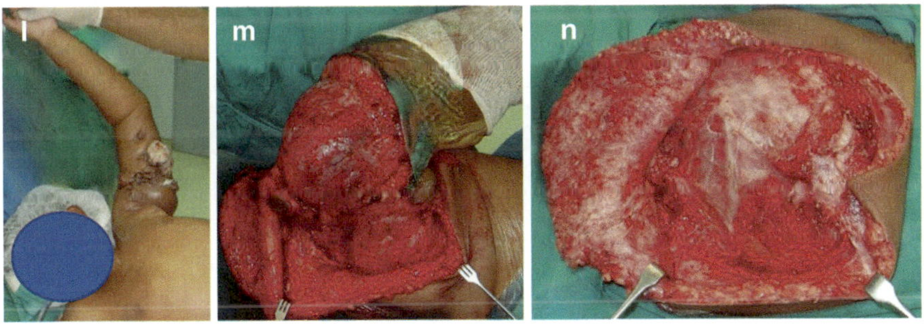

Split skin grafting can be used as composites from amputated limb for large defect (Fig. 4o)

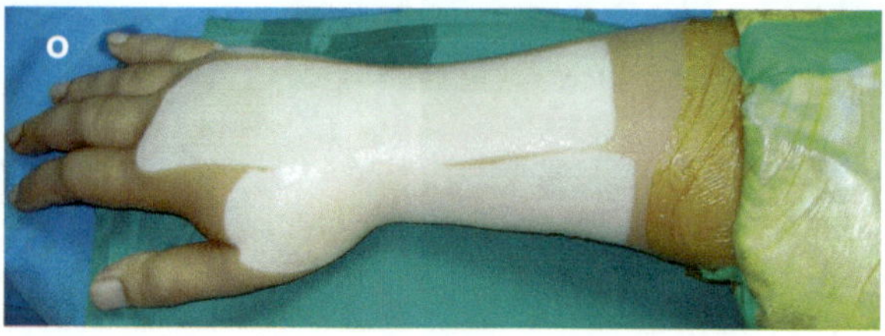

Suggested Reading

1. Karakousis CP. Forequarter amputation atlas of operative procedures in surgical oncology. Springer Nature. p. 103–10.
2. Ehrl D, Wachtel N, Braig D, Kuhlmann C, Dürr HR, Schneider CP, Giunta RE. Defect coverage after forequarter amputation—a systematic review assessing different surgical approaches. J Pers Med. 2022;12:560.
3. Elsner U, Henrichs M, Gosheger G, Dieckmann R, Nottrott M, Hardes J, Streitbürger A. Forequarter amputation: a safe rescue procedure in a curative and palliative setting in high-grade malignoma of the shoulder girdle. World J Surg Oncol. 2016;14(1):1–8.
4. Palmer FT, Karakousis Constantine P. Technique of forequarter (Interscapulothoracic) amputation. Clin Orthop Relat Res. 2004;423:191–5.
5. Kumar A, Naranje S, Gupta H, Khan SA, Yadav CS, Rastoqi S, et al. A single incision surgical new anterior technique for forequarter amputation. Arch Orthop Trauma Surg. 2011;131:955–61.
6. Qadir R, Sidhu S, Romine L, Meyer MS, Duncan SF. Interscapulothoracic (forequarter) amputation for malignant tumors involving the upper extremity: surgical technique and case series. J Shoulder Elb Surg. 2014;23(6):e127–33.
7. Rickelt J, Hoekstra H, van Coevorden F, de Vreeze R, Verhoef C, van Geel AN. Forequarter amputation for malignancy. Br J Surg. 2009;96:792–8.
8. Roubaud MS, Mericli AF, Adelman DM, Hanasono MM, Lewis VO, Moon BS. Reconstruction of forequarter and extended forequarter amputations: indications and outcomes. Plast Reconstr Surg. 2023;152(1):194–205.
9. Faisham WI, Zulmi W, Norazman MZ, Rhendra MZ. Posterior approach for forequarter amputation- technique and operative benefits. Med J Malaysia. Suppl C. 2005.

Resection of Pelvis and Sacrum Sarcoma

Sacrectomy

Wan Faisham Nu'man Bin Wan Ismail

Introduction

Anatomic characteristics make en bloc sacral resections with wide surgical margins a very demanding and challenging procedure in most malignant tumours of the sacrum. Sacral tumours generally respect the nerve sheaths and do not penetrate through them. Instead, they surround the sacral nerves during the growing stages, making it practically impossible to dissect them from the nerves. Ventrally, the tumours also push into the presacral connective tissue layers though they seldom infiltrate the rectum.

Surgical Anatomy

Sacrum is a large triangular bone originating from five separate vertebra that fuses along with the intervening intervertebral discs. The structure is convex dorsally with an apex projecting posteriorly. Sagittal, the sacral base is inclined forward, forming an angulation between the lumbar spine and sacrum is known as the sacral promontory.

Sacrum articulates with four bones:

- Last lumbar vertebra (L5) above via a disc space and facet joint complex.
- Coccyx below with a ligamentous attachment and occasional bony union.
- Ilium via the sacroiliac joint—complex forming a synovial joint anteriorly and strong ligamentous attachments posteriorly.

W. F. N. B. W. Ismail (✉)
Prince Court Medical Center, Kuala Lumpur, Malaysia

Orthopaedic Oncology Reconstructive Unit, Universiti Sains Malaysia, Kubang Kerian, Kelantan, Malaysia

A. Puri, W. F. N. B. W. Ismail (eds.), *Atlas of Orthopedic Oncology Volume 1*, https://doi.org/10.1007/978-981-95-8958-6_14

SIJ (sacroiliac Joint) is formed within the sacral segments S1, S2 and S3 and lies obliquely at an angle to the sagittal plane. The female sacrum is more uneven, less curved and tilted more posteriorly than the male sacrum. The male pelvis is relatively long and narrow, and the iliac crest reaches higher.

These structures must be evaluated for oncological margin in sacral resection. The coccyx is removed in total with the sacrum in all cases.

Ligaments that stabilise the sacrum:

- Sacrotuberus ligament, a thick broad fibrous band, extends from the posterior ilium, lateral sacrum, and coccyx to the ischial tuberosity.
- Sacrospinous ligament, a triangular-shaped structure, is attached to the anterior sacrum (S2–S4) and coccyx to the ischial spine. It forms a boundary of the greater and lesser sciatic foramen.

These ligaments must be detached from the pelvis to free the sacrum for final resection. In large tumour extending laterally to the pelvis closely attached to the ischial spine, resection of the ischial spine together with the tumour will minimise contamination and achieve better oncological margin.

Three muscles originate on the ventral surface of the sacrum:

- Iliacus at the superior lateral aspect.
- Coccygeus along the inferior lateral aspect.
- Piriformis lateral to the ventral sacral foramina.

Muscular attachments on posterior aspect of the sacrum:

- Gluteus maximus is attached below the sacroiliac articulation at the inferior lateral aspect.
- Spinal extensors: multifidus, sacro spinalis and erector spinae muscles originate from the sacral grooves medially.
- Extensor coccyges inferiorly.

The presacral area is a retroperitoneal space, located between the presacral fascia of the sacrum 'Waldeyer fascia' and parietal peritoneum of the posterior abdominal wall. It contains retro rectal fat, areolar tissue, lymph nodes, median sacral vessels, and superior rectal vessels. It extends from the peritoneal reflection at the rectosigmoid junction to the pelvic bottom.

The spinal dura ends at the level of S2 where it becomes a thin cord-like extension (coccygeal ligament or filum terminale) that anchors the dural sac to the sacral periosteum. Care must be taken to ligate the dura in sacrectomy at higher levels to prevent cerebrospinal fluid leak and formation of a fistula.

Level of sacrectomy and functional deficits

- Resection of S1: significantly reduced ambulation, loss of sphincter function and decreased sexual ability.
- Resection of S2: nerve root is associated with long-term urinary and bowel incontinence.

- Preservation of both S2 nerve roots is associated with a 50% probability of normal urinary and bowel function.
- No consensus on the impact of S3 nerve root resection on residual urinary and bowel function.

Common iliac artery is a large artery that originates from the aortic bifurcation at the level of the fourth lumbar vertebra. It ends in front of the sacroiliac joint and bifurcates into the external and internal iliac arteries. The internal iliac artery passes opposite the lumbosacral articulation, and down to the upper margin of the greater sciatic foramen, where it divides into two main branches of the anterior and posterior trunks. It is accompanied by L5 and S1 roots as part of the lumbosacral plexus of the sciatic nerve. The gluteal vessels arising from the posterior branch and supply all the gluteus muscles and it is important to be maintained them for gluteal rotational local flap. In high sacral tumours, these vessels and nerve must be protected anteriorly to prevent injury and massive bleeding.

Median sacral artery arises from the abdominal aorta at the level third lumbar vertebra. It descends in the middle to the fourth and fifth lumbar vertebrae, sacrum, and coccyx. This artery must be ligated for secure haemostasis in sacrectomy.

Assessment

Surgical margin status is the most important prognostic factor. In sacral chordoma en bloc sacral tumour resection is the cornerstone of treatment. Regardless of the approach used, the final goal is to achieve a wide local excision with negative microscopic margins.

Lateral margins strictly correlate with the extent of the muscular resection:

- Gluteus maximus and piriformis muscles around the greater sciatic notch.
- Superior gluteal vessels.
- Sacrospinous and sacrotuberus ligaments.
- In large tumours with lateral extension with postero-inferior margin, both the sacrospinous and sacrotuberus ligaments must be transected by means of an osteotome taking a fragment of the ischial bone en bloc with the ligaments.

Anterior margin

- Tumour invasion of the posterior rectal wall is uncommon. The mesorectum is a loose layer of adipo-lymphatic tissue and though usually sufficient may not always provide a barrier against tumour spread.
- In large or proximally located tumours, the rectum may be displaced anteriorly, along with the common iliac vessels and the hypogastric arteries and veins. Careful preparation of the common iliac vessels, prophylactically ligating the iliolumbar vessels and ischiatic/gluteal branches of the hypogastric arteries and veins is required to reduce the blood supply to the tumour and sacrum.

Superior margin

- Resection of the whole sacral vertebra above the tumour with good marrow margin as well as a meticulous assessment of the spinal canal and para-spinal muscles.

Bowel Preparation and Colostomy

Mechanical bowel preparation for sacral resection aims to reduce stool mass and bacterial count to decrease the rate of surgical site infection. The regimes include:

- Low residual diet 48 hours prior surgery
- Fleet (monobasic sodium phosphate monohydrate, dibasic sodium phosphate heptahydrate) 24 hours prior surgery
- Clear fluid with glucose for 12 hours

No oral antibiotic was added in the regimes, and prophylaxis antibiotics with cefuroxime 1.5 g and additional metranidazole 500 mg were given for 24 hours. The rectum is packed with roller gauze soaked with povidone and liquid parafin. The anus orifices is suture purse string to minimise soiling and surgical wound complication. Postoperatively opsite dressing was used to minimise contamination, and change the dressing every 2–3 days until the wound is healed.

In most cases, colostomy is not necessary except direct involvement of rectum, or in cases in which patients are expected to lose bowel function and for wound hygiene to simplify patient bowel regimens.

Low Sacral Resection: Single Posterior Approach

Sacral chordoma involving S2 and below with ventral extension within the presacral fascia. There is clear plane demarcation with the rectum. Dorsally, there is no tumour extension to the erector spinal and gluteus maximus attachment. There is lateral extension to both the piriformis muscles and these must be included as resection margin. The superior osseous extension is at the mid-level of S2 (Fig. 1a–k). The oncological resection margin is at the upper level of S2.

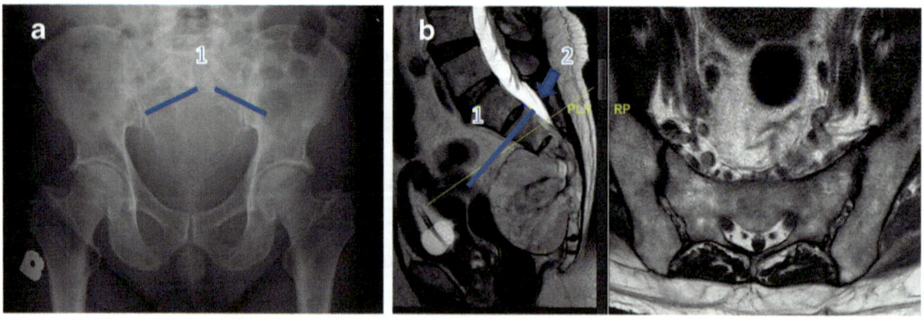

1. Level of osteotomy—transect the dura (must be surgically exposed and ligated)

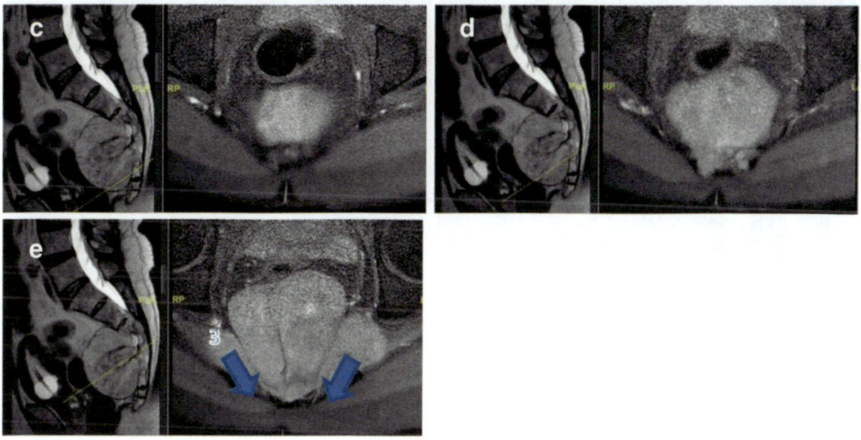

2. Ventral extension tumour with lateral involvement of both the piriformis muscles
3. Gluteus muscle attachment was not involved

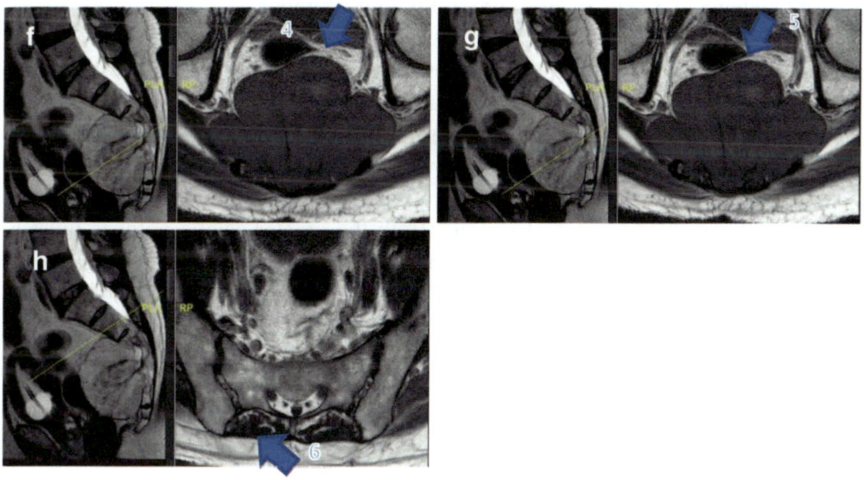

4. Assessment of Waldeyer fascia and presacral fat
5. Fat plane between the tumour and rectum
6. Erector spinae muscle free of tumour extension

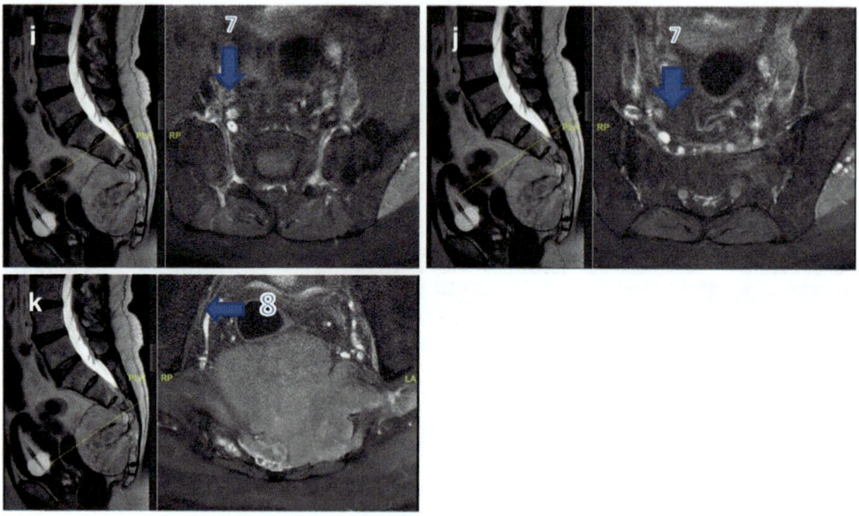

7. Internal iliac vessels are above the planned superior sacral osteotomy
8. Anterior division of the internal iliac vessels, including median sacral vessels and pudendal vessels, in close proximity to the tumour

Anatomical landmark for posterior resection is the L5 spinous process, inferior sacroilliac joint, the sacrotuberus and sacrospinous ligament and Waldeyer space between the rectum and sacrum. Mobilisation of the posterior skin and identification of the gluteus muscle margin followed by transection of both ligaments for lateral exposure (Fig. 1i–n). Piriformis muscle must be transected for mobilisation of the sciatic nerve and gluteal vessels. Both the greater sciatic notches must be cleared from the structures above the superior aspect of the tumour for sacral osteotomy with good margin.

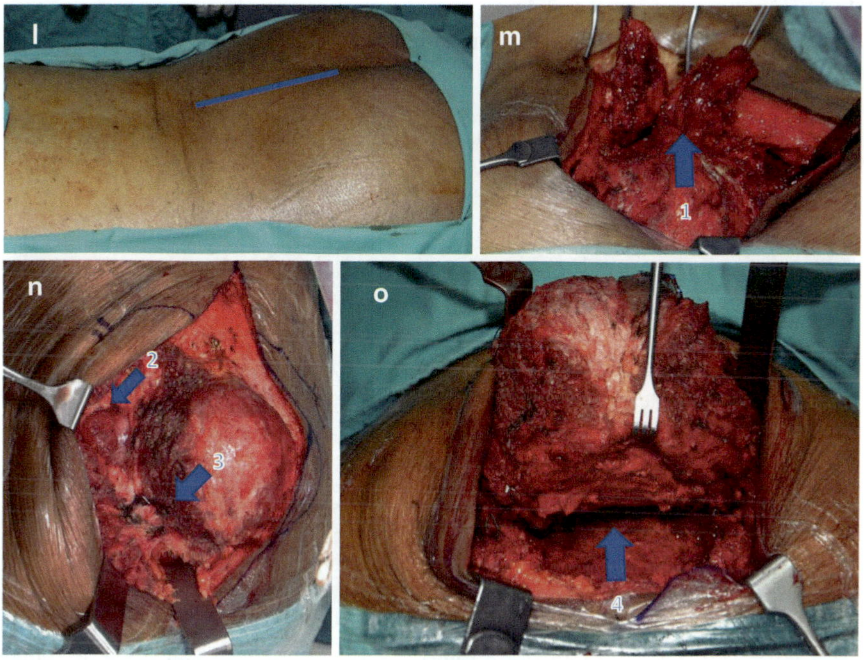

1. Erector spinal muscle elevated from the sacrum
2. Piriformis muscle
3. Sacro tuberous ligament
4. Waldeyer fascia

The gluteus maximus was detached from the lateral border of the sacrum with good margin and identification of the sacrotuberus and sacrospinous ligaments. Both the piriformis tendons were sectioned for visualisation of the greater sciatic foreman and inferior border of the sacroilliac joint. The anal-coccygeal ligament was cut at the inferior border of coccyx and the Waldeyer space created between the anterior border of the sacrum and rectum (Fig. 1m–o).

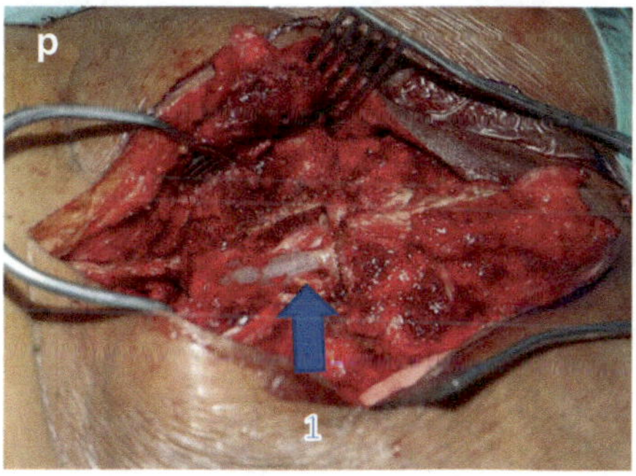

Laminectomy performed for identification of the dura, transected and ligated at the level of mid S2 for final resection (Fig. 1p).

1. Laminectomy and exposed dura
2. Piriformis muscle removed in total with the tumour

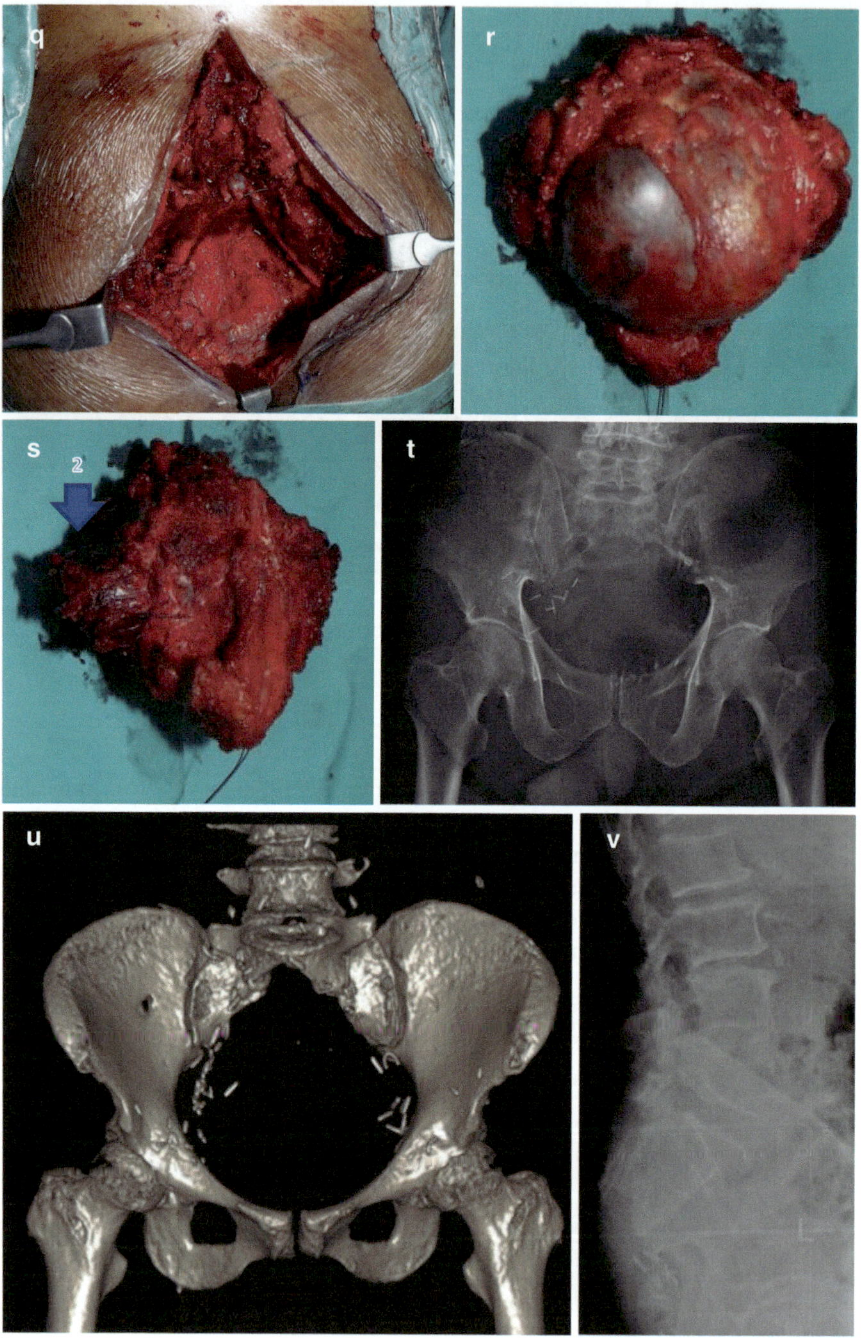

Surgical bed and specimen after resection with X-rays and CT scan follow-up (Fig. 1q–v).

Posterior Extension with Gluteus Maximus Infiltration

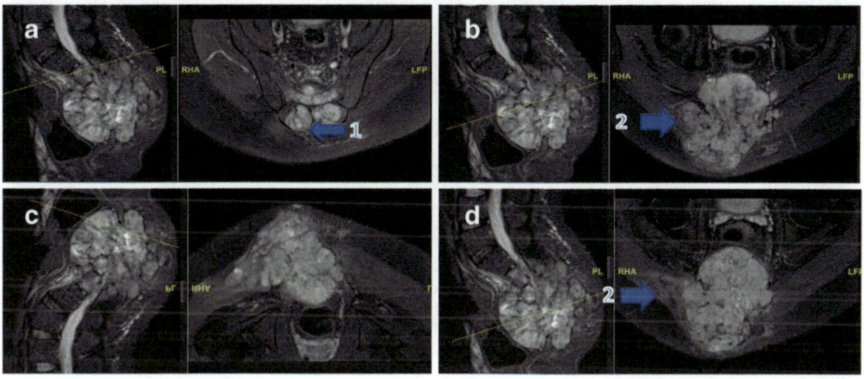

Sacral chordoma with lateral extension to the gluteus maximus muscle and bilateral erector spinal muscle (Fig. 2a–d). Resection with good cuff of muscle margin is important for good oncological margin and local control. The superior margin is at S1S2 level and can be accessed through posterior approach (Fig. 2e–h)

1. Erector spinal muscle involvement
2. Gluteus maximus infiltration

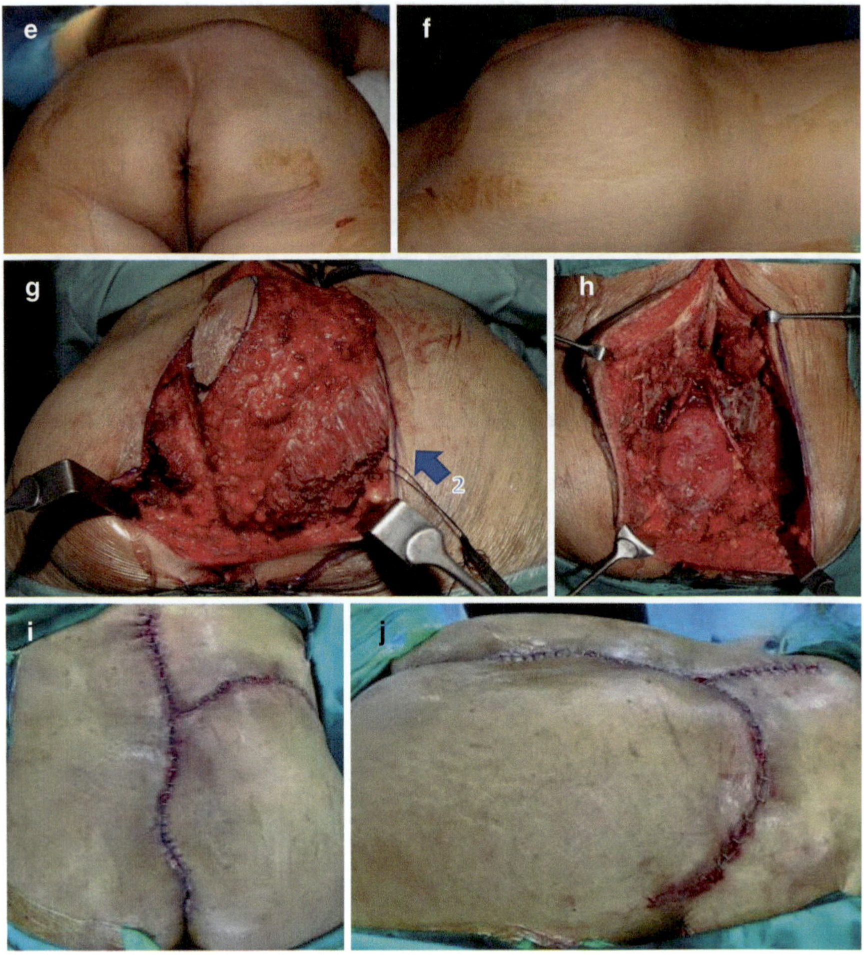

Rotational fasciocutaneous gluteal flap was done to minimise tension at closure and avoid wound complications (Fig. 2i, j).

High Sacrectomy 'Total S1 Resection'

A case of sacral chordoma with tumour extension to the S1 and a huge anterior mass. The tumour occupied half of the S1; however, the S1 nerve root was spared. The sacrospinous and sacrotuberus ligaments were closely attached to the tumour and compressed on the medial border of the acetabulum with minimal space. The posterior structures, gluteus maximus insertions and erector spinal were not involved. There was well-defined space between the anterior mass and the rectum without involvement (Fig. 3a–d).

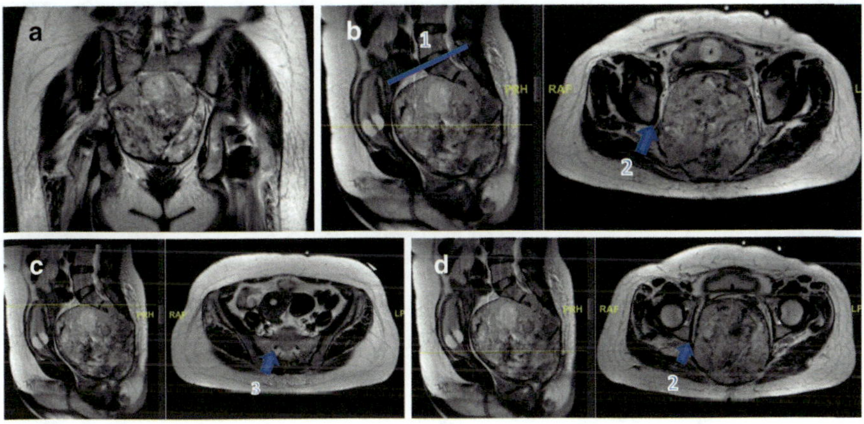

1. Upper border sacral resection trough L5 and S1 intervertebral disc
2. Medial wall acetabulum
3. S1 neural foramina was not involved

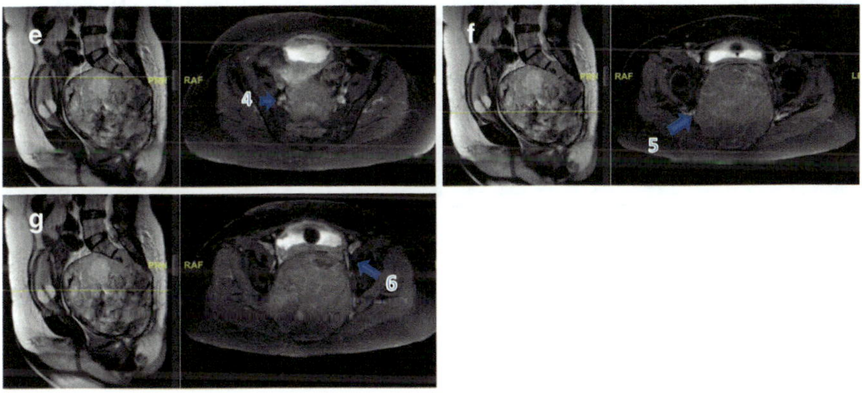

Main internal iliac and its anterior division is closely attached to the tumour and must be ligated to prevent massive bleeding (Fig. 3e–g)

4. Internal iliac vessels
5. Posterior division of the internal iliac vessels—gluteal vessels closely attached to the tumour at greater sciatic notch
6. Anastomosis from the external iliac vessels—obturator vessels

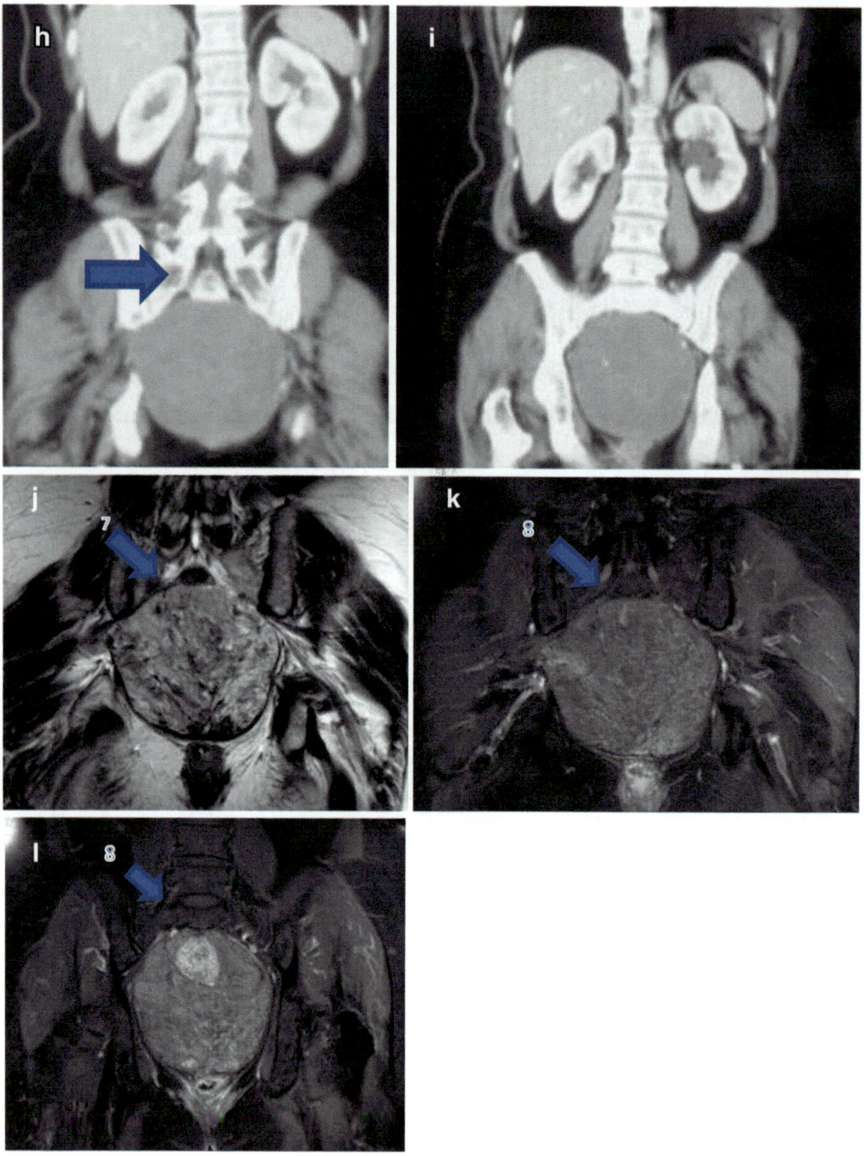

Coronal image of CT and MRI for evaluation of exiting S1 and its correlation with upper tumour border for surgical margin (Fig. 3h–l)

7. S1 root
8. L5 root

Anterior Approach

Resection of the sacrum at the level of S1 and above requires an anterior approach for mobilisation of the anterior structures and securing the haemostasis to prevent major haemorrhage. Retroperitoneal approach for bilateral mobilisation of S1 and L5 root; secure the internal iliac vessels and median sacral artery. Anterior discectomy will destabilise the spine anteriorly. Combining with posterior laminectomy and sacroiliac joint mobilisation will safeguard high sacrum and soft tumour from contamination.

The anterior sacral promontory was identified and cleared bilaterally. The dissection continued distally, and the tumour mass was cleared from the anterior structure and packed. Both the sacroiliac joints were identified and the L5 and S1 root was protected (Fig. 3m–p).

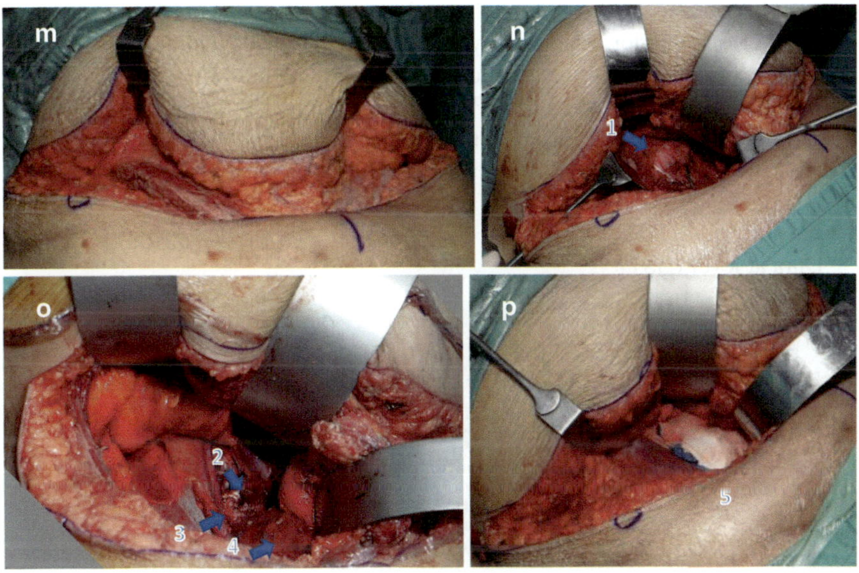

1. Sacral promontory and LS1 intervertebral disc
2. Anterior discectomy
3. Internal iliac vessels
4. Superior border tumour
5. Anterior packing protects—internal iliac vessels, L5 root and rectum

Posterior Approach

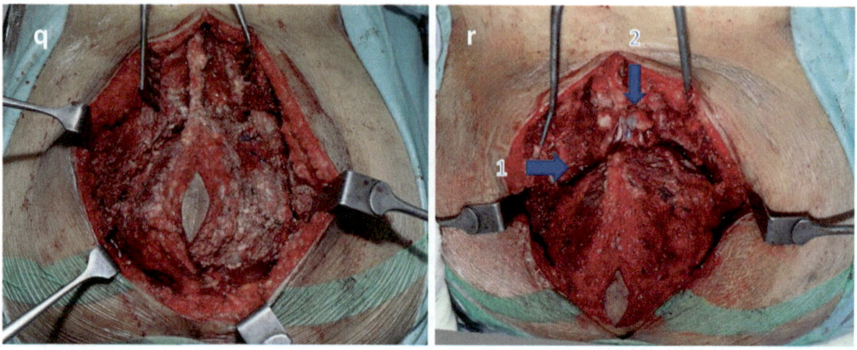

Superiorly, the erector spinae were elevated from the posterior spine and the appropriate level for superior osteotomy was identified. Extensile laminectomy must be done for exploration and protection of S1 root from the posterior to prevent injury during final sacrum osteotomy (Fig. 3q–s). The lower end of the dura below the exit of S1 was ligated, and lower root from S2 was transected for final osteotomy at the L5 and S1 disc level and sacroiliac joint.

1. Lateral exploration of S1
2. Dura at level L5S1

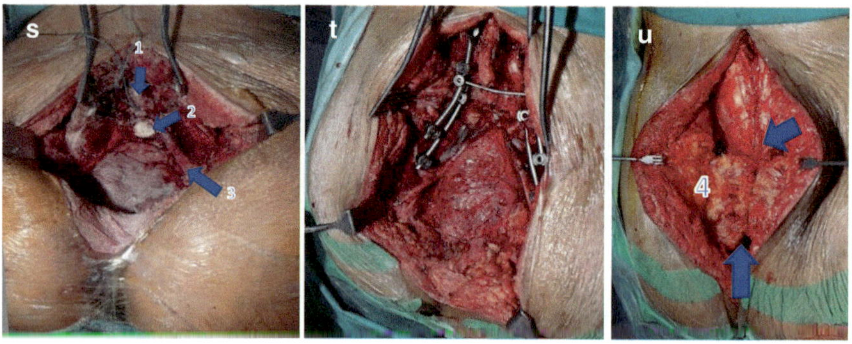

Final post resection of the sacrum, S1 root and L5 were maintained as major branches of the sciatic nerve. The cancellous bleeding from the remnant pelvic and L5 body can be controlled by bone wax or argon diathermy. The entire rectum was exposed for final inspection, spinopelvic stabilisation using two-rod technique to prevent the risk of early failure (Fig. 3t–v). Lateral fusion with bone grafting from transverse process of L5 to the iliac crest. Gluteus maximus and remnant of erector spinal mobilised to cover the spinopelvic implant and final closure.

1. Dura ligated at L5S1
2. L5 disc
3. S1 root
4. Erector spinal and gluteus maximus

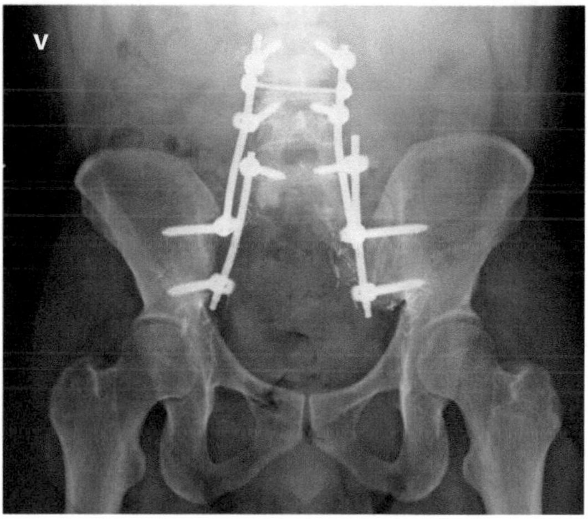

Sacrectomy Spinopelvic Stabilisation Technique

Spinal stabilisation and fusion allowed immediate ambulation as it stabilised the spine to the main torso. Patient would be able to weight bearing immediately without pain. No telescoping of the spine distally that may cause traction injury to the nerve root and lead to chronic pain and instability (Fig. 4a, b).

Single rod Galveston technique or using iliac screw tends to fail due to high stresses over mobile segment of L5 and pelvis. Double rod stabilisation technique using two-iliac screw and three-level lumbar stabilisation is optimum, especially when planning for non-fusion technique and early radiotherapy. Posterolateral fusion using grafting technique of L5 transverse process to remnant ilium is an option, though this technique tends to fail due to high stresses and post-operative radiotherapy.

The best option described is a triangular fibula strut configuration along with spinopelvic screw rod construct to achieve solid fusion in axial and rotation.

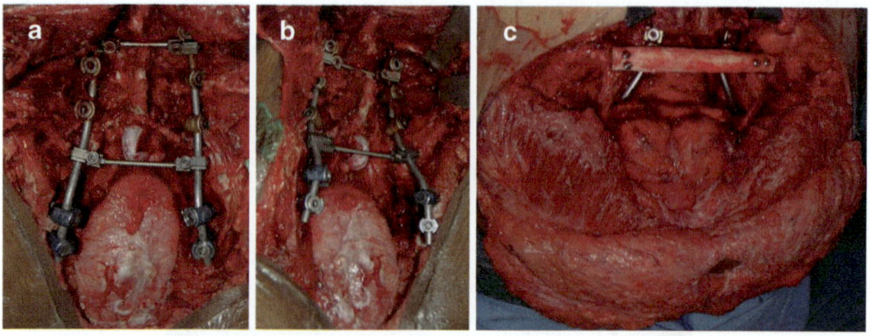

Rod prebend and slotted to the ileum with intrapelvic fusion with fibula graft 'Galveston technique' (Fig. 4c).

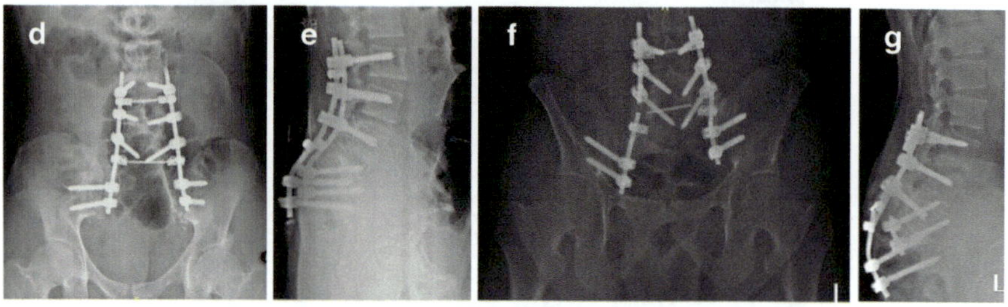

Fracture at six months with single rod reconstruction, revision surgery using double rod and posterolateral fusion technique. Stable with solid fusion (Fig. 4d–g).

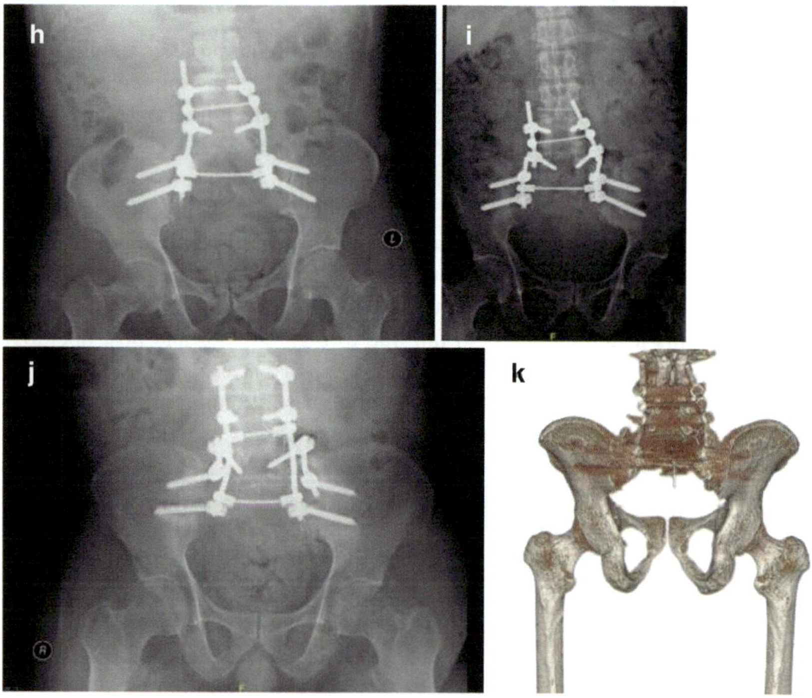

Few methods of spinal stabilisation using two-rod technique to improve stability and minimise the risk of late failure (Fig. 4h–o).

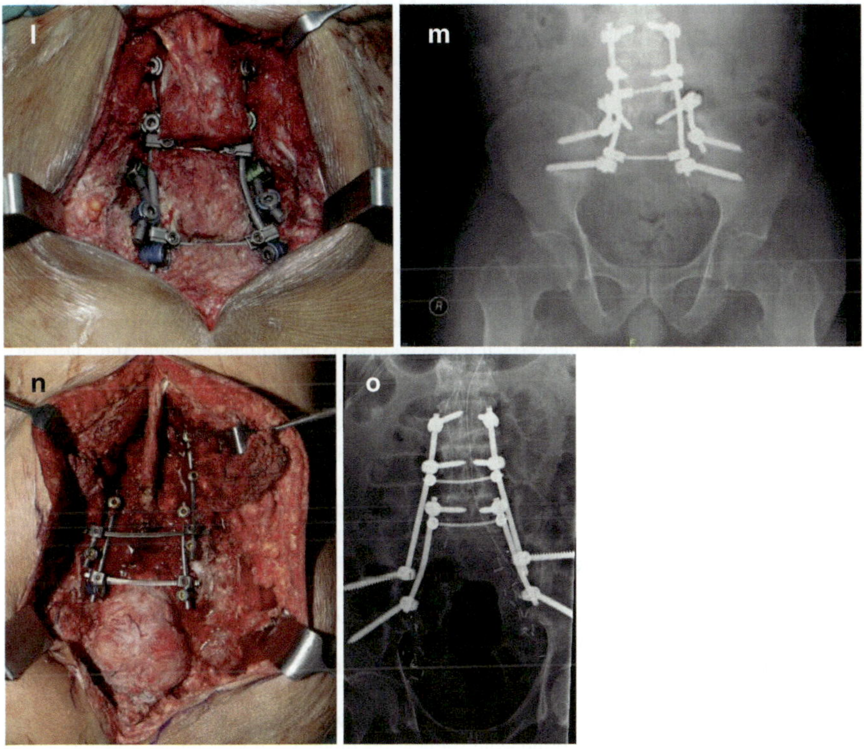

Double head pedicle screw is an option to maintain better stability using both rods to the entire stabilisation (Fig. 4p–r).

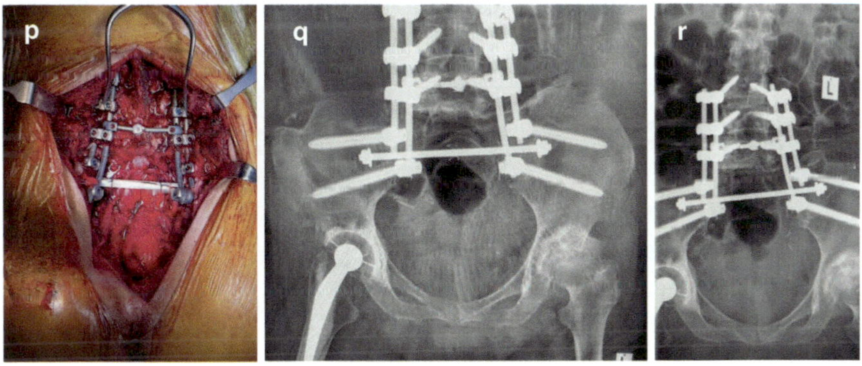

Acknowledgments The author thanks Professor Mohd Imran Yusof, Dr. Joehaimey Johari, Dato' Professor Mohd Hisam Muhammad Ariffin and Dato' Dr. Azmi Baharudin from the spine unit at Universiti Sains Malaysia and National University of Malaysia for their contributions and team member for managing the patients. The spine unit was involved as a combined team approach for sacral resection and spinal stabilisation.

Suggested Reading

1. Dickey ID, Hugate RR Jr, Fuchs B, Yaszemski MJ, Sim FH. Reconstruction after total sacrectomy: early experience with a new surgical technique. Clin Orthop Relat Res. 2005;438:42–50.
2. Glatt BS, Disa JJ, Mehrara BJ, et al. Reconstruction of extensive partial or total sacrectomy defects with a transabdominal vertical rectus abdominis myocutaneous flap. Ann Plast Surg. 2006;56:526–31.
3. Hugate RR Jr, Dickey ID, Phimolsarnti R, et al. Mechanical effects of partial sacrectomy. When is reconstruction necessary? Clin Orthop Relat Res. 2006;450:82–8.
4. Eck JC, Yaszemski MJ, Sim FH. Sacrectomy and spinopelvic reconstruction. Semin Spine Surg. 2009;21:99–105.
5. Houdek MT, Sim FH, Yaszemski MJ, Rose PS. Biological sacral reconstruction 47–52 orthopedic surgical oncology for bone tumors. Springer Nature Switzerland AG; 2022.
6. Papagelopoulos PJ, Mavrogenis AF, Rose PS, Yaszemski MJ. Amputative sacral resections 93–100 master techniques in Orthopaedic surgery orthopaedic oncology and complex reconstruction. Lippincott Williams & Wilkins, A Wolters Kluwer; 2011.
7. Rose PS, Sim FH, Yaszemski M. Sacrectomy 83–93 master techniques in orthopaedic surgery orthopaedic oncology and complex Rreconstruction. Lippincott Williams & Wilkins, A Wolters Kluwer; 2011.
8. Kiatisevi P, Sukanthanak B, Piakong P, Piyaskulkeaw C. Total sacrectomy without spinopelvic reconstruction 53-60 orthopedic surgical oncology for bone tumors. Springer Nature Switzerland AG; 2022.
9. Cheong YW, Sulaiman WA, Halim AS. Reconstruction of large sacral defects following tumour resection: a report of two cases. J Orthop Surg (Hong Kong). 2008;16(3):351–4.
10. Rose PS. The management of sacral tumours. Bone Joint J. 2022;104-B(12):1284–91.
11. Radaelli S, Fossati P, Stacchiotti S, Akiyama T, et al. The sacral chordoma margin. Eur J Surg Oncol. 2020;46(8):1415–22.

Total Sacrum Resection by Posterior Approach

Wei Guo and Haijie Liang

Introduction

Primary malignant sacral tumors are a rare entity and usually require en bloc resection for local control. To avoid injury of the presacral viscera and vessels, most centers adopted a combined anterior/posterior approach to perform sacrectomy above S3 level in a one-stage or two-stage setting, which had been justified for its safety and efficacy but were time-consuming and at risk of massive bleeding. However, we have previously reported the experience of total en bloc sacrectomy via a posterior-only approach that could significantly decrease operative time and hemorrhage. Indications for total en bloc sacrectomy using a posterior approach in our center were as follows: (1) primary malignant sacral tumor involving at least S1–2; (2) tumor not involving the internal iliac vessels and bowel, based on imaging studies and digital rectal examination; and (3) recurrent sacral tumor in patients who had not previously undergone an anterior procedure.

This case involves a patient with sacral osteosarcoma affecting the entire sacrum. The soft tissue mass was not significant, and the tumor's upper limit was below the L5/S1 disc. The sacrospinous and sacrotuberous ligaments were unaffected, but the piriformis muscles were edematous. The posterior structures, including the gluteus maximus insertions and the erector spinae muscles, were not involved. Although there was edema in the presacral fascia, the presacral fatty space remained unaffected (Fig. 1a–d).

W. Guo (✉) · H. Liang
Musculoskeletal Tumor Center, Peking University People's Hospital, Beijing, China

A. Puri, W. F. N. B. W. Ismail (eds.), *Atlas of Orthopedic Oncology Volume 1*,
https://doi.org/10.1007/978-981-95-8958-6_15

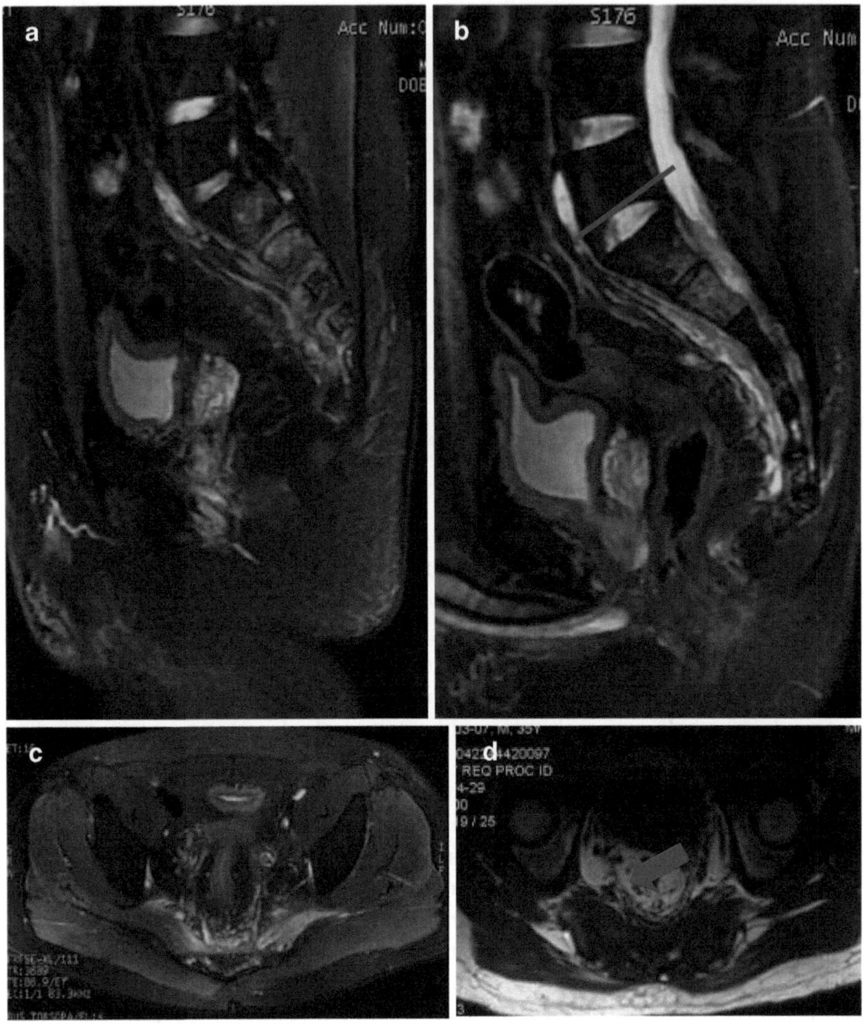

- Osteosarcoma involving the entire sacrum
- Upper border sacral resection through the L5/S1 intervertebral disc. Edema in the presacral fascia was noted
- Edema of the piriformis muscles necessitated their resection
- The presacral fatty space was spared

The one-stage posterior-only total sacrectomy was first proposed by Guo et al. in 2015. The procedure's safety and effectiveness have been demonstrated in selected cases. Intraoperative hemorrhage control is essential, achieved through preoperative selective arterial embolism and intra-aortic balloon occlusion during surgery (Fig. 1e–j).

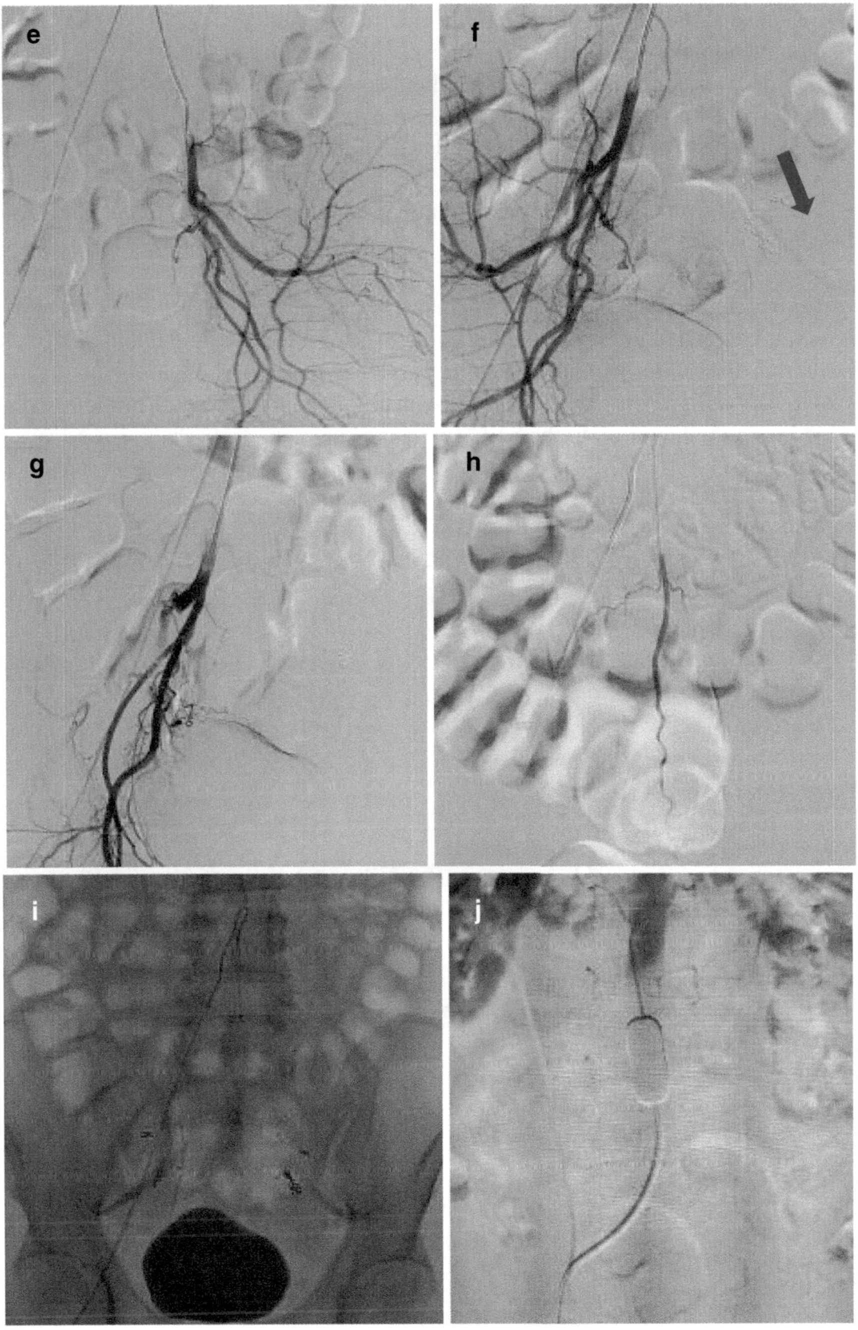
e
f
g
h
i
j

- Selective embolization of the right lateral sacral veins
- Completion of the embolization of the right lateral sacral veins
- Selective embolization of the left iliolumbar vein
- Selective embolization of the median sacral vein
- Completion of the embolization of bilateral iliolumbar veins, lateral sacral veins, and the median sacral vein
- Upon inflation of the intra-aortic balloon, occlusion of the blood flow was achieved

An inverted Y incision was used. The parasacral muscles and the gluteus maximus were dissected to expose the lumbar and sacrum. The rectum could be visualized from the posterior approach after resecting the sacrospinous ligament, the sacrotuberous ligament, and the anococcygeal ligament and was then bluntly dissected from the tumor up to the S1 level via packing gauze into the presacral space (Fig. 1k–m).

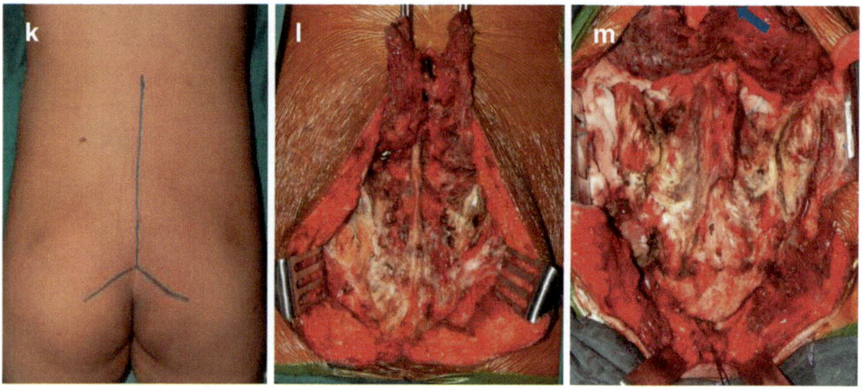

- Skin incision
- Dissection of erector spinal muscle and the gluteus maximus to expose the posterior sacrum
- The presacral space was dissected by packing gauze (arrow) after cutting the sacrospinous, the sacrotuberous, and the anococcygeal ligaments

The transverse process of L5 was removed to facilitate blunt finger dissection from the upper and lower edges of the sacroiliac joints. Gauze was packed into the space in front of the sacroiliac joints to protect the lumbosacral trunks and internal iliac vessels from the osteotomy lines. A silicone tube was introduced through the anterior space of the sacroiliac joint, enabling a wire saw to pass through and cut both sides of the iliac bone (Fig. 1n–p).

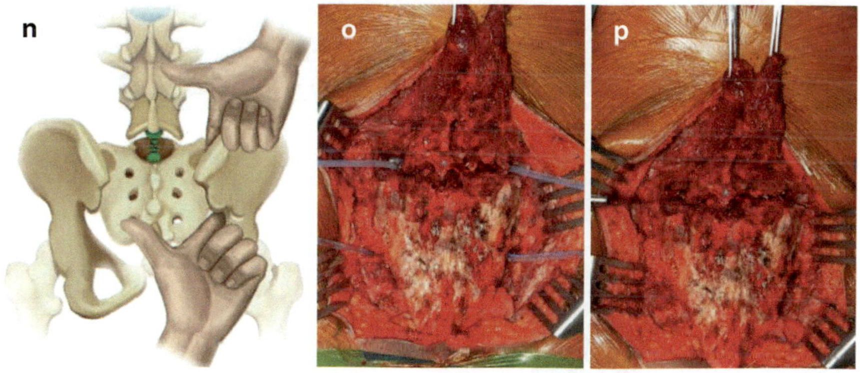

- Scheme of blunt dissection of the pre-sacroiliac space
- A silicone tube was introduced through the anterior space of the sacroiliac joint
- A wire saw was introduced by the silicone tube for osteotomy along the sacroiliac joint

Laminectomy of L5 was performed to expose the dural sac and identify the L5 nerve roots. The dural sac below L5 was ligated and transected. The L5/S1 disc was thoroughly removed using a posterior approach. After bilateral ilium osteotomy, the sacrum was mobilized, allowing visualization of the iliac vessels, lumbosacral trunks, sacral nerves, and rectum by lifting the sacrum. Soft tissue anterior to the tumor was separated, and the sacral nerve roots were cut while preserving bilateral L5 nerves. The remaining part of the L5/S1 disc was removed, and the entire sacrum along with bilateral portions of the ilium were excised (Fig. 1q–u).

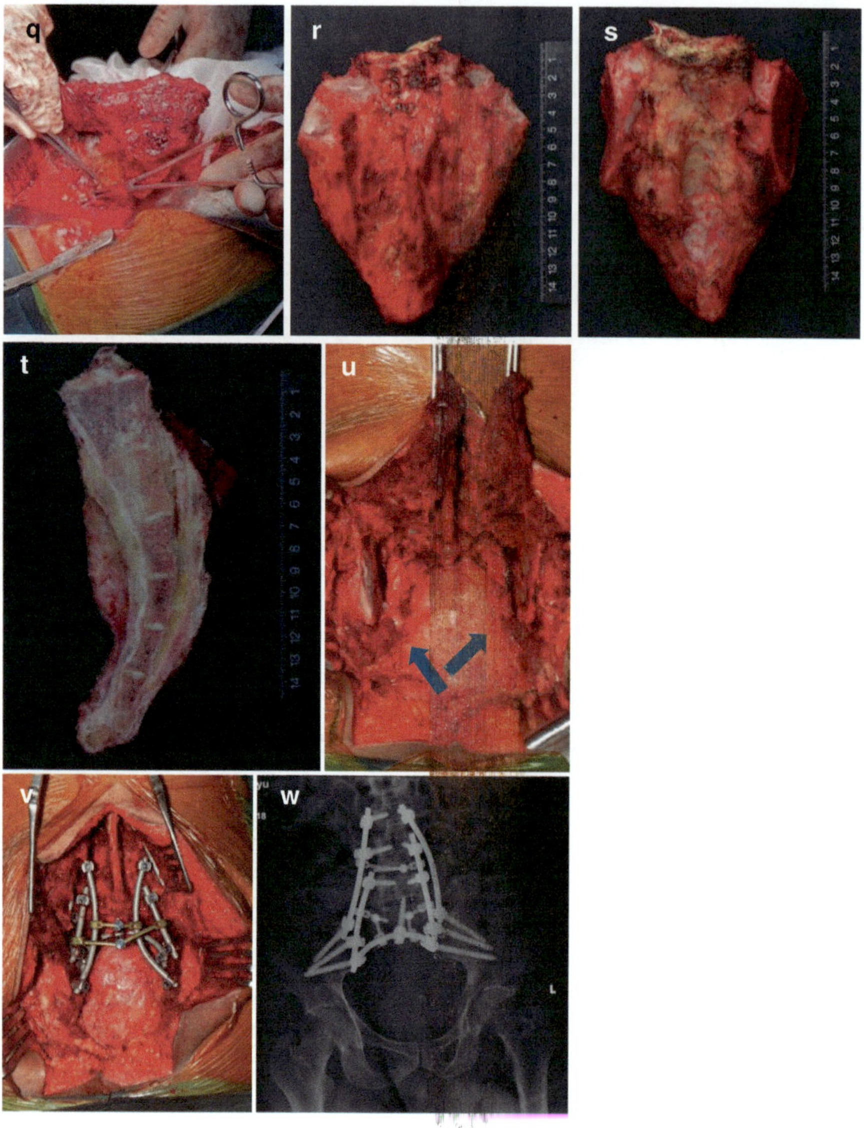
q
r
s
t
u
v
w
L

- After osteotomy, the sacrum could be mobilized and the presacral vessels and nerves could be divided and transected
- Dorsal view of the specimen
- Ventral view of the specimen
- Sagittal view of the specimen
- Bilateral L5 nerves were preserved
- Reconstruction was done using multiple screws and rods (Fig. 1v).
- Postoperative X-ray film (Fig. 1w).

Comments

Potential complications unique to the posterior approach for total sacrectomy includes the injury to the vessels and contamination of the surgical margins. To avoid vascular injury, meticulous preoperative radiological examinations should be performed to rule out those encasing the iliac vessels. If there were signs of vascular invasion or adhesion, a combined anterior-posterior approach would be recommended. Moreover, if the tumor had invaded the sacroiliac joint or extending above L5/S1 disc, an intralesional margin would be expected by this posterior approach. Lastly, attentions should be paid to the recurrent cases as the presacral space might be adhered by fibrous scar derived from the previous surgery. In that case, dissection from the posterior approach would be much more difficult and risky.

Intraoperative Abdominal Aortic Balloon Occlusion

This technique effectively controls intraoperative hemorrhage in sacropelvic tumor resections, particularly for high-level en bloc sacrectomy via a posterior-only approach. The balloon would be inserted just after SAE in the interventional department if preoperative SAE and sacrectomy surgery were done on the same day. This insertion could also be done in the OR if preoperative SAE was finished on the previous day. Coda® balloon catheter (Cook Medical, Bloomington, IN, USA) is commonly used. The common femoral artery is punctured using Seldinger's method, after which a guide wire is introduced through the needle. Following needle withdrawal, an 11-Fr sheath is inserted into the proximal artery (Fig. 2a–c).

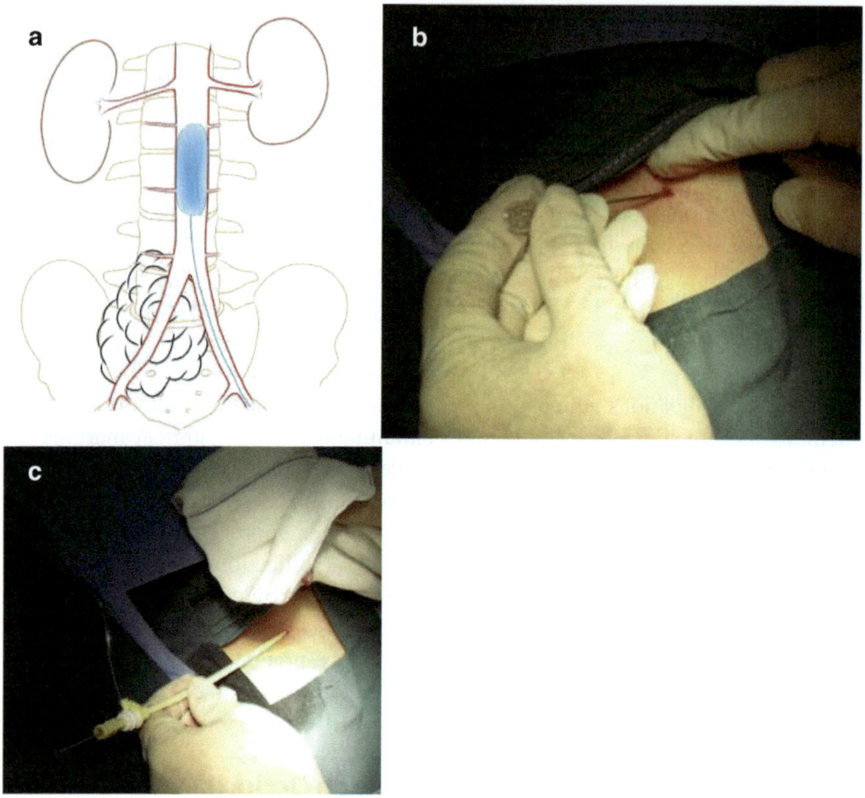

- Scheme of the application of an abdominal aortic balloon (adapted from Clin Orthop Relat Res (2018) 476:490–498)
- Puncture of the common femoral artery
- Insertion of the sheath

The balloon catheter is introduced through the sheath under fluoroscopic monitoring, guided by a long guide wire (RF*GA35153M, Terumo Corporation, Japan). Balloon positioning and desired pressure are achieved in three steps (Fig. 2d–g):

- First, the balloon is filled with the injected contrast (diluted with twofold saline) and determined to be stable at the level just caudal to the renal artery bifurcation.
- Second, angiography of the proximal aorta should show abundant blood flow within both renal arteries after the balloon is inflated.
- Third, the angiogram should show no blood flow in the distal aorta. Constant intraoperative monitoring of the distal femoral arterial pressure and urine volume is obligatory and critical to ensure the balloon is working properly.

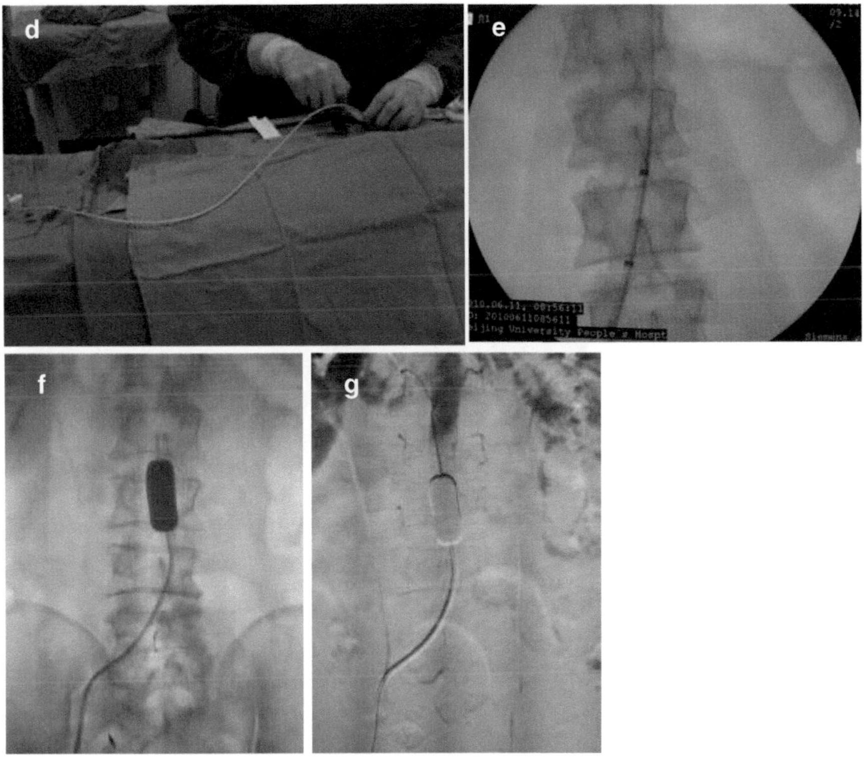

- Insertion of the balloon catheter
- Advancement of the balloon catheter under fluoroscopy
- Inflation of the balloon with diluted contrast until it is stabilized within the aorta
- Angiography of the proximal aorta shows no blood flow in the distal aorta

After confirming the balloon's location and effectiveness, it is deflated by extracting the contrast. The volume of the contrast is recorded, and the balloon catheter and sheath are secured and wrapped. The same volume of saline is used for intraoperative inflation. Aortic occlusion should generally last no longer than 60 min at a time. Therefore, the balloon should be inflated during essential procedures (i.e., just before osteotomy of the sacroiliac joint), and the tumor is expected to be removed before deflation of the balloon. Moreover, bone wax to seal the osteotomic plane, ligation of the lacerated vessels, and compression by gauzes are usual methods to control bleeding after deflation. If the balloon needs to be reinflated, a minimum interval of 20 min should be waited.

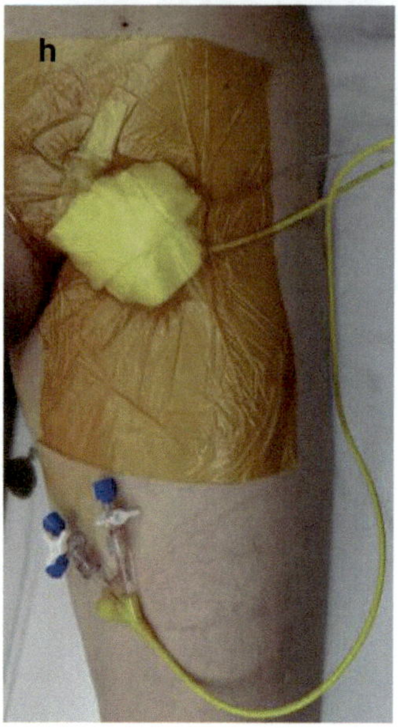

Securing and wrapping the balloon catheter and sheath (Fig. 2h)

Before balloon deflation, the anesthesiologist ensures the patient is stable enough to handle the sudden circulatory change. Rapid and continuous evacuation of the saline is recommended to prevent catheter bending. The balloon catheter and sheath should be promptly removed after the sacral operation to avoid the risk of acute arterial thrombosis.

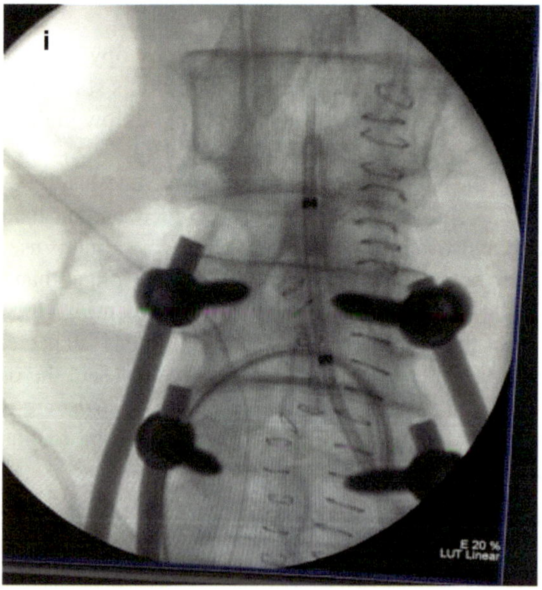

- Bending of the balloon catheter during interrupted deflation (Fig. 2i)

Reconstruction-Sacral Prosthesis

Various reconstruction methods have been reported and can be classified into three concepts according to Bederman et al.: spinal pelvic fixation (SPF), posterior pelvic ring fixation (PPRF), and anterior spinal column fixation (ASCF). Combining these methods achieves optimal stability and minimal stress on the instruments. A 3D-printed modular sacrum prosthesis, synthesizing the biomechanical characteristics of SPF, PPRF, and ASCF, has been designed and applied to simplify combined reconstruction procedures after total sacrectomy.

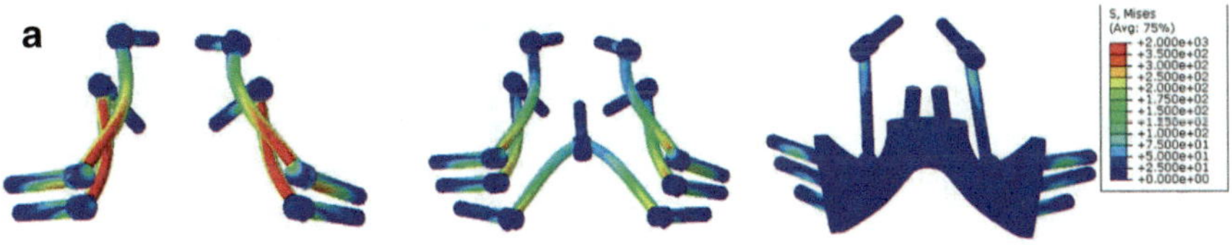

- Biomechanical analysis by finite element analysis indicated that the reconstruction with the total sacrum prosthesis has the biomechanical advantages of a more uniform stress distribution, a lower peak stress, and better stability compared with the rod-screw system (Fig. 3a)

The prosthesis consists of three bone-implant interfaces: the proximal surface fits the inferior endplate of the L5 vertebra to reconstruct the lumbosacral joint, and the surfaces on both flanks match the bilateral iliac osteotomic planes to reconstruct the sacroiliac joints. Screw trajectories are preserved on all bone-contacting surfaces for fixation. The bone-implant interfaces feature a porous trabecular structure to facilitate bone ingrowth and achieve osseointegration.

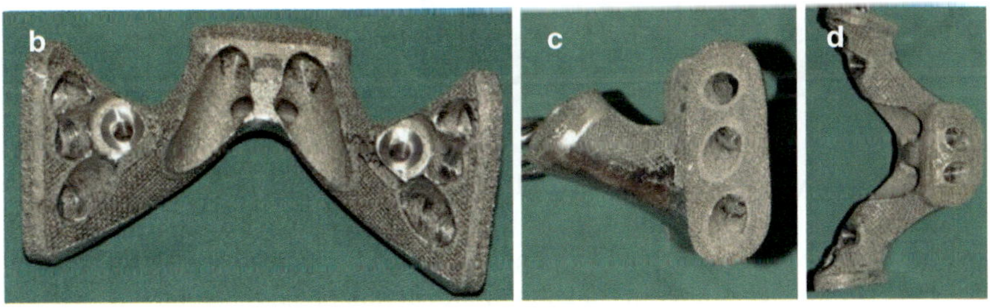

- The posterior view of the prosthesis shows the screw trajectories through the three interfaces. (Fig. 3b)
- The lateral view of the prosthesis shows the three screw trajectories through the porous lateral interface. (Fig. 3c)
- The top view of the prosthesis showed two screw trajectories through the porous proximal interface. (Fig. 3d)
- Rehearsal of the prosthesis installation on plastic model. (Fig. 3e)

After tumor removal, the ilia's osteotomy planes were trimmed to fit the prosthesis, and the L5/S1 disc was resected to expose the inferior endplate. The appropriately sized prosthesis was placed under the L5 inferior endplate and fixed with two screws through the trajectories into the L5 vertebral body. The prosthesis was then fixed sequentially to each ilium with compression at the bone-implant surface. Titanium rods were used to connect the prosthesis to the pedicle screws. Generally, we closed the wound by direct suture without applying any flap. We also would not use prophylactic colostomy unless the rupture of the rectum was identified intraoperatively.

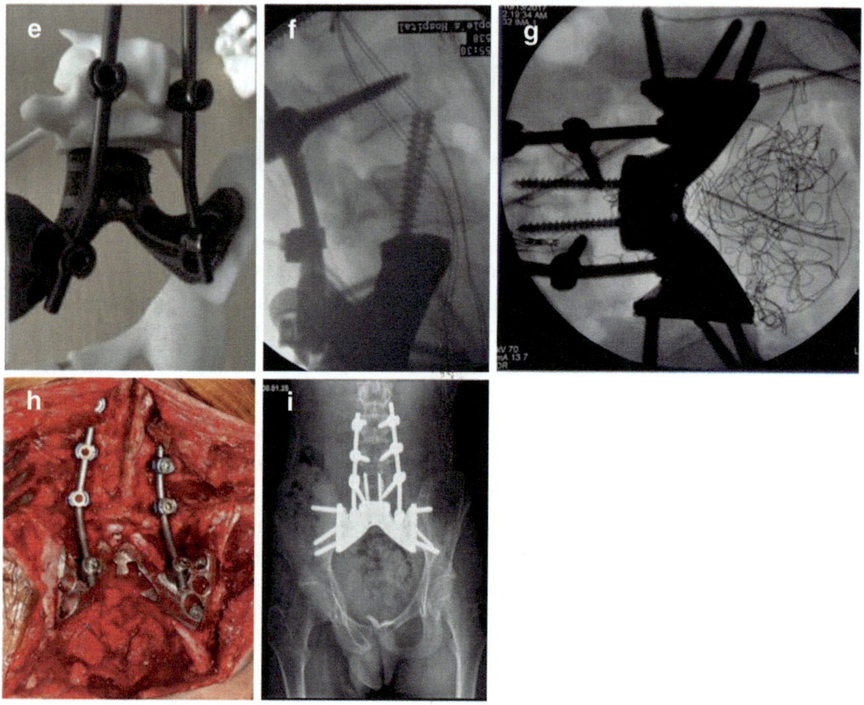

- Intraoperative fluoroscopy showed good fixation through the L5 endplate (Fig. 3f)
- Intraoperative fluoroscopy showed good fixation through bilateral ilia (Fig. 3g)
- Intraoperative view after installation of the sacrum prosthesis (Fig. 3h)
- X ray films showed good fixation of the prosthesis without loosening, breakage, or subsidence (Fig. 3i)

To prevent postoperative infection, two drainage tubes were used and withdrawn when the 24 h drainage volume was below 30 ml. The third-generation cephalosporin was used intravenously during drainage (usually two weeks) and was changed to oral antibiotics for another one week. The patients are recommended to stay in bed for 1 week and then start to mobilize using a walking aid if the srew-rod system is used for reconstruction. Weight bearing should be withheld for 6–8 weeks postoperatively for the 3D-printed prosthesis to allow for initial bone ingrowth and scar formation

Suggested Reading

1. Tang X, Guo W, Yang R, Tang S, Dong S. Use of aortic balloon occlusion to decrease blood loss during sacral tumor resection. J Bone Joint Surg Am. 2010;92(8):1747–53. https://doi.org/10.2106/JBJS.I.01333.
2. Zang J, Guo W, Yang R, et al. Is total en bloc sacrectomy using a posterior-only approach feasible and safe for patients with malignant sacral tumors? J Neurosurg Spine. 2015;22(6):563–70.
3. Wei R, Guo W, Ji T, et al. One-step reconstruction with a 3D-printed, custom-made prosthesis after total en bloc sacrectomy: a technical note. Eur Spine J. 2017;26(7):1902–9.
4. Zhang Y, Guo W, Tang X, Yang R, Yan T, Dong S, Wang S, Zaphiros N. Can aortic balloon occlusion reduce blood loss during resection of sacral tumors that extend into the lower lumber spine? Clin Orthop Relat Res. 2018;476(3):490–8. https://doi.org/10.1007/s11999.0000000000000053.
5. Wang Y, Liang W, Qu S, et al. Assessment of patient experiences following total sacrectomy for primary malignant sacral tumors: a qualitative study. J Surg Oncol. 2019;120(8):1497–504.
6. Huang S, Ji T, Guo W. Biomechanical comparison of a 3D-printed sacrum prosthesis versus rod-screw systems for reconstruction after total sacrectomy: a finite element analysis. Clin Biomech (Bristol, Avon). 2019;70:203–8.
7. Wei R, Guo W, Yang R, et al. Reconstruction of the pelvic ring after total en bloc sacrectomy using a 3D-printed sacral endoprosthesis with re-establishment of spinopelvic stability: a retrospective comparative study. Bone Joint J. 2019;101-B(7):880–8.
8. Zhao Z, Wang J, Yan T, Guo W, Yang R, Tang X, Yang Y. A clinical study of the hemodynamic and metabolic effects of Zone 3 REBOA for sacral and pelvic tumor resections. BMC Surg. 2022;22(1):246. https://doi.org/10.1186/s12893-022-01694-w.

Type I Pelvic Resection

Wan Faisham Nu'man Bin Wan Ismail

Introduction

Malignant tumours of the pelvis remain a challenge for both oncologists and reconstructive surgeons. Type I resection is defined as a resection of the ilium with preservation of the acetabulum. Type I+S is when part of the sacrum is removed together with the sacroiliac joint.

Surgical Anatomy

The ilium is covered by the iliacus muscle that provides good anatomical boundaries for anterior tumour extension. The gluteus maximus and medius origins are posteriorly attached to the ilium and can be infiltrated by the posterior extension of tumour. The sartorius and inguinal ligaments attached to the ASIS must be evaluated prior to resection. Important structures to be evaluated for osseous margins also include:

- The sacroiliac joint—tumours crossing the joint require resection of the ala of the sacrum or part of the sacrum with good osseous margin.
- The supra-acetabulum—for distal resection (marrow margin of at least 1 cm must be achieved for good oncological clearance).

W. F. N. B. W. Ismail (✉)
Prince Court Medical Center, Kuala Lumpur, Malaysia

Orthopaedic Oncology Reconstructive Unit, Universiti Sains Malaysia, Kubang Kerian, Kelantan, Malaysia

A. Puri, W. F. N. B. W. Ismail (eds.), *Atlas of Orthopedic Oncology Volume 1*,
https://doi.org/10.1007/978-981-95-8958-6_16

Major Vessels

- The abdominal aorta bifurcates at the level of L4 to form the common iliac, which travels laterally over the sacrum ala and branches into the internal iliac artery at the sacroiliac joint.
- The internal iliac descends to the greater sciatic notch and branches into several arteries that supply the gluteal muscle. These arteries are important for viability of the posterior flap.
- The external iliac vessels are directly related to medial brim of ilium; however, they are protected by thick iliopectineal fascia.

Major Nerves

- The sciatic nerve arises from L4–5 and S1–3 roots that join the anterior sacroiliac joint and emerge posteriorly through the greater sciatic notch below the piriformis muscle. Clearance of the sciatic notch after mobilisation of the sciatic nerve and internal iliac vessels is a key surgical step for sacroiliac joint and supraacetabular osteotomy.
- The femoral nerve passes between the psoas and iliacus muscles and enters the proximal thigh underneath the inguinal ligament lateral to the superficial femoral artery.
- The obturator nerve descends through the iliopsoas muscle and courses distally over the sacral ala into the lesser pelvis to the medial brim and traverses the obturator foramen into the medial thigh. It can be mobilised and secured for type I resection.

Ureters, intraperitoneal structures, lie on the peritoneal surface and are commonly pushed by a medial iliac tumour. Ureters cross medially at the common iliac bifurcation to the sciatic notch to insert into the trigone of the bladder. Large tumours with medial extension require a ureteric stent for easy palpation during surgery to minimise risk of injury.

Assessment

Assessment of the anatomical boundaries and major neurovascular structures is important to achieve oncological clearance during:

- Sacroiliac joint infiltration
- Distal osseous extension in relation to superior dome of the acetabulum
- Iliopsoas muscle for anterior tumour
- Gluteus origin for posterior tumour extension

Chondrosarcoma Ilium

A 34-year-old gentleman with fast-growing mass over the left ilium for 6 months. Radiography suggested a diagnosis of chondrosarcoma. CT and MRI evaluation revealed that the mass was confined to the ilium approximately 2 cm above the acetabular dome and did not cross the sacroiliac joint. The medial part of the mass pushed the iliopsoas muscle and displaced the common and external iliac vessels. The ala of the sacrum was free; however, it was overhung by the mass, the L5 and S1 roots were visualised and need to be explored and protected to minimise morbidity. Multiple exostoses over the posterior ilium brim needed to be removed in total with the mass (Fig. 1a–o).

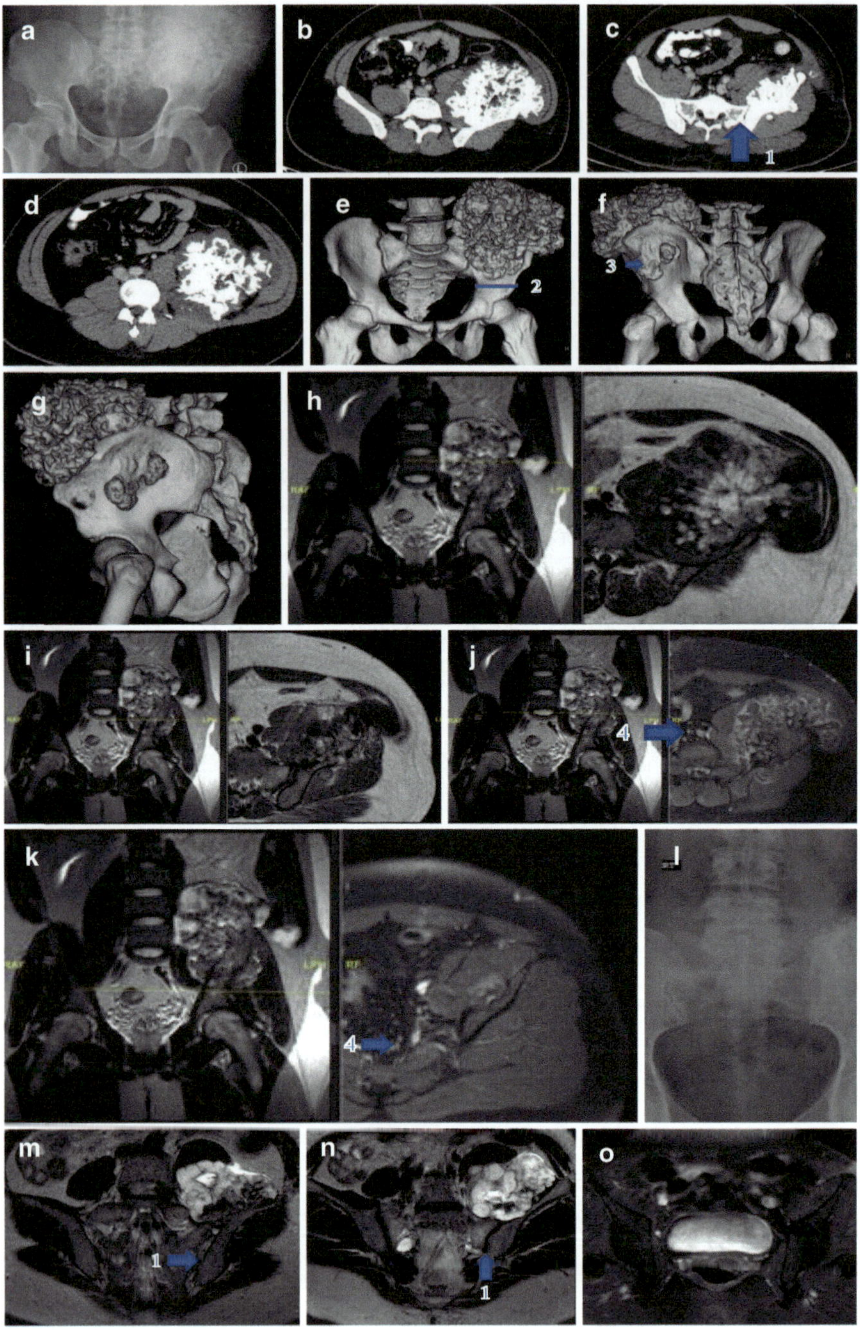
a
b
c
1
d
e
2
f
3
g
h
i
j
4
k
4
l
m
1
n
1
o

1. Sacroiliac joint—free of tumour involvement
2. Supra acetabulum osteotomy
3. Posterior iliac wing extension
4. External iliac artery

Surgical Steps

Utilitarian pelvic incision includes ilioinguinal approach medially to the symphysis pubis and posteriorly to the level of the sacroiliac joint (Fig. 1p, q). The inner pelvis is entered by reflecting all 3 abdominal muscles from the pelvic brim to the posterior superior iliac spine. Sometimes, the quadratus lumborum attachment must be mobilised from the pelvic brim and erector spinae fascia for sacroiliac joint involvement or resection over the ala of the sacrum. The inguinal ligament is elevated medially together with the entire abdominal muscle. Care must be taken to identify and protect the inferior epigastric artery.

Exploration of major vessels and nerves includes:

- Mobilising the external iliac vessels from inguinal region medially from the iliopectineal fascia.
- Identifying the common iliac vessels over the ala of the sacrum.
- Tracing the internal iliac vessels and mobilising them anteriorly from the greater sciatic notch.
- Identification of the S1 and L5 roots over the ala of the sacrum and mobilising them to be free from the sciatic notch.
- Identification of the femoral nerve and mobilising it from the iliacus muscle together with the psoas muscle and tendon.
- Posterior exploration through gluteus maximus splitting approach to identify the sciatic nerve and all the branches of glutei vessels and mobilising them from the sciatic notch.
- Soft tissue margin including the Iliacus anteriorly and gluteal origin posteriorly.
- Using K wire insertion for image guided of iliac osteotomy.

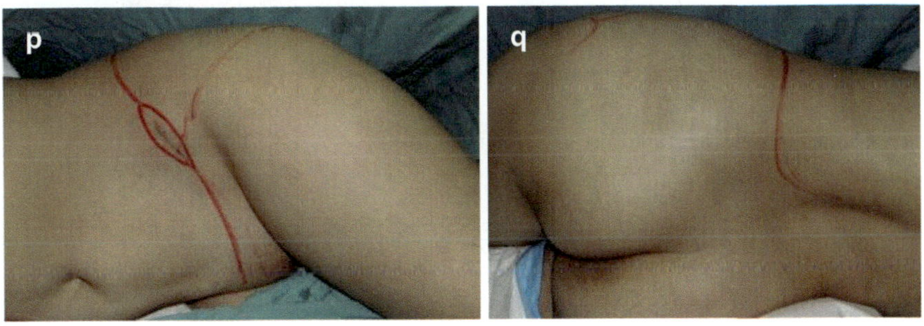

Mobilisation of the external iliac vessels and femoral nerve. The psoas major and iliacus muscles are left as part of the surgical margin (Fig. 1r).

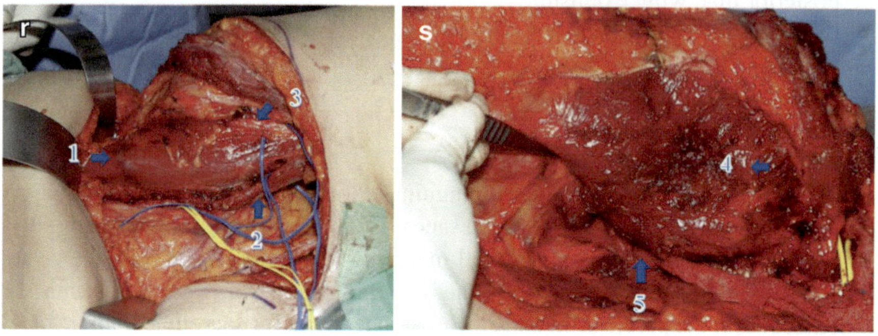

1. Psoas muscle
2. External iliac artery
3. Femoral nerve
4. Gluteus medius
5. Roller gauze passed thru greater sciatic foramen

Gluteus maximus is elevated from pelvic brim; the gluteus medius is maintained as oncological margin. Long roller gauze is passed from the anterior to posterior through the greater sciatic notch (Fig. 1s). Osteotomy over the supraacetabular bone after securing the margin and at the ala of the sacrum (Fig. 1t–w).

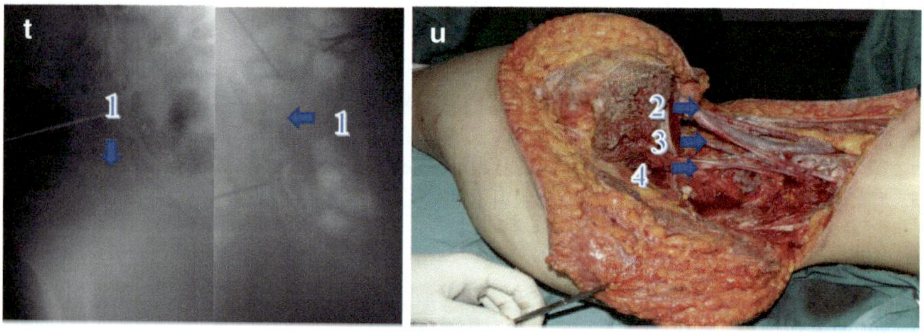

1. K wire—supra-acetabulum & Sacroiliac joint
2. Femoral nerve
3. Obturator nerve
4. Sciatic nerve

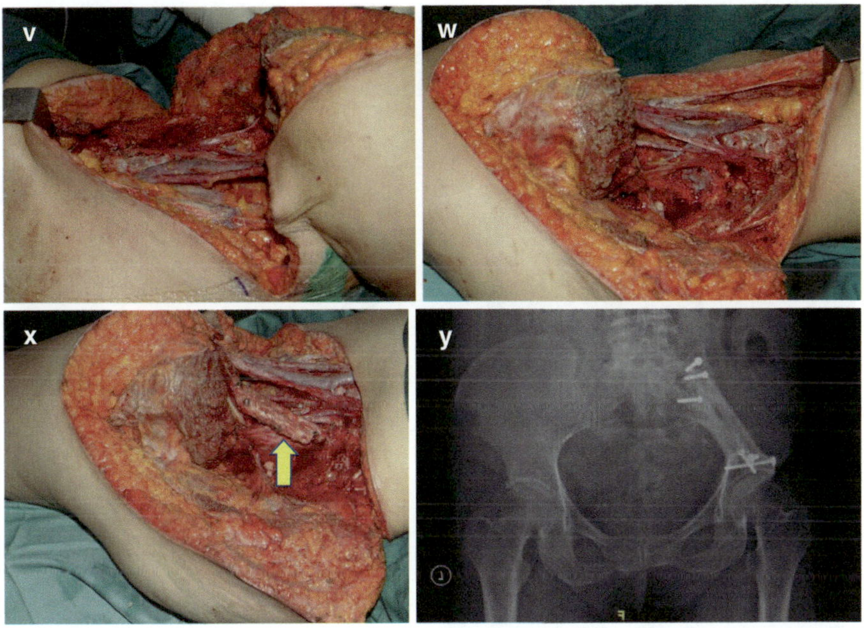

A non-vascularised fibula graft to bridge the defect from the supra-acetabulum to the body of S1 will improve stability and prevent superior translation of the hip joint and chronic pain over the symphysis pubis (Fig. 1x, y)

Soft Tissue Sarcoma with Pelvic Brim Infiltration

Soft tissue sarcoma within the pelvis infiltrated and involved the anterior abdominal wall and pelvic brim (Fig. 2a–g). Wide oncological margin requires partial pelvic resection and abdominal wall resection. A local flap is required to reconstruct the back of the abdominal wall (Fig. 2h).

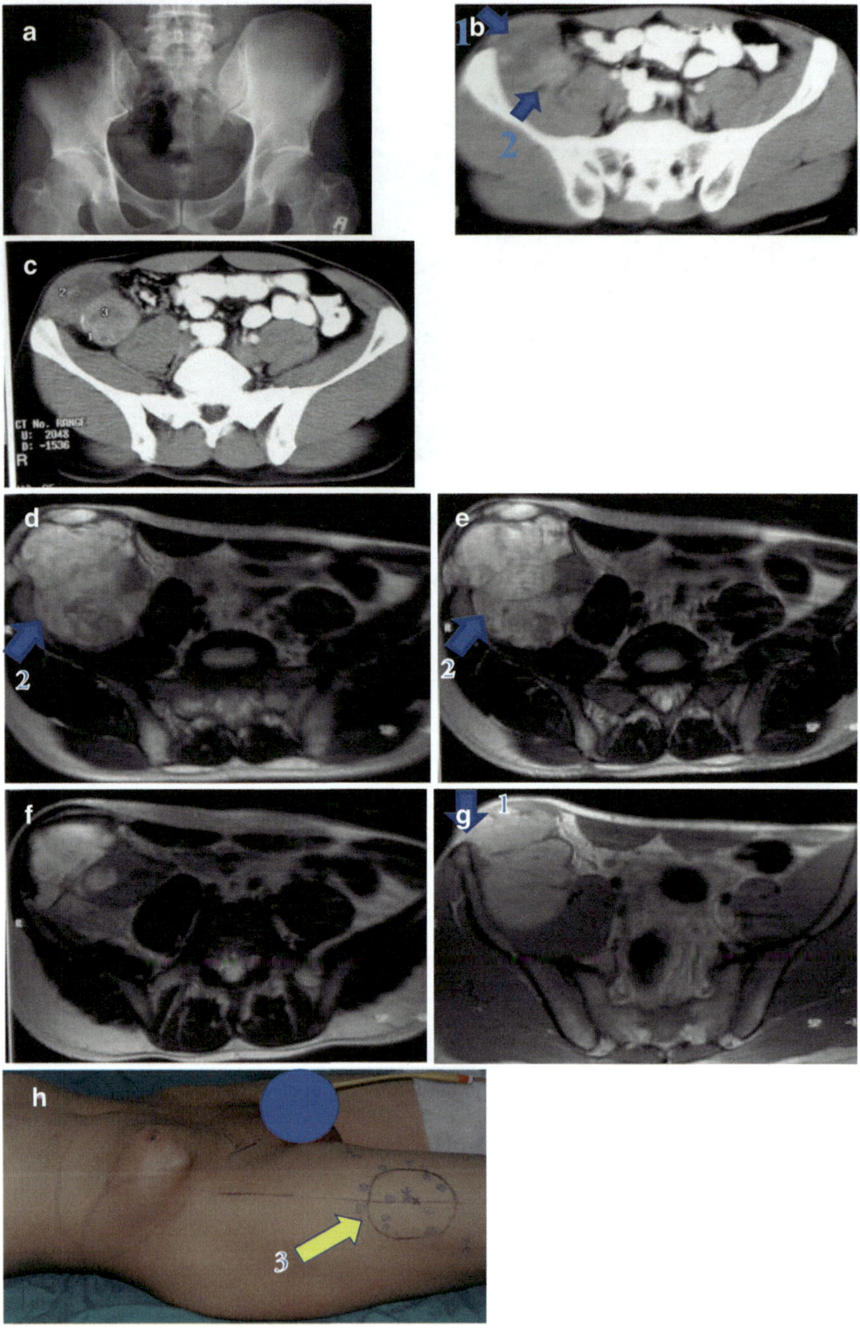

- Sarcoma with involvement
    1. Lateral abdominal wall
    2. Iliac wing infiltration
    3. Lateral thigh flap

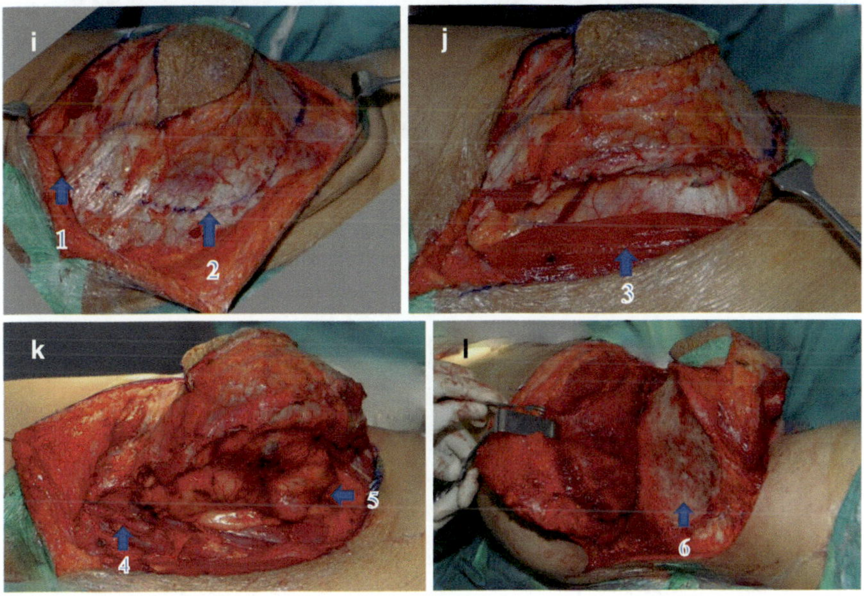

1. Inguinal ligament
2. Plan margin—external oblique aponeurosis
3. Rectus abdominis muscle
4. External iliac vessels
5. Retroperitoneal fat covering iliacus muscle
6. Outer rim pelvis

The surgical margin is lateral to the rectus abdominis. All abdominal muscles attached to the pelvic brim were included in the resection margin. The peritoneum was reflected medially to expose the retroperitoneal structures. Exploration of the external iliac vessels and femoral nerve and mobilisation from the iliacus and psoas major muscle. Both muscles were closely attached to the tumour and removed in total (Fig. 2i–l).

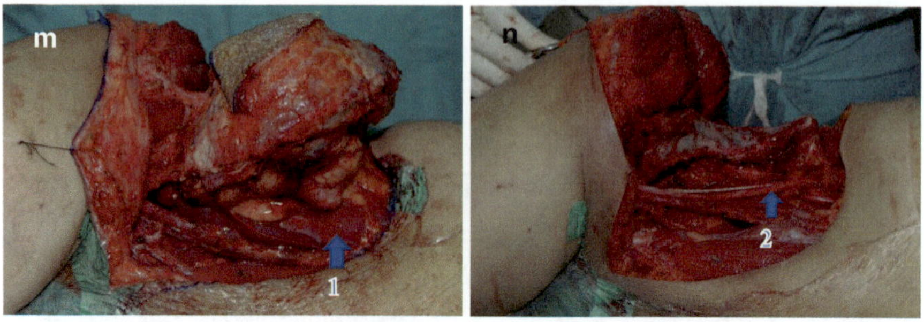

The posterior part of pelvis was free of tumour, and soft tissues were reflected sub-periosteally away from the pelvic brim. The medial pelvis, which was free from tumour infiltration, was maintained for pelvic ring continuity and stability (Fig. 2m–q).

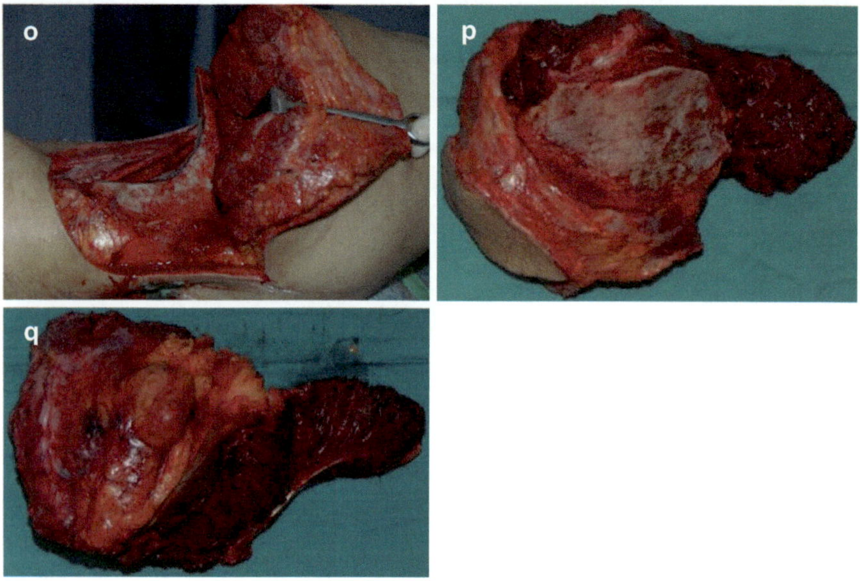

1. Psoas muscle
2. Femoral nerve

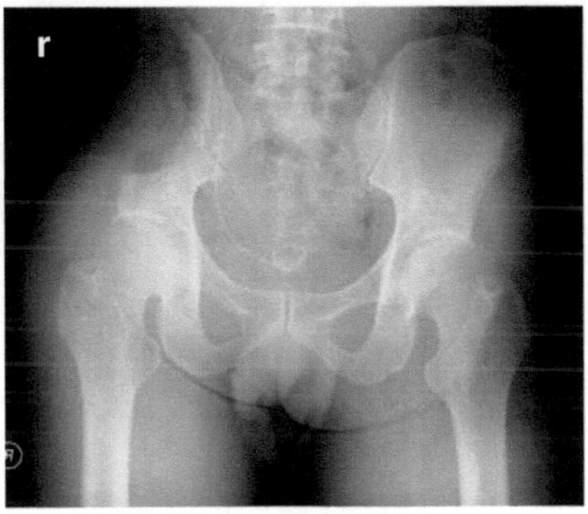

Ureteric stent was kept post-operatively and is usually removed after the completion of 8–10 weeks of local radiation (Fig. 2r)

PNET Sacroiliac Joint with Anterior Posterior Involvement

A case primary neuroectodermal tumour (PNET) of the entire gluteal muscle and iliopsoas that crosses the sacroiliac joint up to the root of S1 and L5 (Fig. 3a–h). Mobilisation of both roots and marginal resection of the sacrum and local radiotherapy are options to minimise functional morbidity and control the disease.

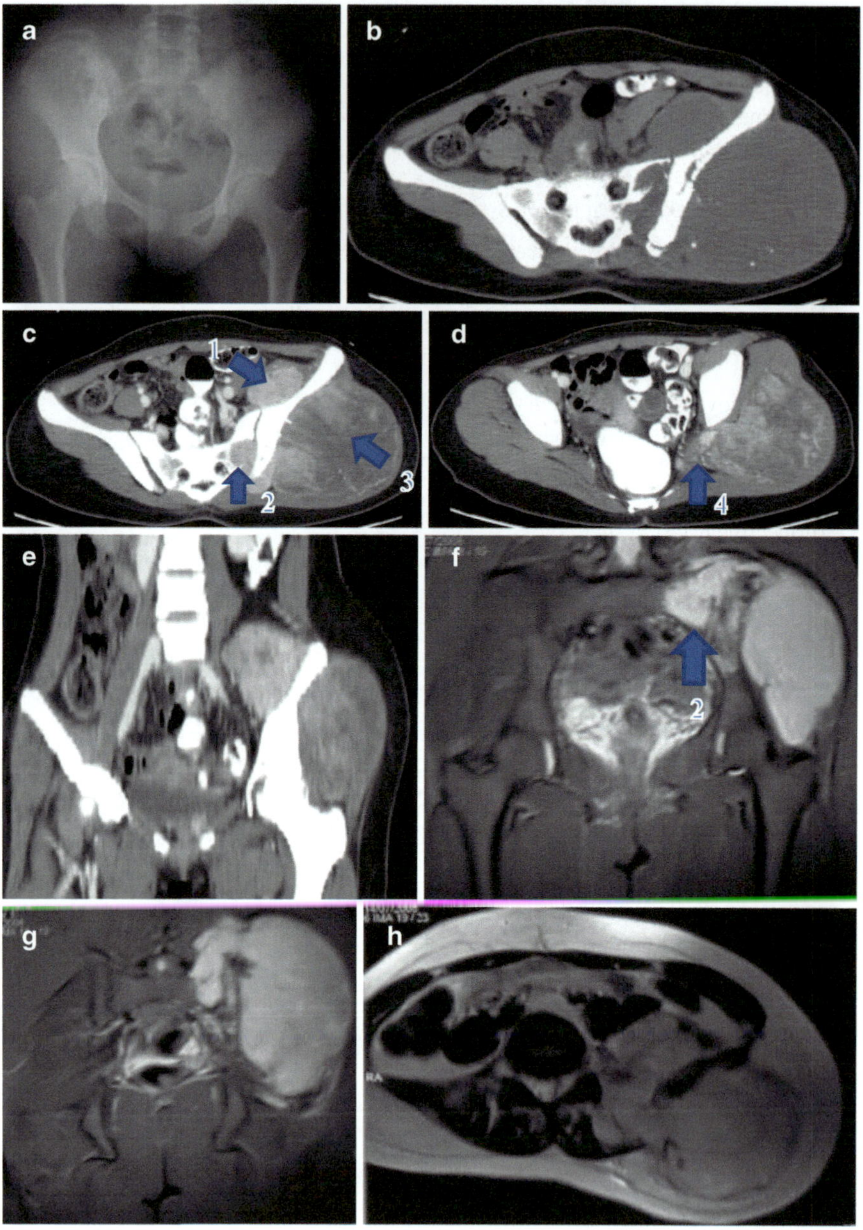

1. Psoas muscle
2. Alar of the sacrum and sacrum neuroforamina
3. Gluteal muscle involvement
4. Sciatic foramen/sciatic nerve

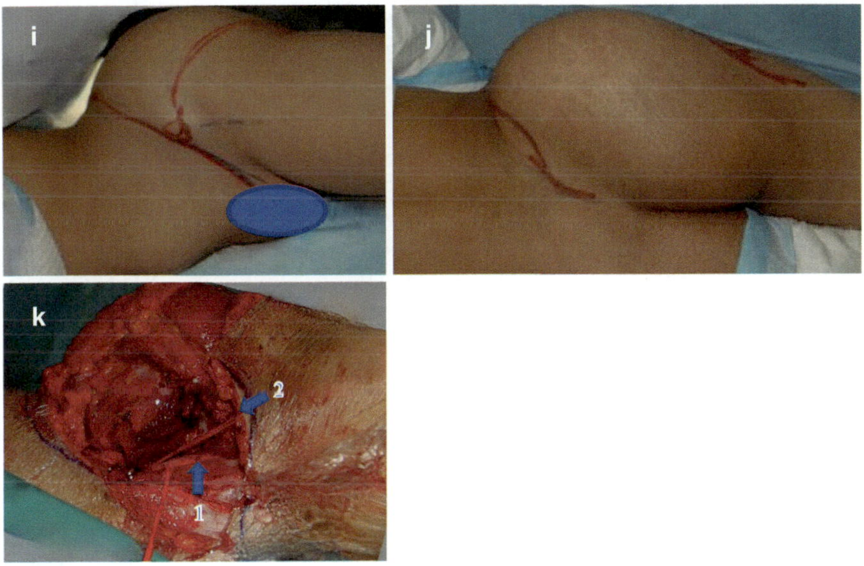

1. Femoral nerve
2. Lateral cutaneous nerve of the thigh

Correlation sacroiliac joint, vessels, and L5&S1 root (Fig. 3l–n)

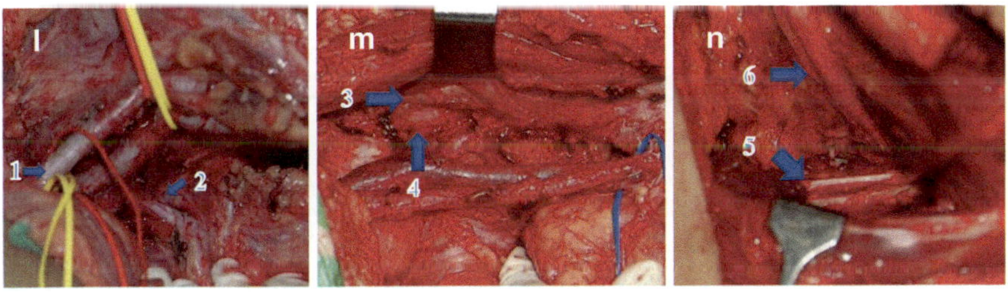

1. Common iliac vessels
2. Internal iliac artery
3. Sacroiliac joint
4. L5 root
5. L5 & S1 root
6. Roller gauze passed through greater sciatic foramen

Anterior mobilisation of the femoral nerve and external iliac vessels. The iliopsoas was removed completely with the entire ilium (Fig. 3i–n). Posterior mobilisation of the fasciocutaneous flap and entire gluteus muscle exposed to the sacrum origin for partial sacrectomy (Fig. 3o, p). The osteotomy level is at the foramen of S1 after mobilisation of the L5 root (Fig. 3q).

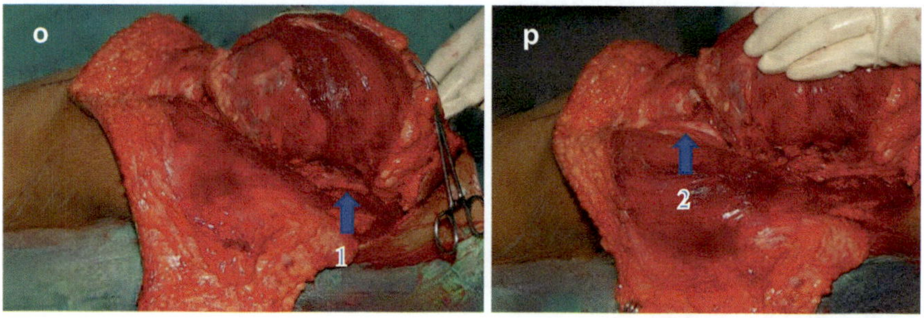

1. Sacrum lateral to the foramina
2. Sciatic nerve
3. External iliac vessels
4. Femoral nerve

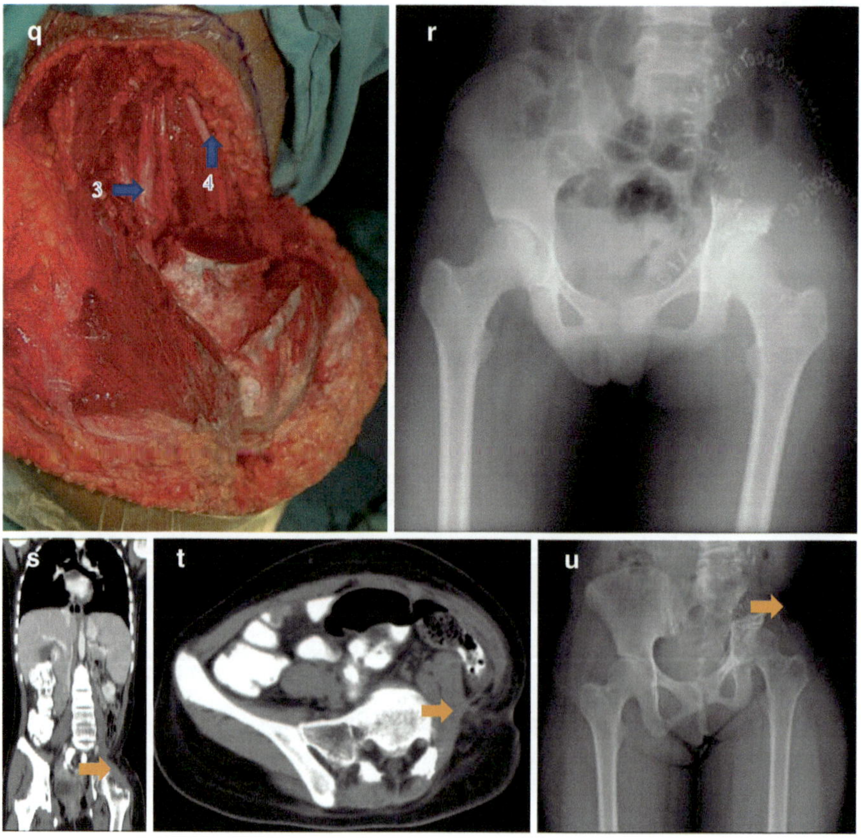

No bony reconstruction was done as adjuvant radiotherapy was planned. There was no local recurrence at 10 years; however, there was superior translation of the hip joint with a 3 cm limb length discrepancy (Fig. 3r–u).

Sacroiliac Joint Resection (Type I + S)

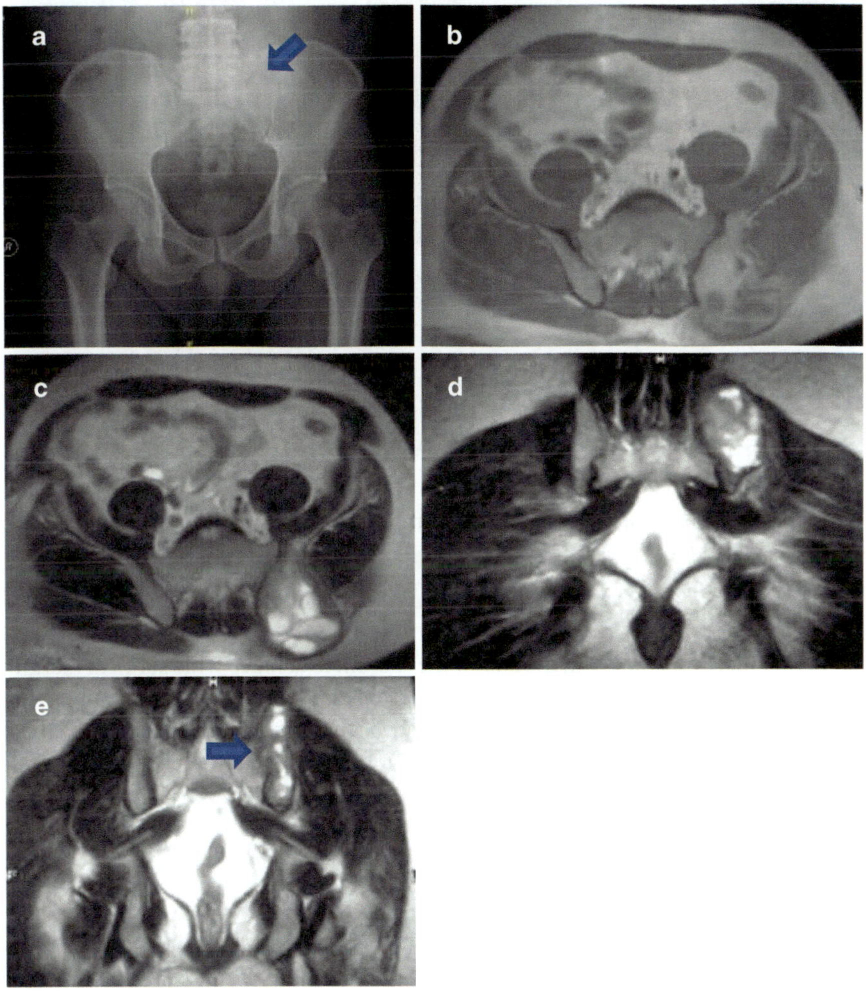

A case of sarcoma sacroiliac joint with posterior ilium soft tissue in close proximity to the erector spinae. No anterior soft tissue extension (Fig. 4a–e). The alar of the sacrum was removed in total with the mass to achieve the oncological margin. Part of the erector spinal also was included in the margin (Fig. 4f–i).

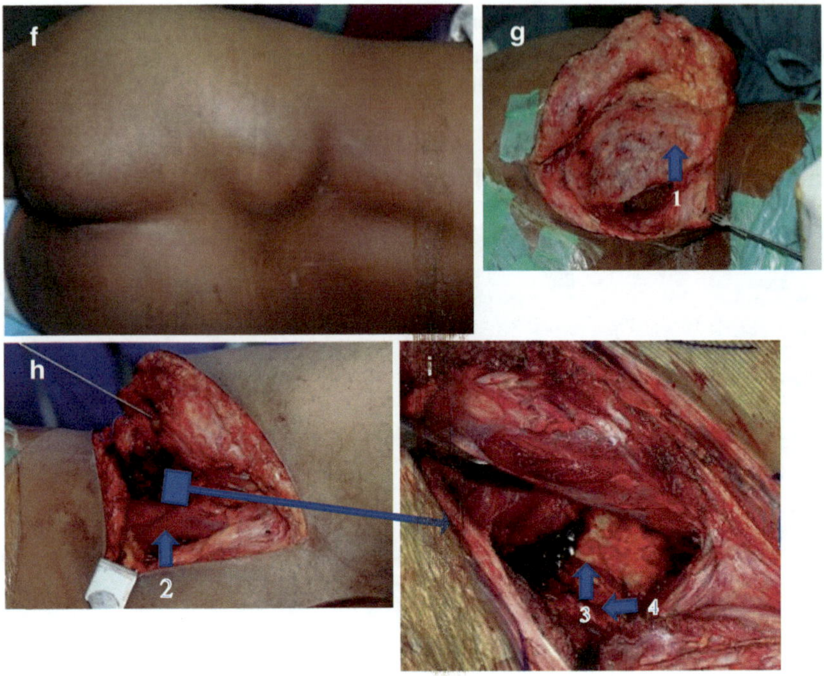

1. Gluteus maximus and erector spinal muscle
2. Psoas muscle
3. Sacroiliac joint
4. Alar of sacrum

Partial iliac resection with the alar of the sacrum to achieve wide surgical margin. Reconstruction for resection of the entire sacrum alar in cases of sarcoma involving the sacroiliac joint is difficult due to limited bone for screw stabilisation. Pedicle screw with iliac wing stabilisation is an option for early stability of the fibular graft strut (Fig. 4j–l).

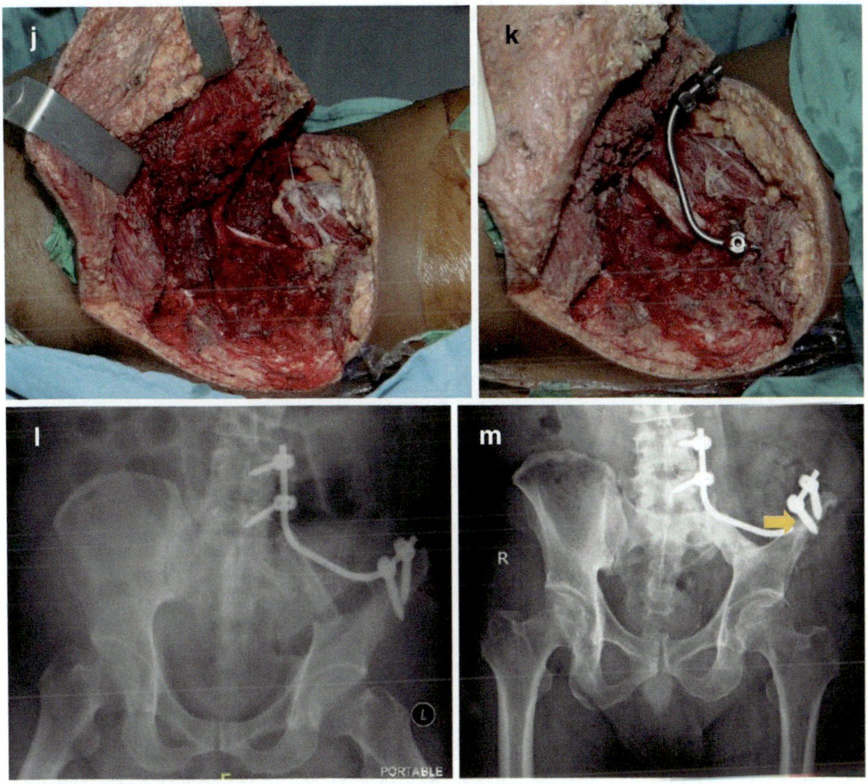

Fibula hypertrophy and solid bone bridge over the sacrum and pelvic wing despite rod failure (Fig. 4m).

Iliac Wing with Partial Acetabulum Resection

Aggressive bone tumour iliac wing supra-acetabulum

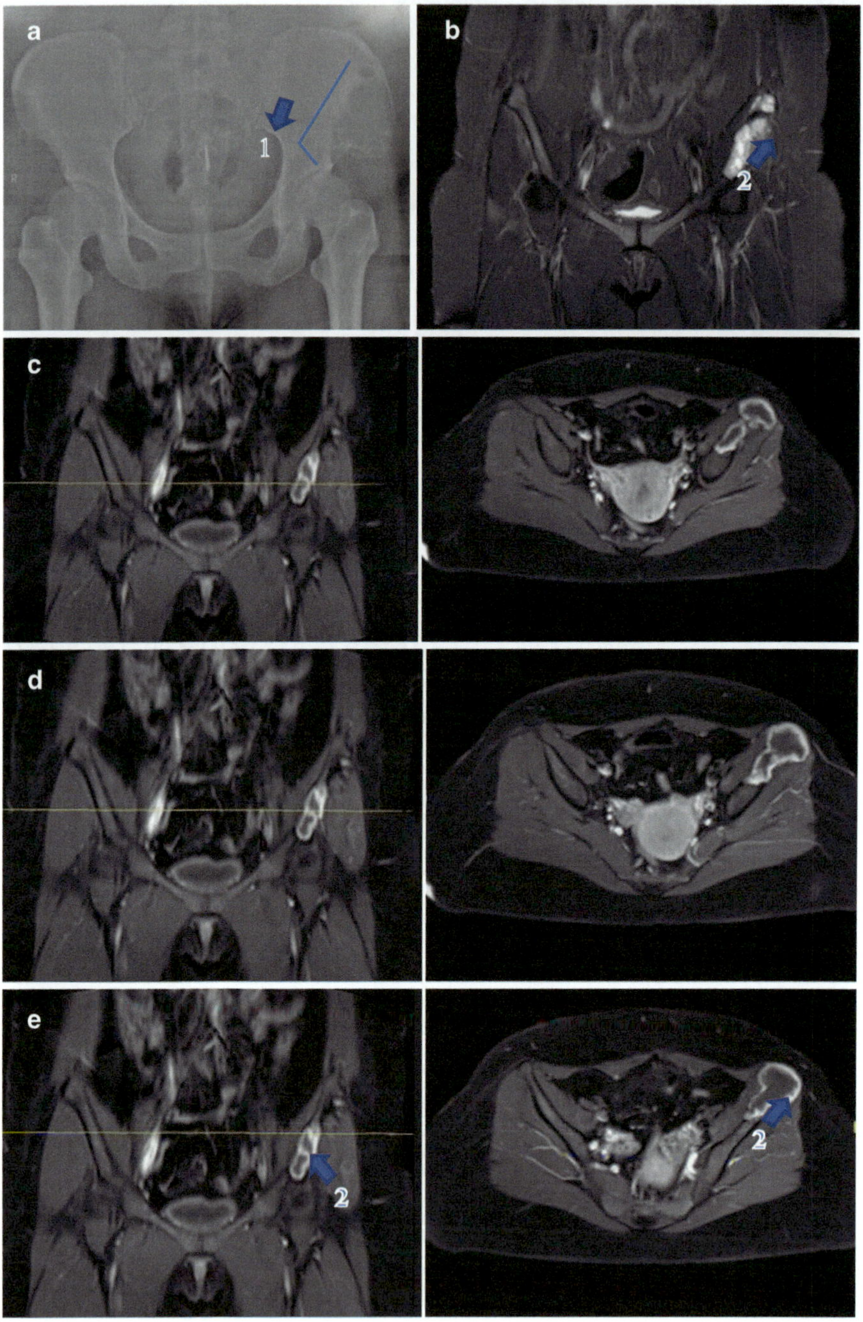

1. Plan bone resection
2. Intraosseous lesion with no soft tissue extension

An aggressive bone tumour fibro myxoid chondroma involving illiac wing with subchondral anterolateral supra-acetabulum extension (Fig. 5a–e). Resection of mainly the lateral iliac wing thru retroperitoneal approach for inner pelvic brim exposure. The gluteus, sartorius and tensor fascia latae origin were detached for lateral iliac rim visualisation prior to resection of ilium and supra-acetabulum region (Fig. 5f–j).

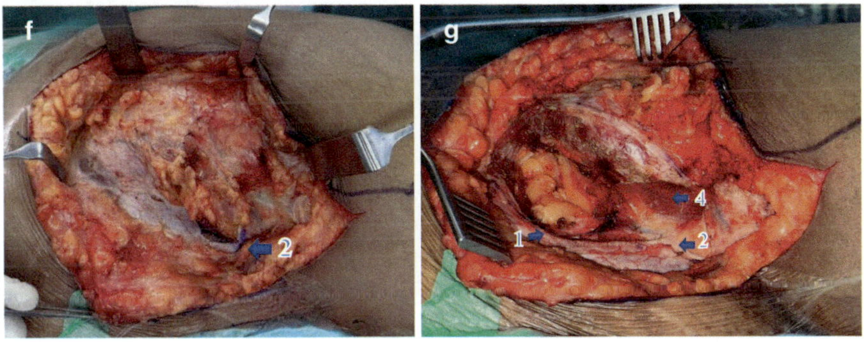

1. Inguinal ligament
2. ASIS
3. Lateral abdominal wall muscle and aponeurosis
4. Ilio-psoas muscle

Retroperitoneal space exposed by elevating abdominal muscle and inguinal ligament from iliac crest and femur fascia

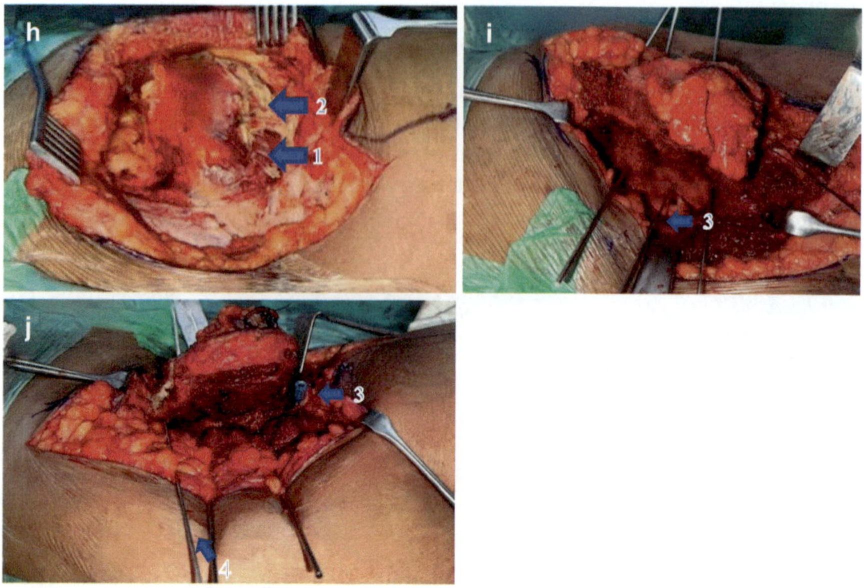

1. Sartorius insertion at ASIS
2. Tensor fascia latae origin
3. Hp joint needle guide
4. Multiple K-wire inserted for final confirmation with image intensifier

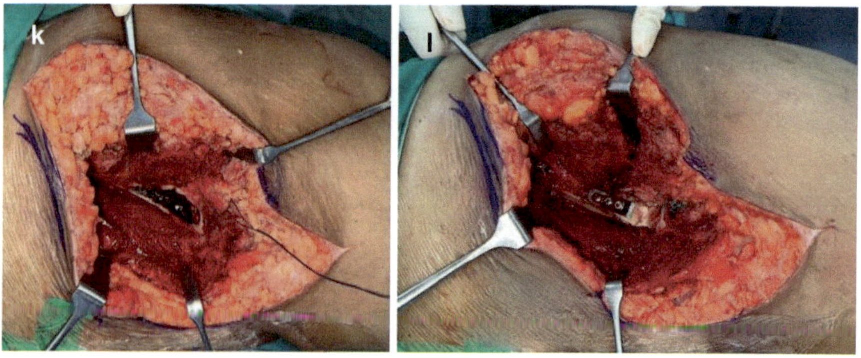

Anterolateral part of resected acetabulum was reconstructed with allograft femoral head and stabilised with acetabulum spring plate (Fig. 5k, l).

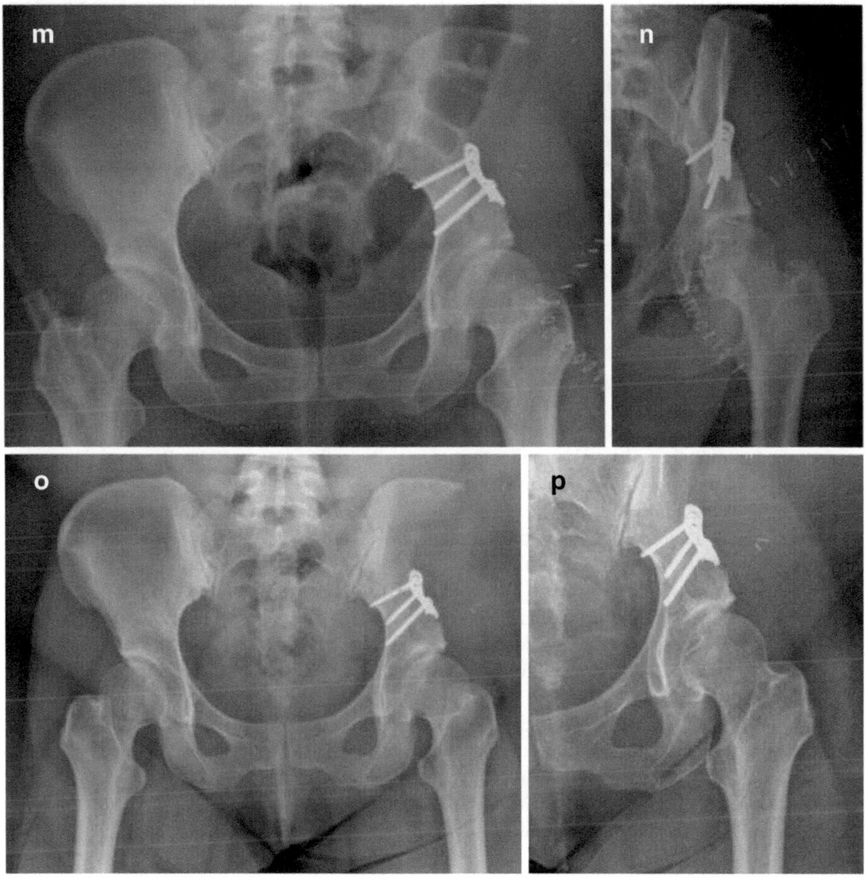

Allograft reconstruction of anterolateral defect showed full incorporation at 1 year (Fig. 5m–p).

Suggested Reading

1. Akiyama T, Clark JC, Miki Y, Choong PF. The non-vascularised fibular graft: a simple and successful method of reconstruction of the pelvic ring after internal hemipelvectomy. J Bone Joint Surg Br. 2010;92(7):999–1005.
2. Mavrogenis AF, Papadopoulos D, Tsantes AG, Angelini A, Papagelopoulos PJ, Ruggieri P. Reconstruction vs. no reconstruction for pelvic resections. In: Surgery for pelvic bone tumour. Springer Nature; 2021. p. 165–83.
3. Arif S, Nawaz AH, Nur Azman MZ, Zulmi W, Faisham WI. Outcome of surgical treatment of pelvic osteosarcoma. MOJ. 2013;7(1)
4. Aratani A, Chan CM, Parker Gibbs C, Scarborough M. Principles of pelvic surgery. In: Surgery for pelvic bone tumour. Springer Nature; 2021. p. 113–22.

5. Karakousis CP. The T or L incision in resection of tumors of the pelvis/Tumour along the femoral vessels. In: Atlas of operative procedures in surgical oncology. Springer Science; 2015. p. 233–236/311–322.
6. Conrad Ill EU, Weisstein J, Lisle J, Stemheim A, Martin M. Malawer overview on pelvic resections: surgical considerations and classifications. In: Operative technique in orthopaedic surgical oncology. Lippincott Williams & Wilkins, A Wolters Kluwer; 2012. p. 161–79.
7. Evrard R, Schubert T, Paul L, Docquier PL. Resection margins obtained with patient-specific instruments for resecting primary pelvic bone sarcomas: a case-control study. Orthop Traumatol Surg Res. 2019;105(4):781–7.
8. Özger H, Alpan B, Karaaltın MV. Biological reconstruction of the pelvis: I: liquid-nitrogen treated autograft and onlaid free vascular fibula. In: Orthopedic surgical oncology for bone tumors. Springer Nature Switzerland; 2022. p. 71–85.
9. Park H, Shah AA, Hornicek FJ. Innovative techniques in pelvic reconstructions. In: Surgery for pelvic bone tumour. Springer Nature; 2021. p. 123–34.
10. Mayerson JL, Wooldridge AN, Scharschmidt TJ. Pelvic resection: current concepts. J Am Acad Orthop Surg. 2014;22:214–22.
11. Karim SM, Colman MW, Lozano-Calderón SA, Raskin KA, Schwab JH, Hornicek FJ. What are the functional results and complications from allograft reconstruction after partial hemipelvectomy of the pubis? Clin Orthop Relat Res. 2015;473:1442–8.
12. Khan M, Wilkerson H, Vassos N, Hannay JA, Thway K, Messiou C, Hayes AJ, Strauss DC, Smith MJ. Oncologic outcomes of surgically managed primary pelvic soft tissue sarcoma; tumour biology or surgical constraints of the true pelvis? Eur J Surg Oncol. 2023;49(5):941–9.
13. Laitinen MK, Parry MC, Albergo JI, Jeys LM, Grimer RJ. Resection of the ilium in patients with a sarcoma: should the pelvic ring be reconstructed? Bone Joint J. 2017;99(4):538–43.
14. Peter FM. Choong General Considerations Pelvis. In: Master techniques in orthopaedic surgery orthopaedic oncology and complex reconstruction. Lippincott Williams & Wilkins, A Wolters Kluwer; 2011. p. 3–13.
15. Puchner SE, Funovics PT, Böhler C, Kaider A, Stihsen C, Hobusch GM, Panotopoulos J, Windhager R. Oncological and surgical outcome after treatment of pelvic sarcomas. PLoS One. 2017;12(2):e0172203.
16. Faisham WI, Zulmi W, Aidura M, Yazid MD, Sallehuddin AY, Norazman MZ. Partial resection of the pelvis and salvage of the lower limb in the treatment of malignant pelvic tumour. Med J Malaysia. 2001;56(2)

Type II Pelvic Resection

Wan Faisham Nu'man Bin Wan Ismail

Introduction

Periacetabular or Type II pelvic resection is oncological resection of the acetabular component of the hip joint with surrounding anatomical boundaries. The entire acetabulum is removed through supra-acetabular ilium, superior pubic rami, and ischium osteotomy. The femoral head and hip joint capsule are included together with the resection in case of hip joint contamination. Reconstruction of periacetabular defects after periacetabular resection is a challenging procedure and is associated with high complication rates and morbidity.

Surgical Anatomy

Anatomical relations to the periacetabular region

- Anterior—covered by the iliacus muscle, iliopsoas tendon and thick iliopectineal fascia that covers the medial brim. The external iliac vessels traverse through the inguinal canal to form the femoral vessels together with the femoral nerve. All these structures must be mobilised for superior pubic rami osteotomy. The anterior acetabulum and capsule must be exposed for extraarticular hip resection.
- Posterior—the short rotator tendons and muscles: piriformis, superior gemellus, obturator internus, inferior gemellus and obturator externus. The sciatic nerve travels from the greater sciatic notch below the piriformis above all these ten-

W. F. N. B. W. Ismail (✉)
Prince Court Medical Center, Kuala Lumpur, Malaysia

Orthopaedic Oncology Reconstructive Unit, Universiti Sains Malaysia, Kubang Kerian, Kelantan, Malaysia

A. Puri, W. F. N. B. W. Ismail (eds.), *Atlas of Orthopedic Oncology Volume 1*,
https://doi.org/10.1007/978-981-95-8958-6_17

dons. The greater sciatic notch must be exposed and free for supraacetabular osteotomy, and the sciatic nerve must be mobilised posteriorly for ischium osteotomy.
- Medial—obturator internus covers the medial wall of the acetabulum, and posteriorly the sacrospinous ligament is attached to the spinous process and pelvic floor muscles iliococcygeus and ischiococcygeus. The obturator artery runs at the medial acetabulum together with the obturator nerve to the obturator fossa.
- Corona mortis is an anastomosis of the external iliac, inferior epigastric, and obturator vessels located in the retropubic region and must be carefully dissected and ligated as it can cause excessive bleeding

Assessment

The bony and marrow extension is an important part of the assessment to determine the level of osteotomy for clear margins. Traditionally, osteotomy level is determined by an MRI image and subsequently intraoperatively based on the surgical anatomy of bony reference points. Multiple K-wires with image guidance can be used for final osteotomy level confirmation. Recently, 3D real-time guided images are used intraoperatively for accurate levels of resection.

Structures to be evaluated for direct infiltration by the tumour:-

- Hip joint contamination
- Sacrospinous ligament
- Obturator internus muscle
- Short external rotator muscles and tendons
- Pelvic floor muscle attachments

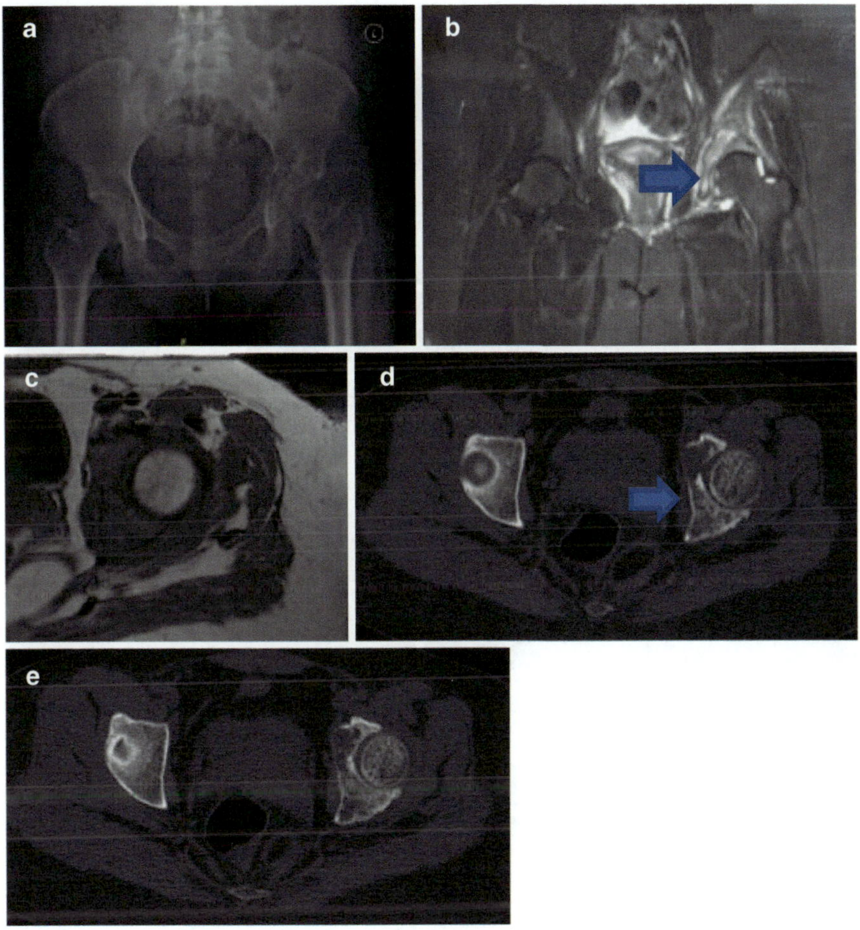
a
b
c
d
e

- Obturator internus covering medial acetabulum wall

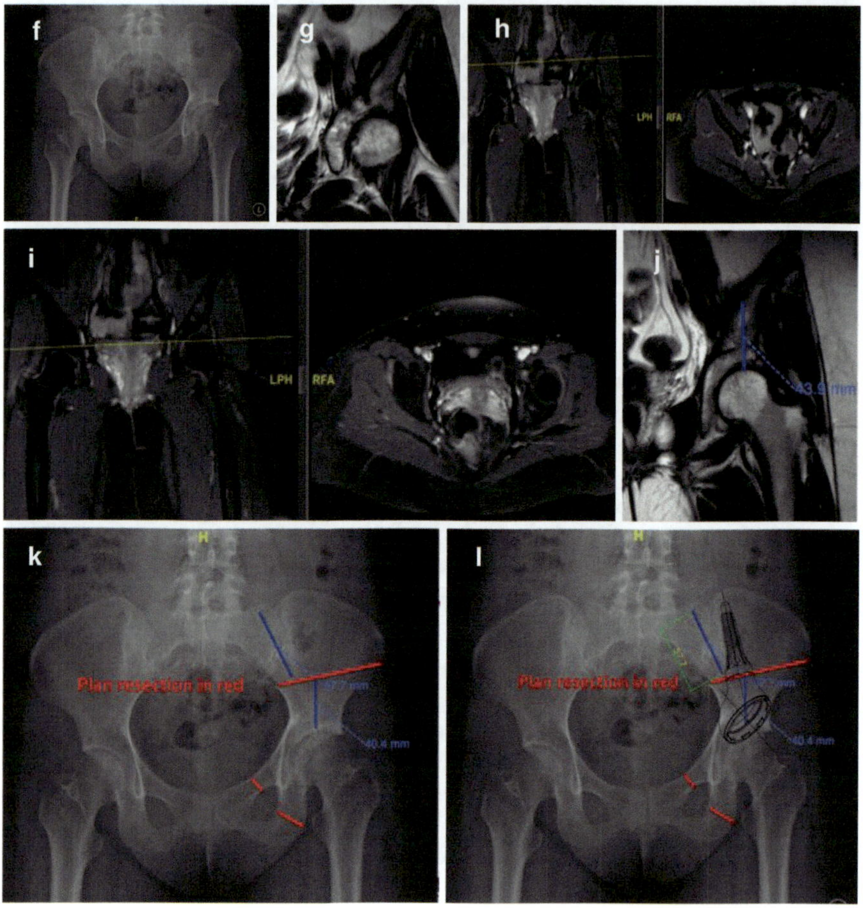

A case of osteosarcoma that responded well to chemotherapy in a 17-year-old lady. The tumour was confined to the intraosseous component with suspicious medial break and infiltration of the obturator internus muscle. The anterior neurovascular structures and iliopsoas had a good plane from the tumour. All posterior short rotator muscles were free without infiltration. Surgical osteotomy plan was based on MRI and CT imaging. Final implant with Lumic cup for hip reconstruction (Fig. 1a–l)

Surgical Steps

- Anterior ilioinguinal approach is planned for retroperitoneal approach for the iliac vessels, femoral nerve exploration and mobilisation of the iliopsoas tendon up to level of superior pubic rami for anterior osteotomy.
- The medial wall acetabulum with obturator internus muscle can be visualised and is normally included as a surgical margin
- Posterior flap utilised gluteus maximus flap for mobilisation of the sciatic nerve, securing the gluteus medius and 360° control of supra-acetabulum osteotomy
- Gluteus maximus is detached posteriorly for large posterior approach of the entire acetabulum. The sciatic nerve is mobilised posteriorly, and the short rotator tendons and muscles are mobilised to expose the entire posterior acetabular wall to the ischial spine
- Sacrospinous ligament can be transacted through this approach.
- Trochanteric osteotomy and mobilisation of the gluteus medius and nerve supply to retain the abduction function were done prior to femoral neck osteotomy or femoral head dislocation. It is important for hip stability. This step is important for complete evaluation over supraacetabular bony area
- Obturator vessels and corona mortis vessels must be identified and ligated prior to osteotomy

Triple osteotomy

- Supra-acetabulum
- Ischium
- Superior pubic rami

Chondrosarcoma Peri Acetabulum with Saddle Prosthesis Reconstruction

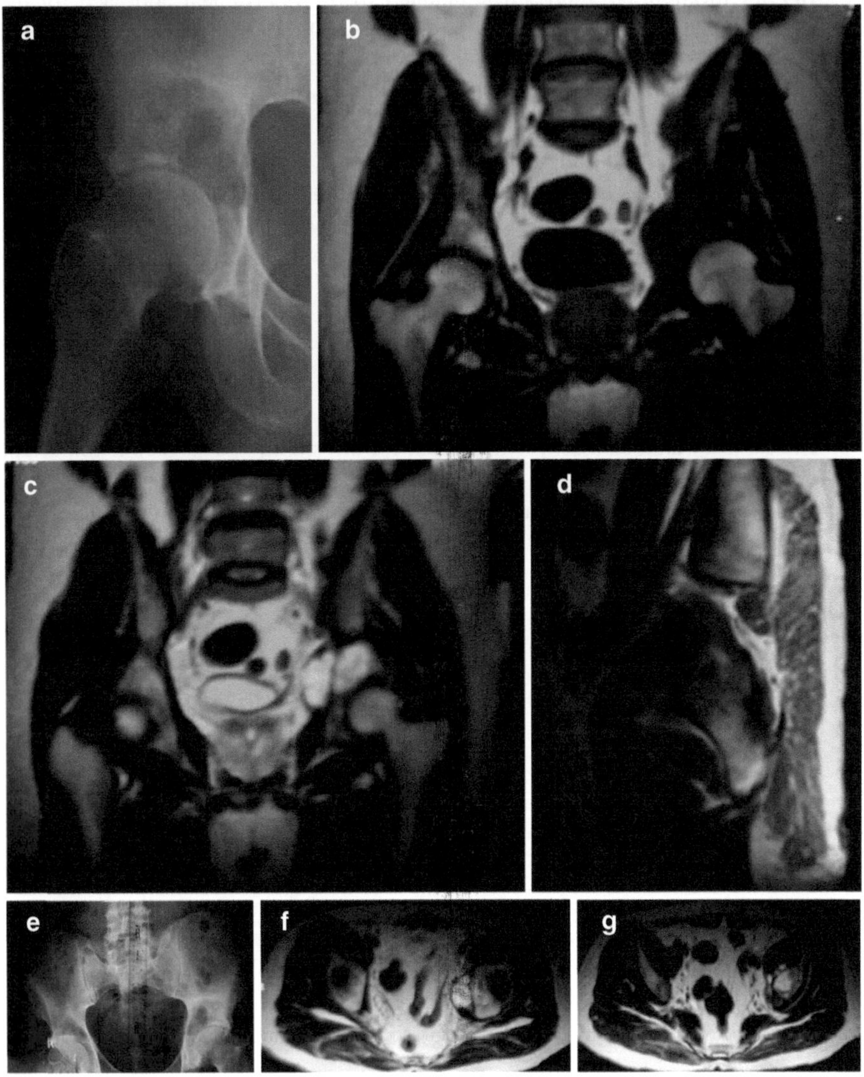

A case of intraosseous chondrosarcoma peri-acetabulum with minimal soft tissue extension. X-ray was used for resection planning and supra-acetabulum margin planning (Fig. 2a–g).

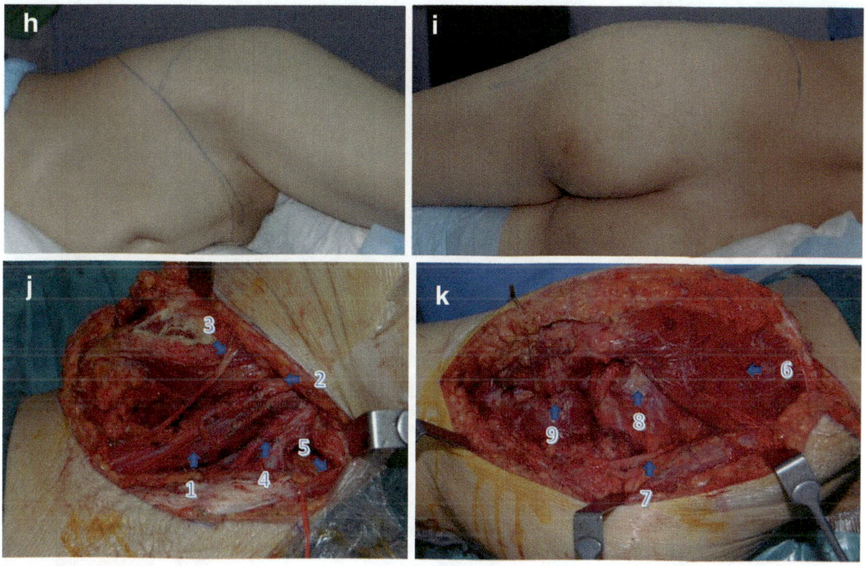

1. Psoas muscle
2. Femoral nerve
3. Lateral cutaneous nerve of the thigh
4. External iliac artery
5. Spermatic cord
6. Gluteus medius
7. Sciatic nerve
8. Piriformis tendon
9. Quadratus femoris

Incision is planned for retroperitoneal approach for the iliac vessels, femoral nerve exploration and anterior osseous osteotomy. The gluteus maximus is flipped posteriorly to expose the sciatic nerve and all short rotators for evaluation of the entire posterior column of acetabulum, including the greater sciatic foramen and ischium, for pelvic osteotomy (Fig. 2h–k).

The gluteus medius attachment is detached through trochanteric osteotomy. The gluteus minimus muscle is a good anatomical boundary for oncological barrier. The base of the neck femur is osteotomised to mobilise the femur for final removal of the acetabulum (Fig. 2l–n).

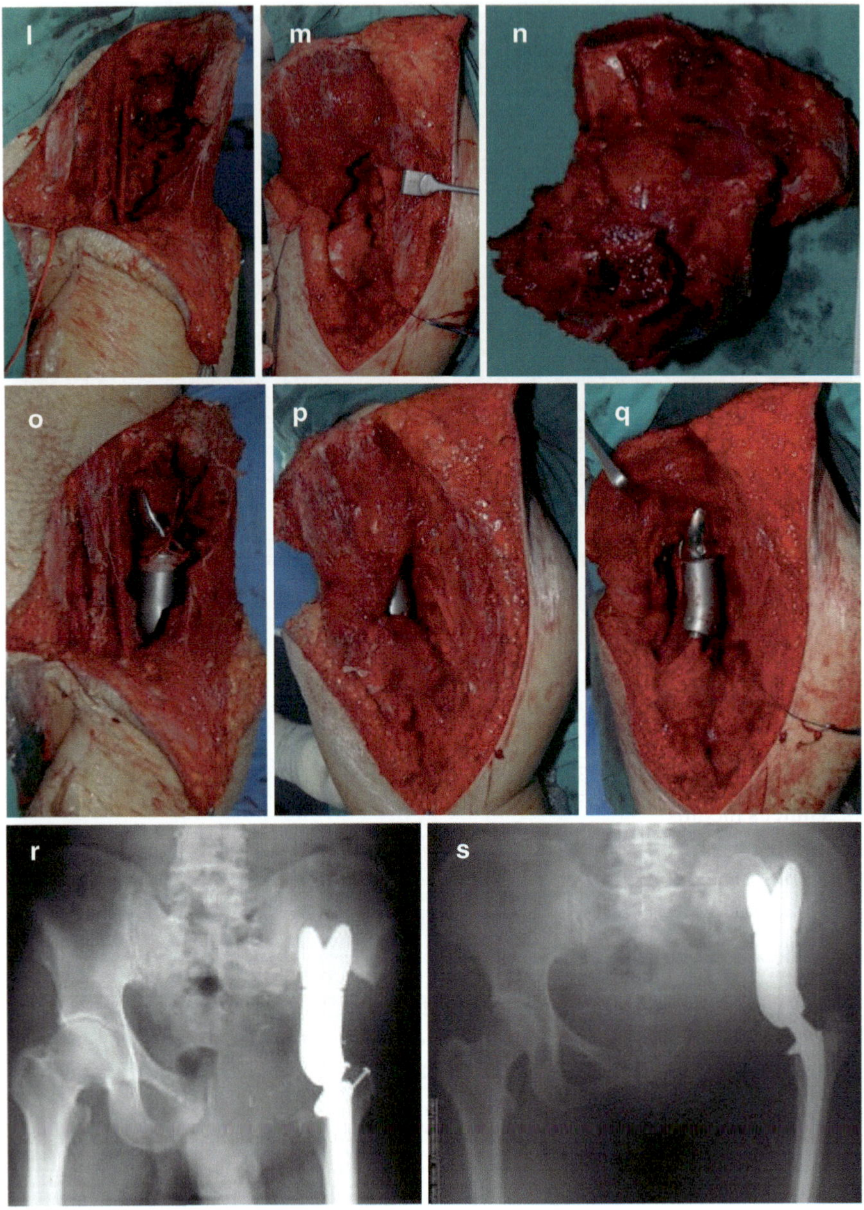

Final reconstruction with saddle prosthesis. The abductor is reattached to the greater trochanter for better function. Bony reaction over the saddle prosthesis after three years of mobility (Fig. 2o–s). The functional outcome with saddle prosthesis deteriorates significantly after a few years and is currently not an option for reconstruction.

Type II Acetabulum Resection and Lumic Pelvic Reconstruction

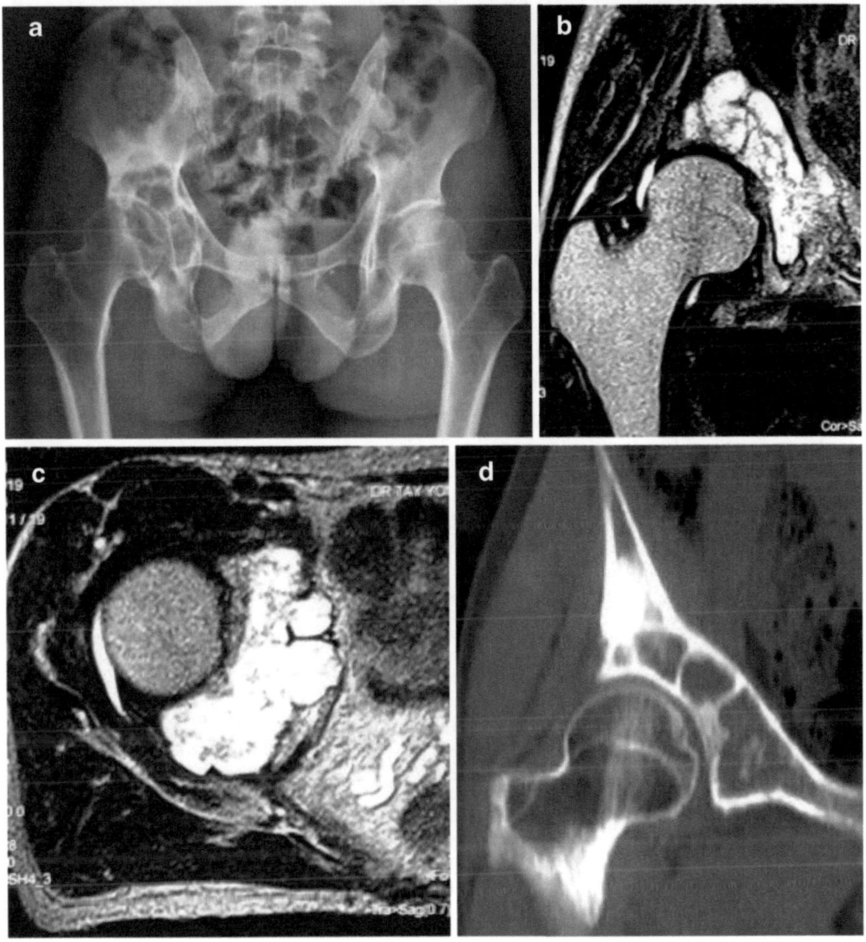

A case of peri-acetabulum chondrosarcoma involving the supra-acetabulum and both columns of the acetabulum, including the medial wall of the quadrilateral plate. The superior pubic rami and ischium were involved, and to achieve wide bony margin, the bony cut is planned at the level of symphysis pubis and supra-acetabulum (Fig. 3a–d).

The incision is shown for exposure of both the anterior and posterior aspects of the pelvis. The ilioinguinal incision is used to develop the retroperitoneal space, and the posterior gluteus maximus flap is used to exposed the retro gluteal space (Fig. 3e, f).

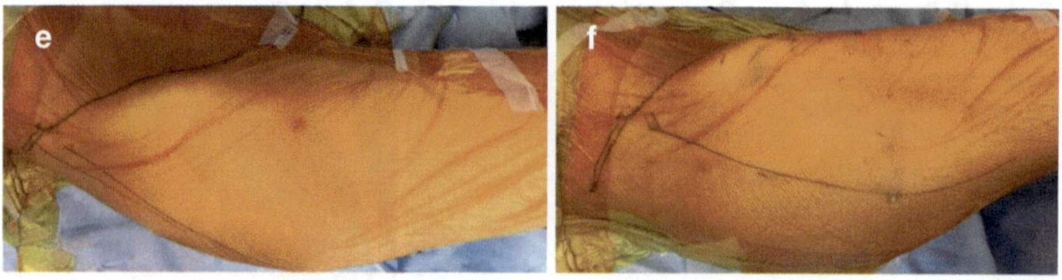

Floppy lateral positioning for anterior and posterior approach for Type II resection. Mobilisation of the anterior neurovascular structures and psoas muscle as well as spermatic cord from anterior margin of the ilium and pubic rami. The Iliacus muscle was retained with the ilium as part of surgical margin. The entire gluteus maximus was mobilised posteriorly for complete exposure of the sciatic nerve and short rotator muscles. The sciatic foramen must be evaluated from the anterior to posterior and the sciatic nerve and branch of the internal iliac mobilised freely from the bone for final bone osteotomy (Fig. 3g–i).

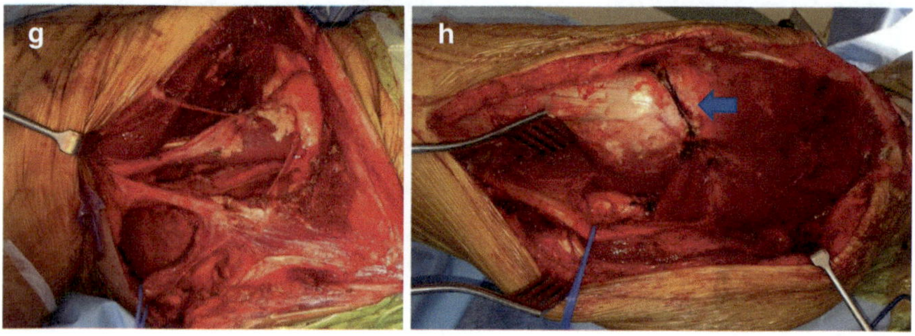

- Trochanteric osteotomy for mobilisation gluteus medius

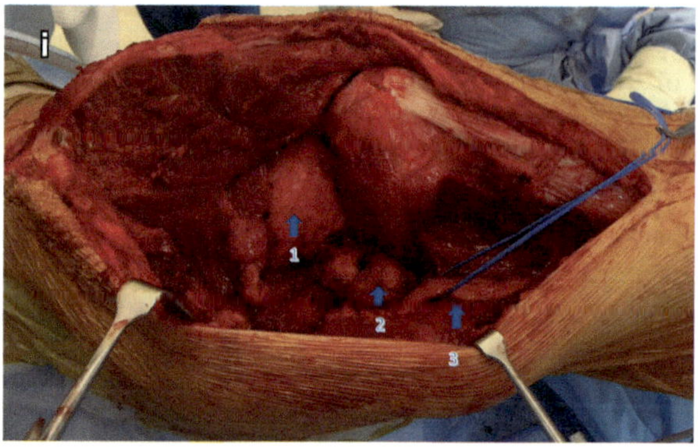

1. Hip capsule
2. Ischium
3. Sciatic nerve

Mobilisation of the gluteus medius by trochanteric osteotomy will expose the entire lateral acetabulum area for direction of supra-acetabulum osteotomy (Fig. 3j, k).

Preparation for Acetabulum Osteotomy and Pedestal Implants

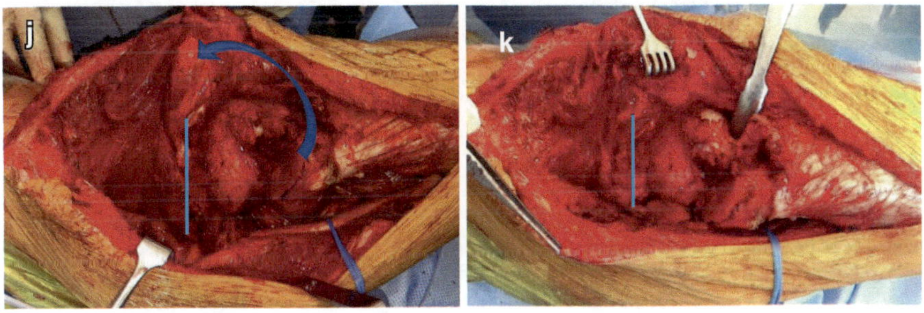

- Trochanter flip for mobilisation gluteus medius and visualisation supra-acetabulum for osteotomy (Fig. 3j)
- Osteotomy neck for free mobilisation of femur shaft (Fig. 3k)

The trochanteric osteotomy and entire gluteus medius and minimus were elevated to expose the entire supra-acetabulum brim, anteriorly the psoas muscle together with the external iliac vessels and the femoral nerve were protected. The entire pelvis was free entirely for osteotomy and 2 K wire inserted for final confirmation (Fig. 3j–n).

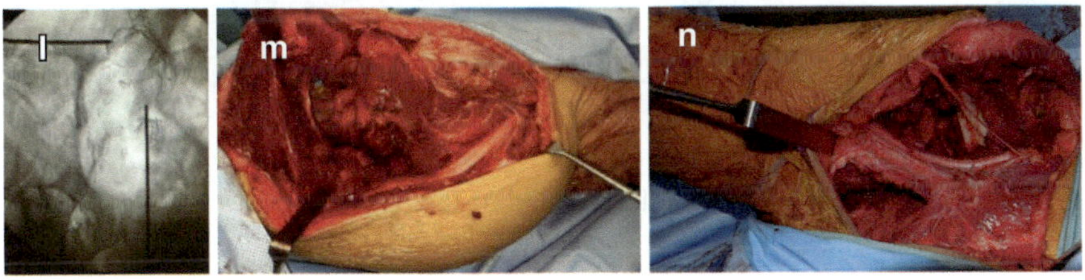

Pedestal cup insertion and its position is confirmed by image intensifier. The correct acetabulum coverage and version is confirmed by testing flexion and rotation of the hip. Soft tissue tension and hip implant offset is determined after reduction of trochanteric osteotomy and gluteus medius tension (Fig. 3o–u).

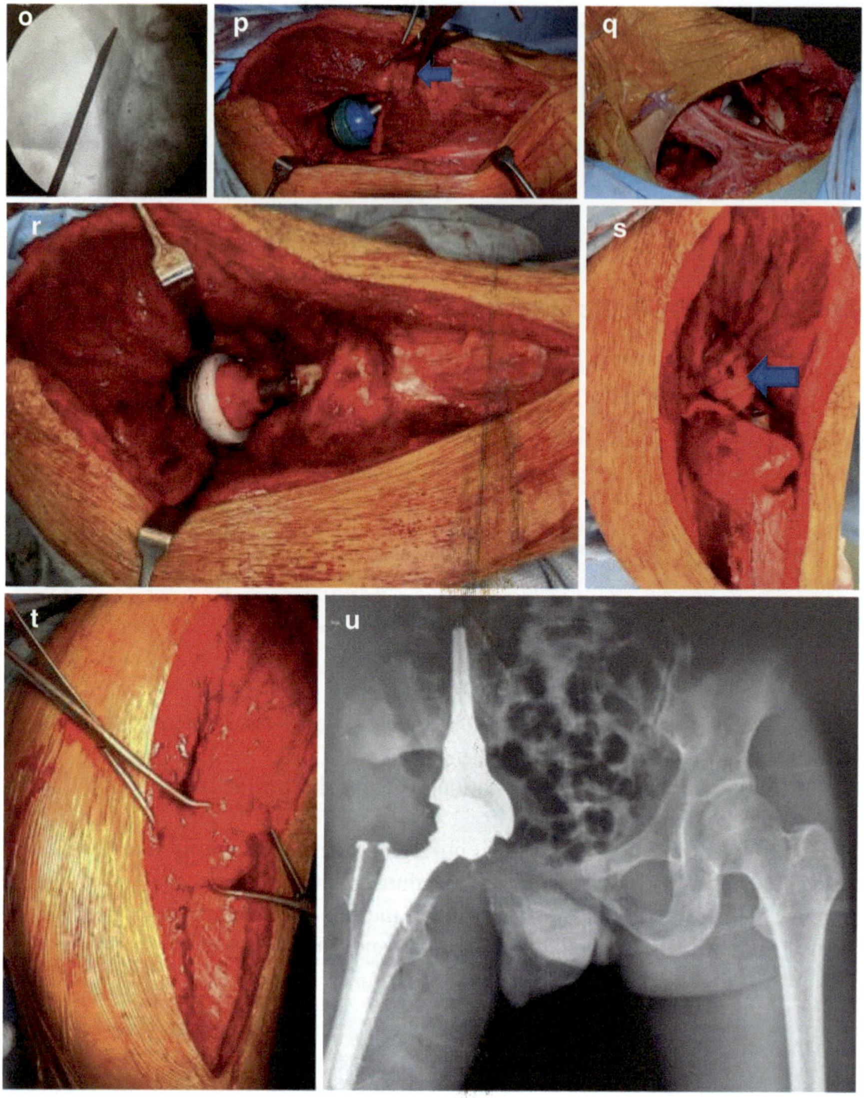

- Apposition of trochanter for gluteus medius tension (Fig. 3p)
- Trevira tube (Fig. 3s)

The hip is reinforced with purse-string Trevira tube to allow soft tissue attachment and fibrosis, mainly with remnants of the Iliacus and psoas muscles anteriorly and gluteus medius posteriorly. The trochanteric osteotomy was stabilized by simple compression screw.

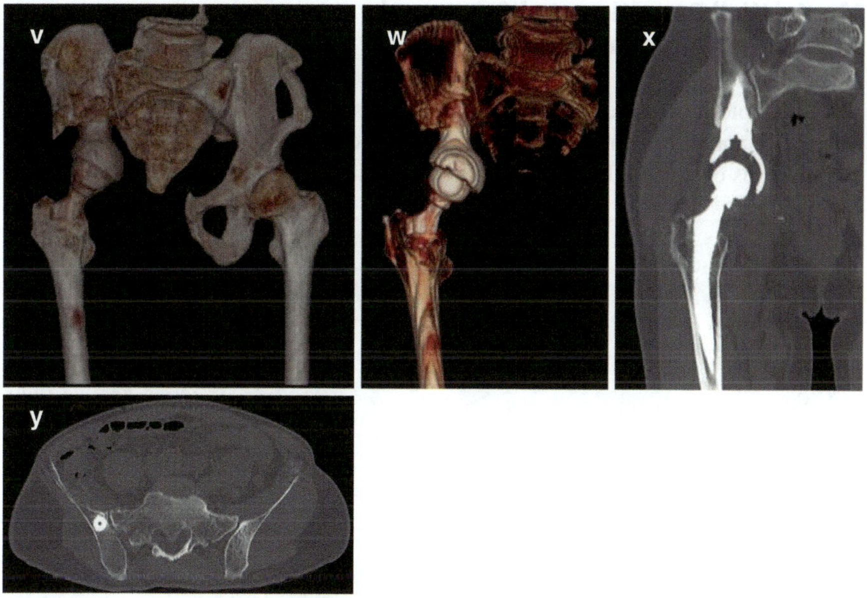

The use of acetabular lumic pedestal cup is a reliable reconstruction option which provides a stable hip joint. The hip centre of rotation, version and inclination of the acetabulum, and accurate offset must be accurately restored to achieve stability. Center position of the surface coatings stem must be aimed at the posterior column towards the sacroiliac joint parallel to the sacroiliac bar to provide fixation in the residual ilium (Fig. 3v–y).

Medial Wall Resection and Advanced Arthroplasty Reconstruction

A 40-year-old lady presented with a 6-month history of hip discomfort upon exertion. MRI and CT scans revealed lytic lesion confined to the medial wall with extraosseous extension. Biopsy confirmed chondrosarcoma grade II (Fig. 4a–j).

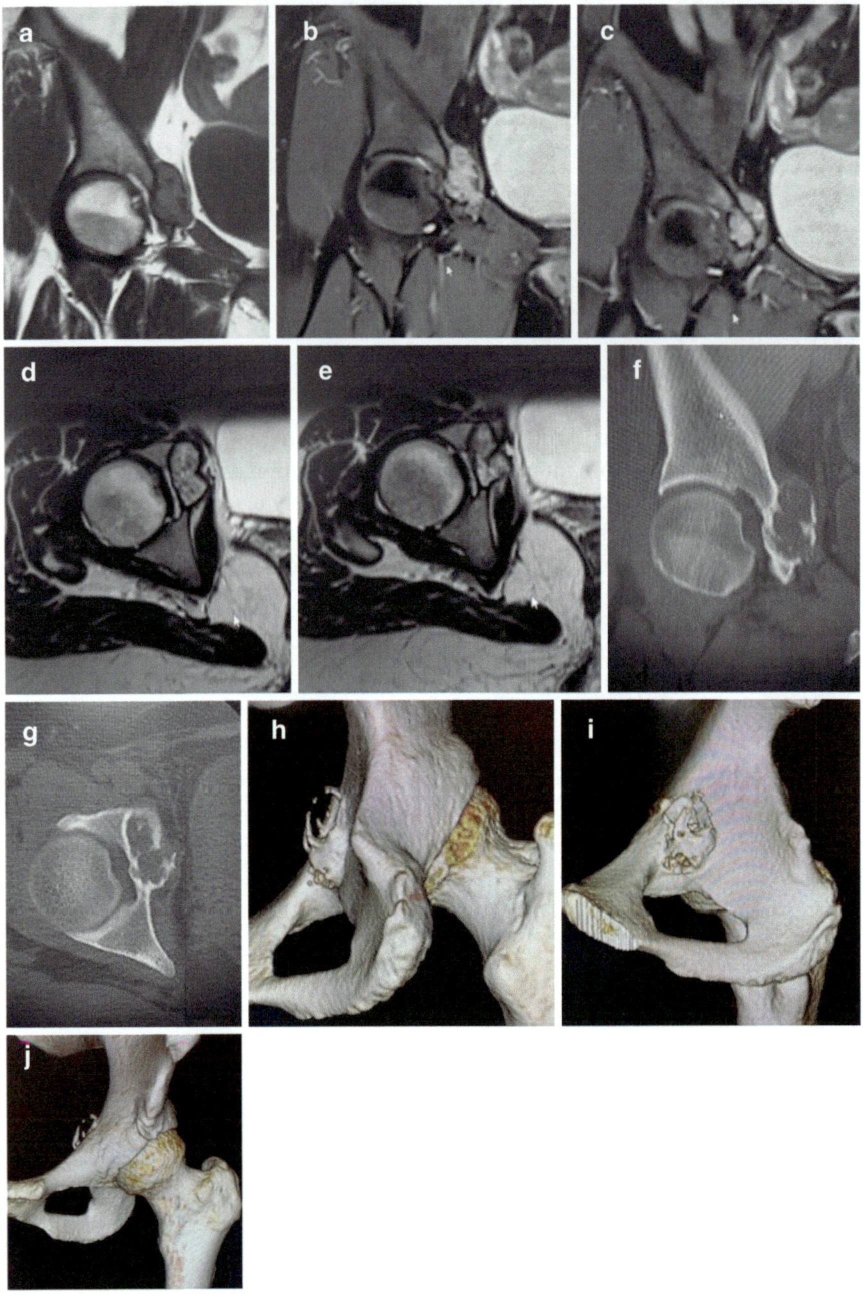

Sarcoma confined to the medial wall with preservation of the anterior and posterior columns of the acetabulum. In view of the findings, medial wall resection and hip joint reconstruction are planned by reusing the femoral head for impaction grafting and protection with cage.

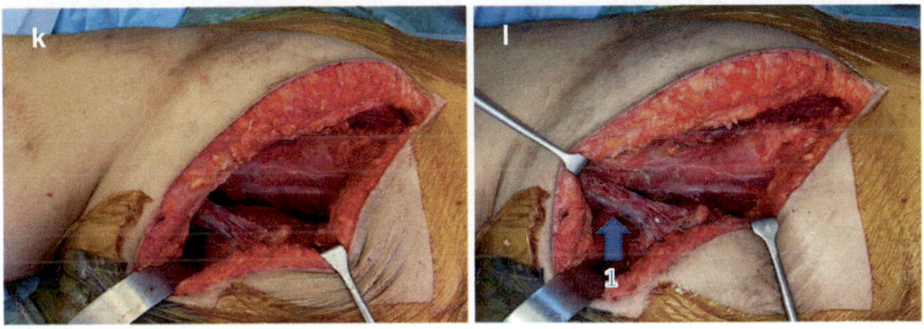

Creation of a mobile window by mobilisation of the external iliac vessels to approach the medial wall "quadrilateral plate" acetabulum. The obturator vessels and nerve mobilised prior to osteotomy were confirmed by image intensifier with surrounding osseous margin (Fig. 4k–n).

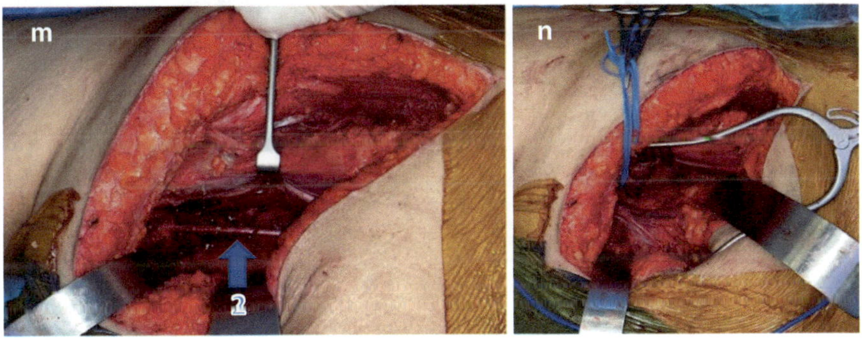

1. External iliac vessels
2. Obturator vessels and nerve

Impaction bone grafting using the remaining femoral head and protection with mesh wire and cages for cemented acetabulum replacement (Fig. 4o–r).

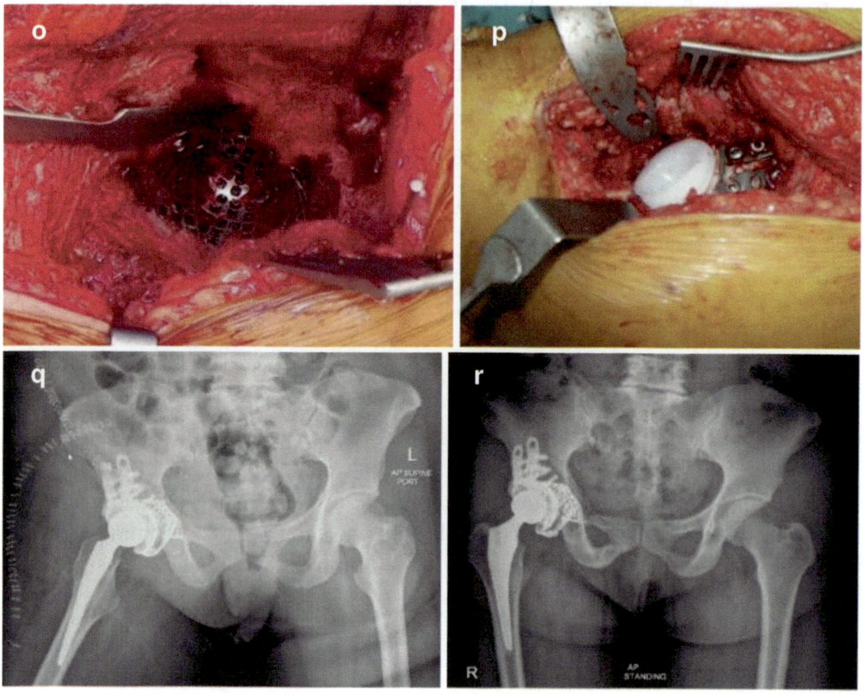
o
p
q
L
r
R

Peri-acetabulum GCT with Extensive Adductor Muscle Extension and Involvement

A 56-year-old lady with giant cell tumour peri acetabulum with proximal adductor involvement that responded well to 6 cycles of denosumab and was planned for resection (Fig. 5a–g).

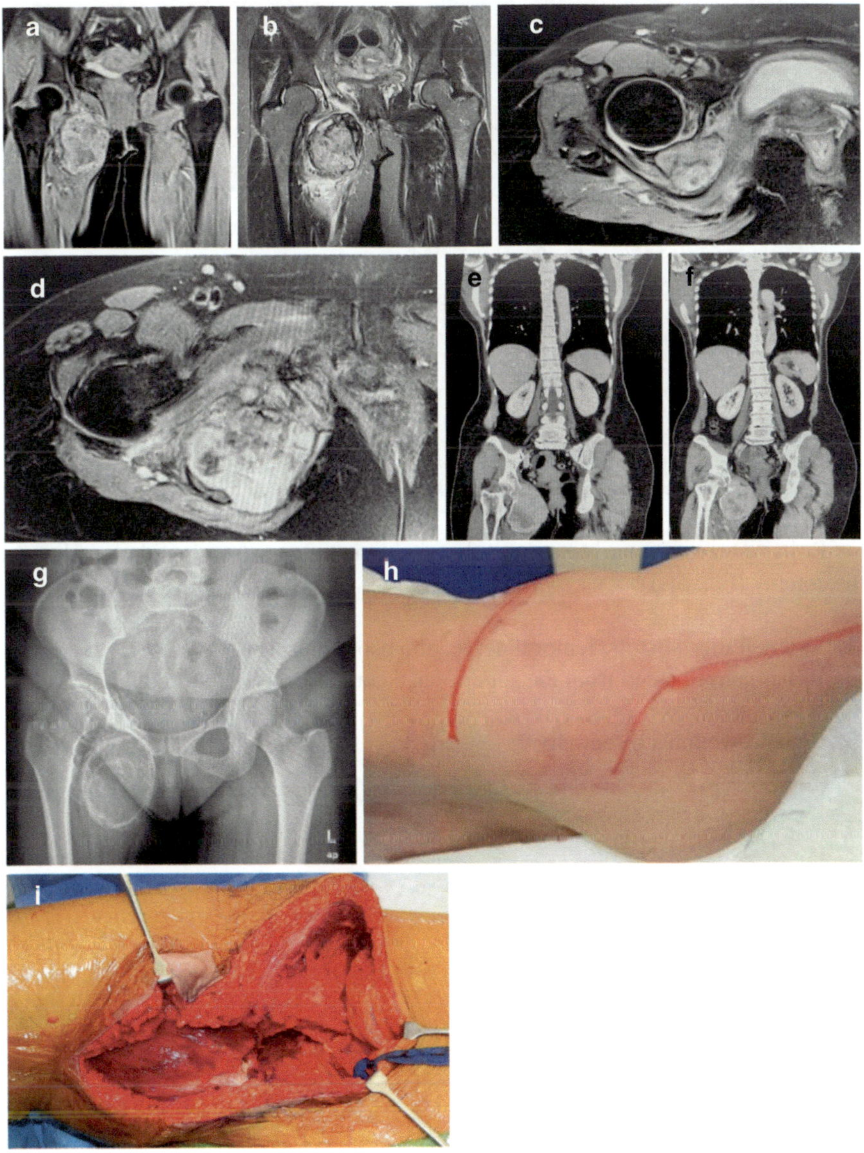

Incision was designed to expose the entire inner pelvis and proximal adductor muscle group. The proximal adductor was planned to be removed in total with the pubic rami at the symphysis pubis and the entire ischium (Fig. 5h–i).

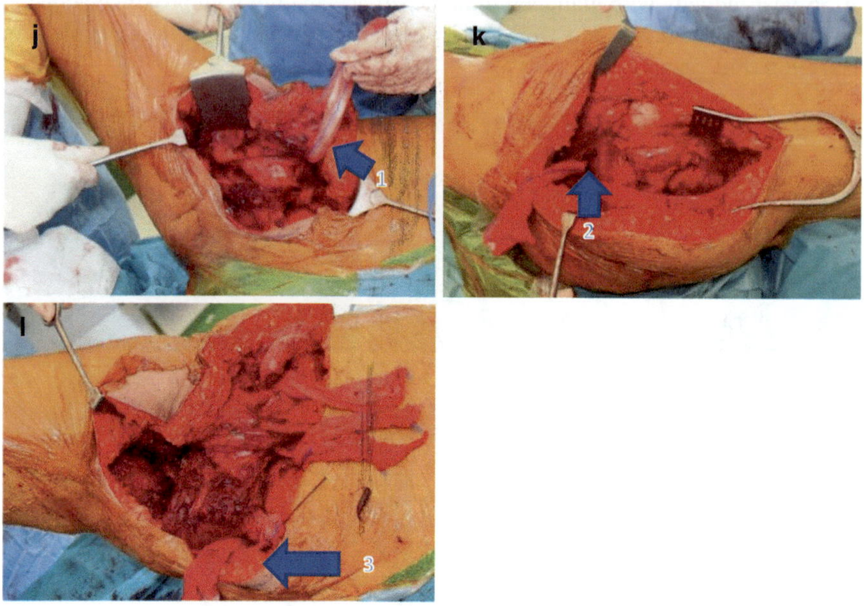

Roller gauze was used to protect the vital structures and as a guide for planned osteotomy (Fig. 5j–l)

1. External iliac vessels, femoral nerve, and psoas muscle
2. Roller gauze passed from the superior acetabulum anteriorly through the greater sciatic notch
3. Symphysis pubis osteotomy

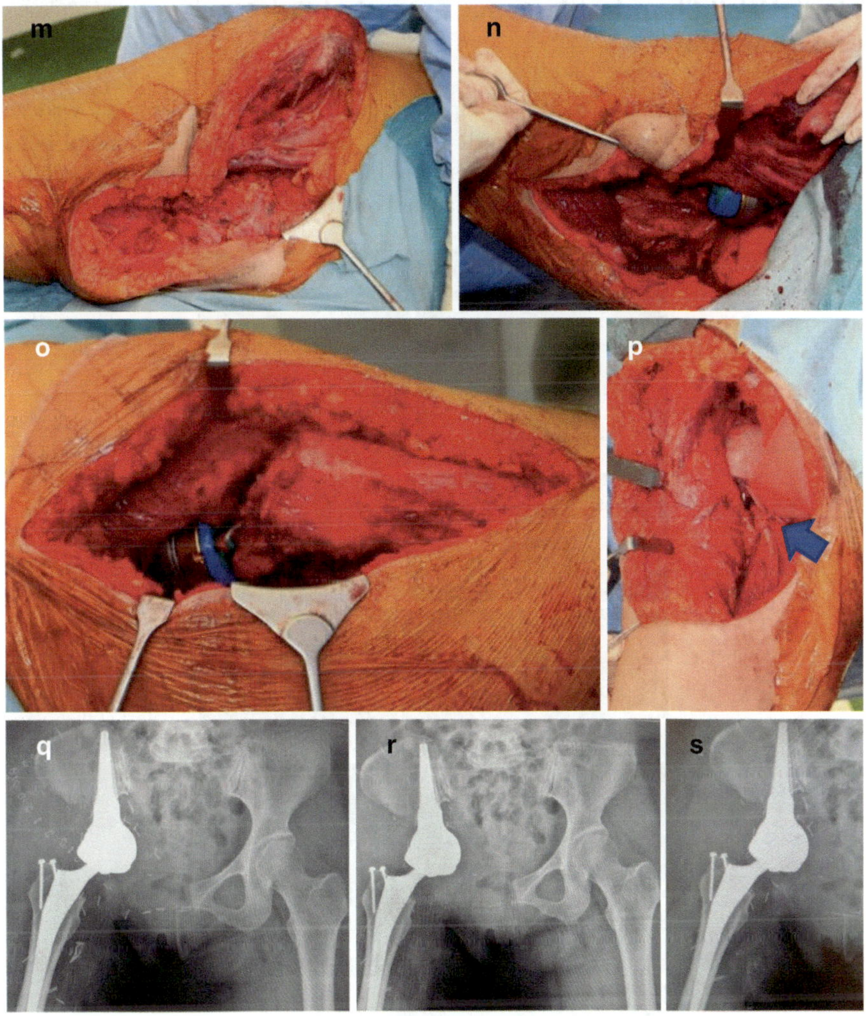

Evaluation of neurovascular, soft tissue tension and hip stability with trial implant is important step for good hip functional outcome and minimize nerve and vessels complication secondary to over distraction (Fig. 5m–o). Trevira 'soft tissue attachment' tube use to wrapped Lumic articulation and reconstruction of the pelvic floor over the adductor origin defect (Fig. 5p). Cementless prosthesis with symmetrical centre of hip rotation X-ray and stable implant on 5-years follow-up (Fig. 5q–s)

Medial Wall Chondroblastoma: Extended Curettage and Bone Graft

A 23-year-old man with a painful hip on weight bearing; an x-ray showed an expansile lesion over the medial wall of the acetabulum. The subchondral bone remained intact, with no soft tissue extension (Fig. 6a–h). The surgical approach for extended curettage is within external iliac and obturator vessels (Fig. 6i–l).

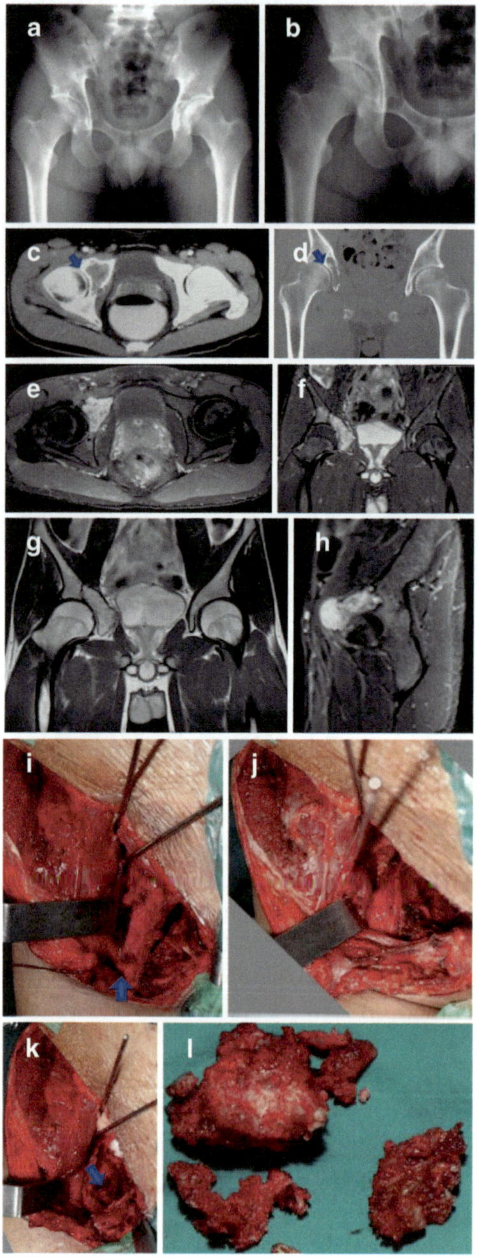

- External iliac vessels
- Subchondral bone after extended curettage

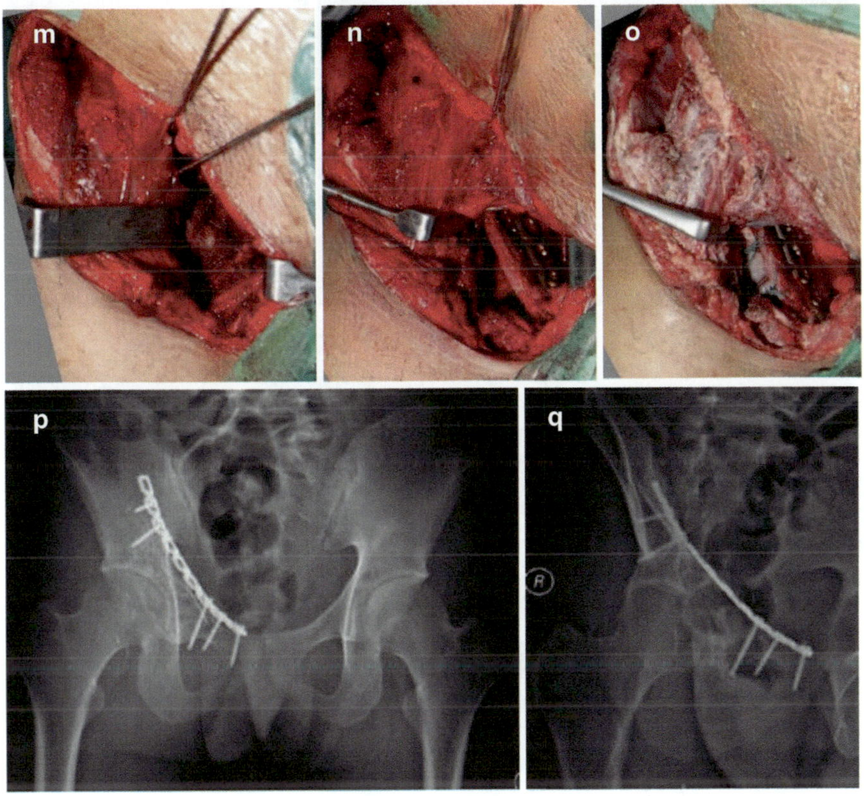

Adjuvant over tumour bed at subchondral bone using argon diathermy and 100% alcohol pack with gauze to minimise irritation of the pelvic organ. Medial wall was recreated by unicortical pelvic autograft and stabilised with plate and screw. The bone defect was packed with combination of allograft and autograft (Fig. 6m–q). 10 years after surgery, x-rays showed equal joint space, and he had no limitation of function (Fig. 6r–v).

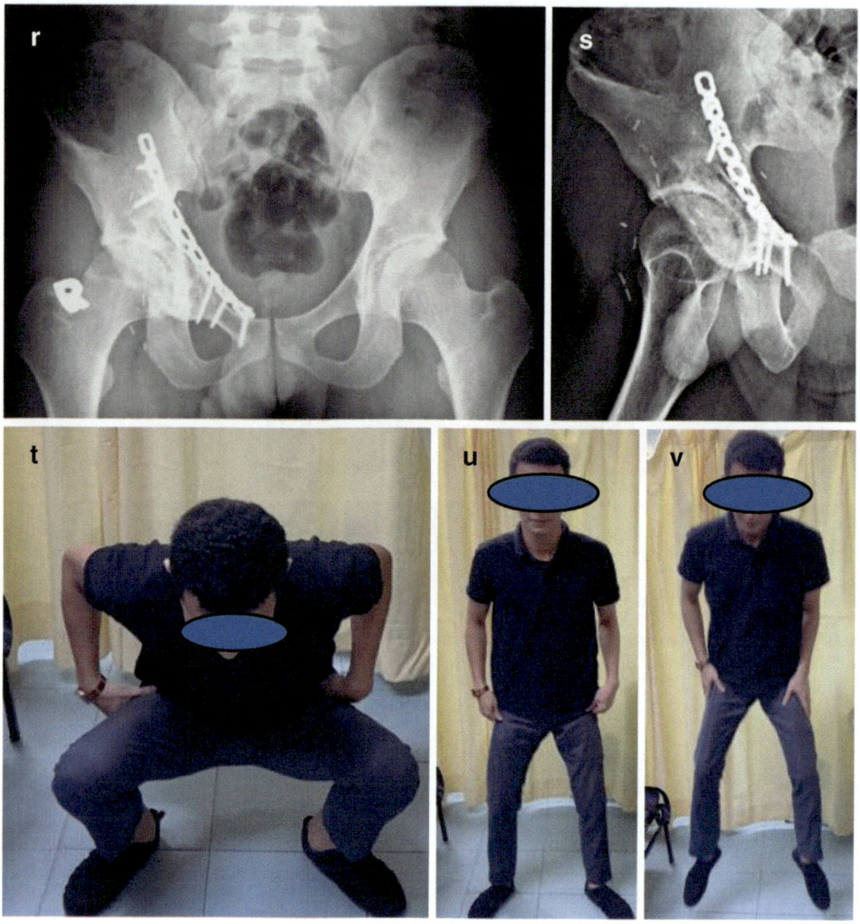
r
R
s
t
u
v

Acknowledgement The author thanks Professor Zulmi Wan, Dr Suryasmi Duski, Dr Lim Chiao Yee, Dr Mohd Salahuddin Abdul Latif and Dr Choong Chee Leong from Hospital Kuala Lumpur for their contributions and team members for management of the patients in this chapter.

Suggested Reading

1. Hipfl C, Stihsen C, Puchner SE, Kaider A, Dominkus M, Funovics PT, Windhage R. Pelvic reconstruction following resection of malignant bone tumours using a stemmed acetabular pedestal cup. J Bone Joint J. 2017;99-B:841–8.
2. Park H, Shah AA, Hornicek FJ. Innovative techniques in pelvic reconstructions. In: Surgery for pelvic bone tumour. Springer Nature; 2021. p. 123–34.
3. Kristy L. Weber Saddle Prosthesis. In: Master techniques in orthopaedic surgery orthopaedic oncology and complex reconstruction. Lippincott Williams & Wilkins, A Wolters Kluwer; 2011. p. 55–67.
4. Bus MPA, van de Sande MAJ. Implant reconstruction of the pelvis: II: modular pedestal cup prosthesis. In: Orthopaedic surgical oncology for bone tumors. Springer Nature Switzerland; 2022. p. 105–11.
5. Dominkus M, Katz R. Pelvic prosthesis. In: Master techniques in orthopaedic surgery orthopaedic oncology and complex reconstruction. Lippincott Williams & Wilkins, A Wolters Kluwer; 2011. p. 43–55.
6. Michaël PA, Szafranski A, Sellevold S, Goryn T, Jutte PC, Bramer JAM, Fiocco M, Streitbürger A, Kotrych D, van de Sande MAJ, Dijkstra PDS. LUMiC endoprosthetic reconstruction after periacetabular tumor resection: short-term results. Clin Orthop Relat Res. 2017;475:686–95.
7. Lackman RD, Crawford EA, Hosalkar HS, King JJ, Christian M. Ogilvie internal hemipelvectomy for pelvic sarcomas using a T-incision surgical approach. Clin Orthop Relat Res. 2009;467:2677–84.
8. Brown TS, Salib CG, Rose PS, Sim FH, Lewallen DG, Abdel MP. Reconstruction of the hip after resection of periacetabular oncological lesions a systematic review. Bone Joint J. 2018;100-B(1 Supple A):22–30.
9. Niu X, Hairong X. Biological reconstruction of the pelvis: II: femoral head plus total hip replacement. In: Orthopaedic surgical oncology for bone tumors. Springer Nature Switzerland; 2022. p. 85–95.

Modified Olier Approach for Type II and Type III Pelvic Resection and Reconstruction

Kumaran Rasappan, Danielle Maes, Vineet Kurisunkal, and Lee Jeys

Introduction

Ollier was the first to describe the lateral trans-trochanteric approach to the hip joint in 1881, which was subsequently popularised by Sir John Charnley and was primarily used for revision arthroplasty, which required a good exposure of the hip joint. Internal hemipelvectomy refers to the resection of all or part of the innominate bone whilst preserving the ipsilateral lower limb. We aim to describe a modified Ollier's approach to the hip and pelvis which enables the surgeon to perform wide and safe type II and type III resections for bone and soft-tissue tumours while providing to offering excellent exposure and allowing safe dissection of the neurovascular structures.

Surgical Anatomy

- In 1978, Enneking and Dunham published a classification system for the resection of pelvic sarcomas, based on the margins of the resection (wide or radical) and the fragment or fragments of bone removed.
- They described three types of resections: the iliac bone (Type I), the periacetabular region (Type II) and the pubis (Type III).
- Surgery was performed through a utilitarian incision that provided adequate exposure but could not avoid delayed wound healing or infectious complications.

K. Rasappan (✉)
National University Hospital, Singapore, Singapore

D. Maes
Queen Elizabeth Hospital NHS Trust, Birmingham, UK

V. Kurisunkal · L. Jeys
Royal Orthopaedic Hospital NHS Trust, Birmingham, UK

A. Puri, W. F. N. B. W. Ismail (eds.), *Atlas of Orthopedic Oncology Volume 1*,
https://doi.org/10.1007/978-981-95-8958-6_18

- Later on, the "reverse Y" approach and the lateral T-incision approach were described, aiming to provide a more extensile view and safer dissection by keeping the neurovascular bundle away from the surgical field.
- However, the complication rates using these approaches remain high, and the intersection of the two incisions appears to be particularly prone to wound complications.
- The modified Ollier's approach consists of a single, curved incision with pedicle-based flaps to ensure adequate wound healing and minimise the risk of wound necrosis.

Indications

- Primary bone sarcomas, soft tissue sarcomas and metastatic bone disease involving the periacetabular bone, superior pubic ramus, inferior pubic ramus, ischium and proximal femur, either separately or as a combination of segments as described by Enneking and Dunham, as well as selected cases for which extra-articular hip resections are required.
- Segments of this approach could be used for cases of severe trauma or osteomyelitis.

Contraindications

- Isolated type I pelvic resection
- Combined pelvic resections where type I and/or type IV resections are required
- Total hemipelvectomy (types I, II, and III +/– type IV)

Two cases where the modified Ollier's approach was utilised for resection of bone tumours. (Figure 1a–c): Pre-op X-ray, MRI scan and post-op X-ray of a patient with right periacetabular chondrosarcoma. (Figure 2a–c): Pre-op X-ray, MRI scan and post-op X-ray of a patient with osteosarcoma of the right proximal femur with intra-articular extension into the hip joint.

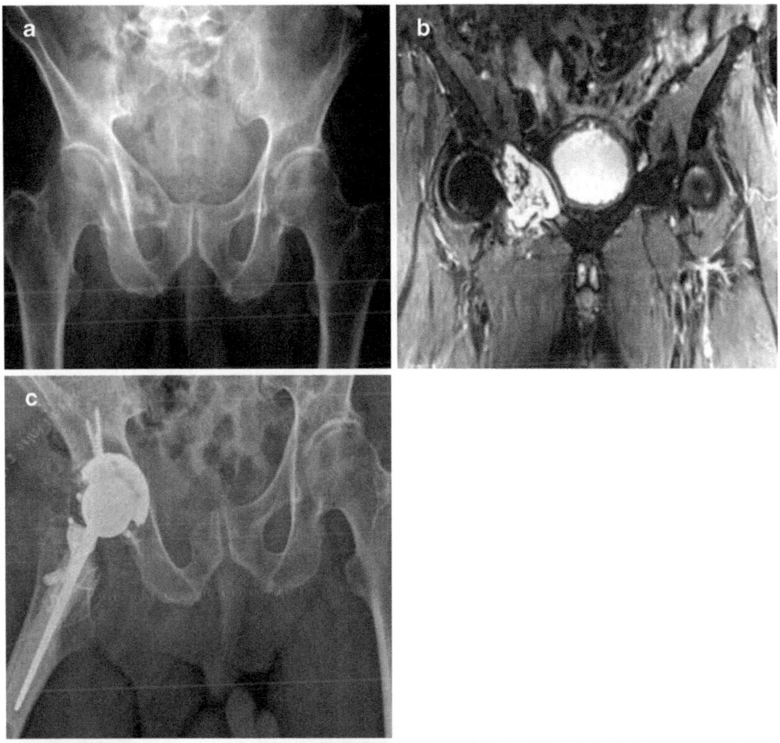
a
b
c

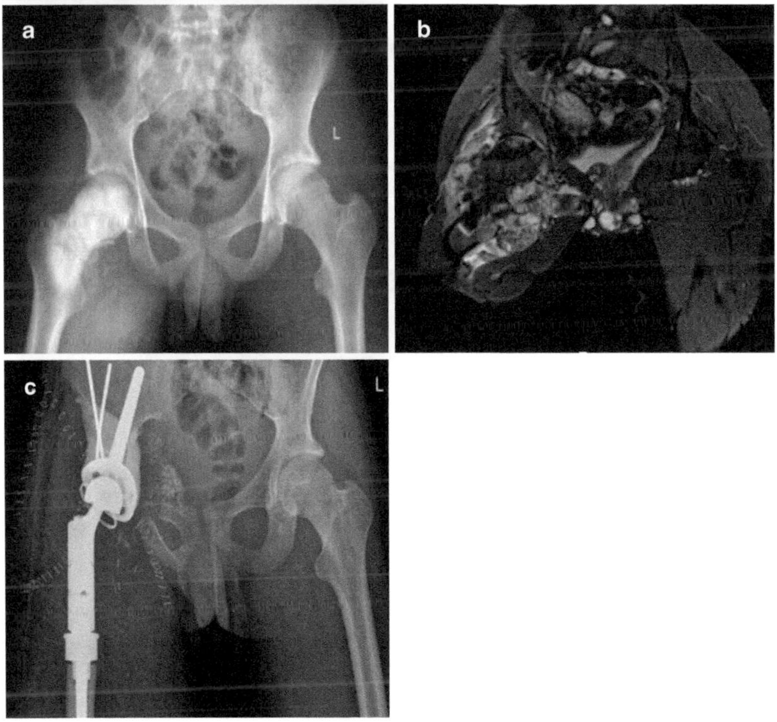
a
b
L
c
L

Surgical Technique

Setup

Adequate anaesthesia in combination with spinal anaesthesia and/or the insertion of an epidural catheter, to ensure adequate postoperative pain relief, is carried out prior to patient positioning. It is recommended to discuss the positioning of the epidural catheter with the anaesthetist in charge to prevent indwelling epidural catheters from intruding into the surgical field. The hypotensive epidural anaesthesia technique should be considered throughout surgery for less blood loss and the need for fewer transfusions. A urinary catheter is always inserted to monitor urinary output during and after the procedure. It can also provide guidance during the procedure to prevent any unintended laceration of the urinary tract. Prophylactic intravenous antibiotics are administered thirty minutes prior to skin incision and are continued until five days postoperatively, in line with the local hospital's policy.

Position

The patient is positioned in a floppy lateral position to be able to access both the anterior and posterior columns of the pelvis. This involves using a secured sandbag anteriorly at the level of the umbilicus and a secured bolster posteriorly at the thoracolumbar junction. Adhesive exclusion drapes are placed from the groin to the umbilicus to the lumbar region and to the natal cleft, thus isolating the affected limb and hemi pelvis for surgery. The contralateral leg is well padded at the level of the fibular head to prevent neurapraxia, and between the knees, this leg can be strapped to the operation table to secure the patient during surgery.

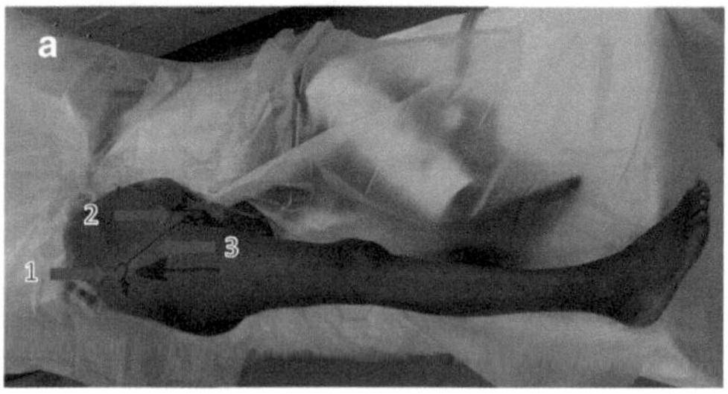

Patient in floppy lateral position with exclusion drapes in place and landmarks drawn for the modified Ollier approach (Fig. 3a)

1. ASIS
2. Pubic Tubercle
3. Inguinal Ligament

Incision

The incision is planned based on bony as well as soft tissue landmarks. The bony landmarks to be identified are the posterior superior iliac spine (PSIS), the greater trochanter (GT), the anterior superior iliac spine (ASIS), and the pubic tubercle (PT). The soft tissue landmark is the course of the adductor longus muscle along the medial thigh if there is a significant mass in the adductor compartment. In case of an oncological diagnosis, the biopsy tract is integrated and excised through the planned skin incision. Anteriorly, the skin incision runs along the groin from the ASIS to the PT and then curves medially along the course of the adductor longus muscle. Lateral and posterior, the incision runs from the ASIS towards the GT and can be extended in the direction of the PSIS to obtain access to the ischium (Fig. 3a). It is important to avoid sharp corners in the incision, and a sweeping, curved incision in an 'S' shape rather than a 'Z' shape is used to prevent flap necrosis at the tips of the flaps. The authors believe this is an advantage of this approach over the extended ilioinguinal approach with a T-incision or 'Mercedes Benz' incision popularised by Malawer and colleagues.

Approach

Anterior Limb of the Approach, Superficial Dissection

Firstly, the anterior or inguinal limb of the skin incision is made. The skin is raised in one layer together with the subcutaneous fat in order to avoid problems with wound healing. The first layer encountered is the abdominal wall fascia (aponeurosis of external oblique). The fascia is opened in line with the skin incision. Identifying the external iliac ring in a male is an important landmark. Performing the dissection in the plane of the spermatic cord can aid safe dissection in a plane away from the external iliac vessels. After dividing the external oblique in line with the muscle fibres, the rectus abdominis muscle is identified medially and transected at its origin on the superior pubic ramus. Laterally, the abdominal muscles are cut in layers i.e. external oblique, internal oblique muscle and rectus abdominis, and detached from the iliac crest. Hereafter, the inferior epigastric artery, a branch of the external iliac artery, can be found traversing the surgical field to anastomose with the superior epigastric branch, which can be isolated and ligated. In the depth of this layer, the round ligament of the uterus in female patients or the cord structures in male patients can be identified, as well as the external iliac vessels. The relationship between the inguinal ligament and the neurovascular bundle can be visualised at this point (Fig. 3b).

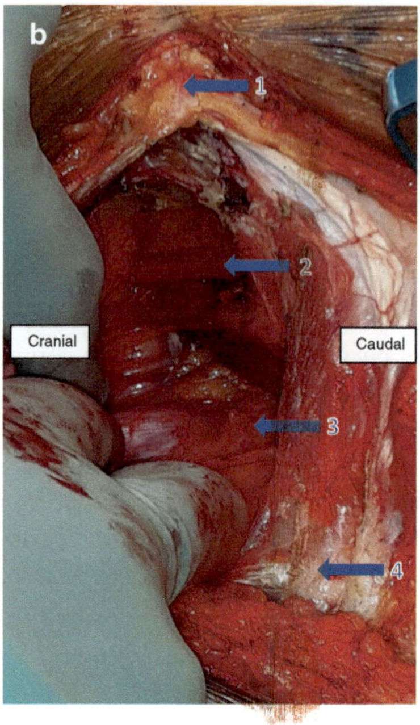

Anterior limb of the approach (superficial dissection)

1. ASIS
2. External Iliac Vessels
3. Round Ligament of Uterus
4. Pubic Tubercle

Posterior Limb of the Approach, Superficial Dissection

Secondly, the skin incision is extended from the ASIS to below the GT and further curved posteriorly in the direction of the PSIS. Fasciocutaneous flaps are raised on both sides of the incision, and the gluteus maximus can be released at its femoral insertion. A plane can be developed between the gluteus maximus and gluteus minimus muscles anteriorly. If additional access to the anterior column of the pelvis is required, the gluteus minimus muscle, and if needed the gluteus medius muscle, can be released from their origins on the posterior surface of the ileum. Subsequently, a plane is developed between the gluteus minimus/medius muscle posteriorly and the sartorius and rectus muscle anteriorly. After applying a stay suture, the inguinal ligament, sartorius and the straight head of the rectus femoris muscles can be detached from their origin i.e. the ASIS and anterior inferior iliac spine (AIIS), respectively (Fig. 3c). This manoeuvre gives access to the iliopsoas muscle, which can be found exiting the pelvis to insert onto the lesser trochanter, as well as access to the femoral sheath. Underneath lies the reflected head of the rectus muscle, in close relationship to the anterior capsule of the hip joint. Either a stay suture can be applied, and the muscle can be retained, or it can be transsected and kept as a margin on the resection specimen. The femoral vessels are located medial to the iliopsoas muscle belly.

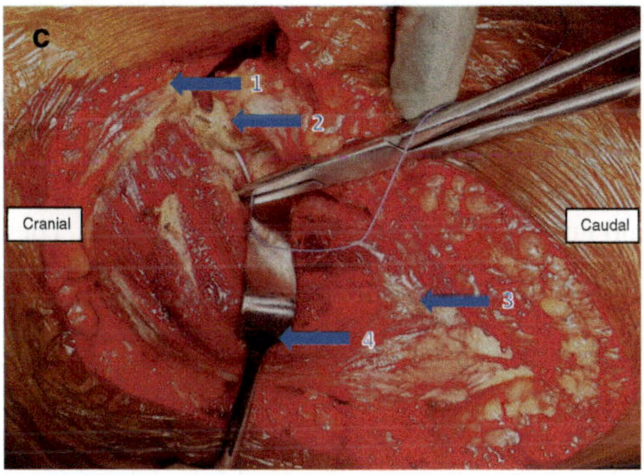

Posterior limb of the approach (superficial dissection)

1. ASIS
2. Inguinal ligament and sartorius attachment to ASIS
3. Greater trochanter
4. Gluteus maximus

Anterior Limb of the Approach, Deep Dissection

Returning to the anterior limb of the incision, the iliopsoas muscle can be mobilised in order to identify the femoral nerve between the two muscle bellies, and a plane can be created between the psoas and iliacus muscles or between the iliacus muscle and the inner table of the ilium, depending on the planned resection margins on the tumour. Usually, the iliacus muscle is regarded as an oncological surgical margin, to be resected along with the specimen if the tumour is involving the iliac bone and/or the periacetabular bone. Deeper dissection involves retracting the external iliac vessels laterally, which gives access to the obturator nerve and vessels, which can be ligated at this point if required based on the extent of the tumour. Mobilising the external iliac vessels can be undertaken in two ways, depending on the tumour position. If a close margin is acceptable on the superior pubic ramus, then the vessels (within the femoral sheath), nerve and iliopsoas can be mobilised en bloc by creating a tunnel utilising the psoas bursa. A loop is tunnelled around the femoral vessels and nerve, including the iliopsoas muscle, in order to be able to localise and mobilise these important structures at all times (Fig. 3d). This technique allows safe mobilisation of the structures but provides only a narrow margin on the bone. If there is soft tissue mass directly underneath the vessels, then the vessels need to be mobilised by incising the inguinal ligament and the superficial femoral sheath, mobilising the vessels out of sheath and leaving the deep structures as a margin on the tumour. This is more technically challenging, and the surgeon needs to be aware of branches from the posterior aspect of the femoral vessels which would need to be ligated prior to mobilising the vascular bundle. The vessels can then be mobilised laterally or medially, depending on which part of the dissection is being performed.

The medial limb of the anterior incision can then be further developed in line with the posterior border of the adductor longus muscle. The adductor muscles are dissected free and transsected either at their origin on the pubis or distally depending on whether there is a tumour mass in the adductors. In the proximal thigh, the obturator vessels and nerve are identified and can be ligated. These steps ensure that the obturator foramen is gradually being freed up. Medially, further dissection is carried out to expose the pubic symphysis or contralateral pubic ramus, depending on the preoperative planning. Often the resection planning is confined to the pubic symphysis, which may be identified intraoperatively with blunt dissection and is separated using a Gigli saw or an osteotome (Fig. 3e). At this point, the urinary bladder, urethra and abdominal viscera are at high risk of inadvertent injury, and care must be taken to protect these structures by palpating the catheter and then placing abdominal mops and abdominal retractors. As the pubis is now more mobile, the inferior pubic ramus can be exposed as well and can be resected as per planned margins, using either a Gigli saw or osteotome. This step must be carried out cautiously, protecting and retracting the urinary bladder and urethra, which are structures at risk during pelvic oncology surgery. These structures can often be found close to or abutting the tumour medially, hence getting stretched and inadvertently injured during the resection.

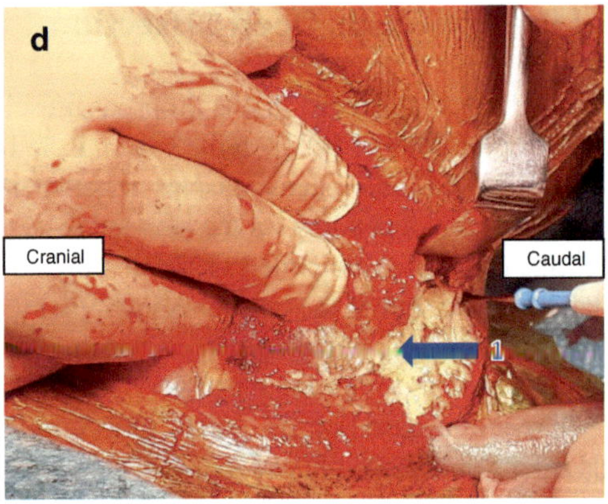

Anterior limb of the approach (deep dissection)

1. Posterior border of adductor longus muscle

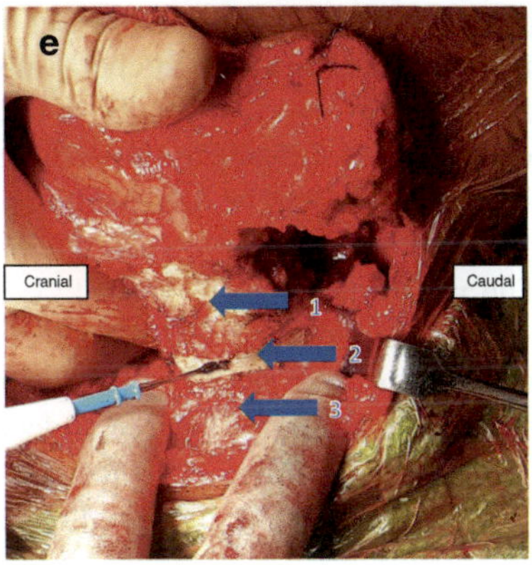

Anterior limb of the approach (deep dissection) (Fig. 3e).

1. Contralateral pubic ramus
2. Pubic symphysis
3. Ipsilateral pubic ramus

Posterior Limb of the Approach, Deep Dissection

In order to gain access to the posterior column of the pelvis in the periacetabular area, the surgical approach is like the posterior approach to the hip as described by Moore, releasing the piriformis muscle, the obturator internus muscle and short external rotator muscles from the posterior border of the femur after applying a stay suture, thereby protecting the sciatic nerve by mobilising it more posteriorly. If a more extensive exposure of the iliac bone is required in this area, the gluteus medius and minimus muscles can be detached either from their origins on the surface of the ileum or by performing a trans-trochanteric osteotomy remaining extra-articular if required (Fig. 3f). The authors recommend using a Gigli saw for more control and accuracy—moving the saw in a direction away from the joint—in performing a Chevron osteotomy, as first described by Charnley, which helps for subsequent trochanteric reattachment. Alternatively, osteotomes or an oscillating saw blade can be used. Depending on the extent of the tumour, the periacetabular osteotomy can be performed through the inner table of the pelvis, using the plane between the iliacus muscle and iliac bone. In case the tumour extends into the acetabular roof, without joint involvement, it is safer to dislocate the hip and to perform the osteotomies through the acetabular cartilage or proceed to an extra-articular hip resection if the joint is involved. In case the proximal femur is equally involved by tumour, resection of the proximal femur can also be performed through this approach, with or without a trochanteric slide osteotomy.

If the extent of the tumour requires resection of the ischiopubic ramus and ischial tuberosity, the posterior limb of the incision can be extended towards the sacrum, in the direction of the PSIS, as per a Kocher-Langenbeck approach. The gluteus maximus, already partially everted, is split in line with its muscle fibres and everted posteriorly, up to the level where the pedicle of the inferior gluteal vessel allows it. A greater exposure can be achieved by mobilising the abductor muscles, either by performing a trochanteric slide osteotomy or a standard trochanteric osteotomy. The piriformis muscle, already detached from the femur when performing the posterior approach to the hip, can be mobilised proximally, providing access to the sciatic notch (greater sciatic foramen) through which the sciatic nerve, superior and inferior gluteal nerves, vessels and pudendal nerve exit the pelvis. A blunt retractor is placed with caution within the foramen in order to protect the neurovascular bundle. The ischial spine can be traced distally, and the sacrospinous ligament can be released from the bone or the ligament can be released by cutting a little sliver of bone from the ischial spine by using a small osteotome. This manoeuvre gives access to the lesser sciatic foramen. Care must be taken not to injure the pudendal nerve exiting the greater sciatic foramen and re-entering the lesser sciatic foramen. The sacrotuberous ligament is then released from the ischial tuberosity. The superficial transverse perineal muscle and ischiocavernosus muscle are released from the inner aspect of the ischiopubic ramus, and the semitendinosus muscle, semimembranosus muscle and long head of the biceps femoris muscle are detached at their origins on the ischial tuberosity, allowing resection of the ischiopubic ramus. When performing dissection in proximity to the ischiorectal fossa, care must be taken to avoid damage to the rectum.

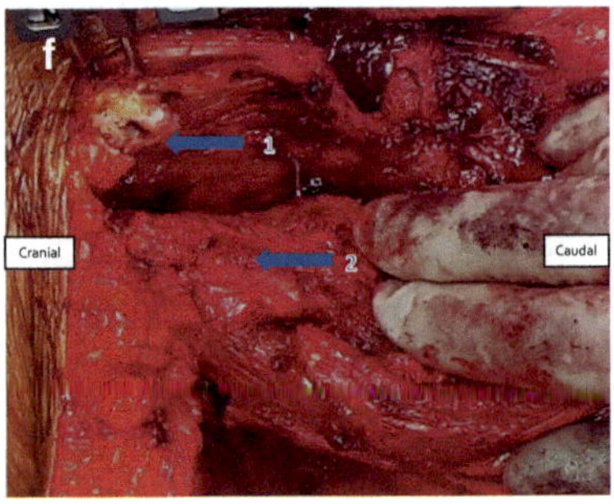

Posterior limb of the approach (deep dissection)

1. Outer table of iliac crest
2. Gluteus medius

Reconstruction

Reconstruction of the pelvic defect is highly dependent on the extent of the bony resection. If the osteotomy in the acetabular area was performed from the inner table of the pelvis and the femoral head has been preserved, limited medial wall acetabular defects can be biologically reconstructed by use of a human acellular dermal regenerative tissue matrix (Graftjacket; Wright Medical Technology, Hertfordshire, UK) which is fixed to the inner table of the pelvis using bone anchors. If the femoral head has been resected and a sufficient amount of acetabular bone has been preserved, a primary total hip replacement can be used to reconstruct the defect. In case the acetabulum has been completely resected, a pedestal cup or ice cream cone can be inserted in the remaining ilium. A dual mobility cup or a constrained acetabular liner could be used together with a femoral intramedullary stem or proximal femoral endoprosthesis to restore leg length. This could be coupled with additional stabilisation by suturing the soft tissues to a Trevira tube (MUTARS® attachment tube, Mutars® Implantcast). Other reconstruction options include performing a hip transposition or the use of a custom-made hemipelvis prosthesis or total acetabular allograft along with a total hip replacement.

Closure

After reconstruction, the gluteus medius and minimus muscles are reattached to their origins on the ilium, if possible, and the sartorius and rectus femoris muscles to the ASIS and AIIS, respectively, using transosseous sutures. If the bone has been removed, then these can be reattached to the abdominal wall to increase function and stability. The inguinal ligament is sutured to the residual gluteal and abdominal muscles, and the wound is closed in layers over two negative suction drains (Fig. 3g). A Vacuum Assisted Closure (VAC) dressing is applied for a minimum of 5 days, and the wound is reviewed after this time (Fig. 3h).

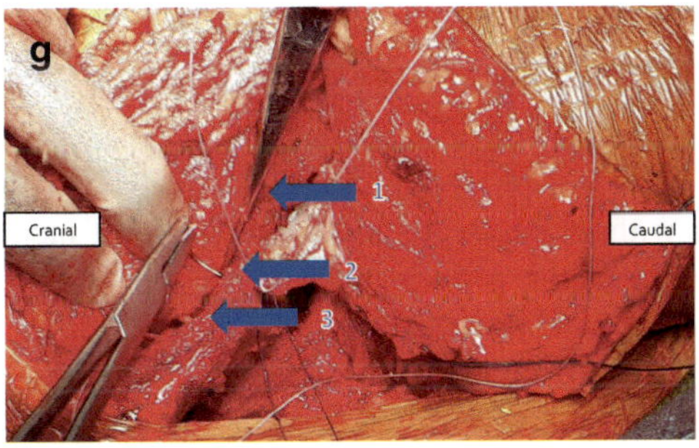

Closure

1. AIIS
2. Inguinal ligament and sartorius
3. ASIS

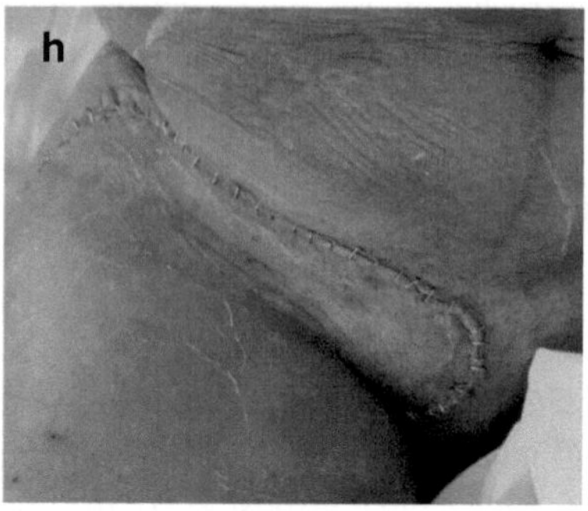

Status on wound review at 5 days post-operatively

Post-operative Care

Post-operatively, vital parameters should be monitored closely for at least 24 h in an intensive care or high dependency unit. Thromboembolic prevention is prescribed according to the hospital's guidelines. Initially, dietary intake is restricted to fluids only until proof of adequate bowel sounds, after which intake of solid food can be resumed gradually. Patients should be reviewed by a dietician during the perioperative period to ensure dietary requirements are met. Patients are prescribed five days of bed rest after which they are gradually mobilised. Weight-bearing status is dependent on the nature of the pelvic reconstruction. Regular wound reviews, in the first instance after 5 days, are required to ensure adequate wound healing is steadily being achieved.

Pearls

- Single incision
- Curved incision without intersecting incisions (i.e. no T-incision)
- Adequate exposure of the periacetabular bone, superior pubic ramus, inferior pubic ramus, ischium and proximal femur
- Pedicle-based flaps allowing for excellent wound healing

Pitfalls

- Limited exposure of the proximal iliac bone: not recommended for isolated type I pelvic resections, combined pelvic resections where type I and/or IV resections are required or total hemipelvectomies (type I, II and III +/- type IV)

- Potential for damage to the superior or inferior gluteal vessels exiting the notch, by excessive retraction or following an inadvertent injury, often associated with flap-related complications
- Familiarity with reattachment of GT required when performing trans-trochanteric osteotomy

Summary

From our experience, this surgical approach provides an extensile access to perform complex resections and reconstructions for the periacetabular area of the pelvis, pubic rami and ischium.

Suggested Reading

1. Ko JY, Wang CJ, Lin CF, Shih CH. Periacetabular osteotomy through a modified Ollier transtrochanteric approach for treatment of painful dysplastic hips. J Bone Joint Surg Am. 2002;84(9):1594 601.
2. Enneking WF, Dunham WK. Resection and reconstruction for primary neoplasms involving the innominate bone. J Bone Joint Surg Am. 1978;60:731–46.
3. https://sarcoma.surgery/pdf/approach_anterior_pelvis_enneking_type_III_resection.pdf

Type III Pelvic Resection

Wan Faisham Nu'man Bin Wan Ismail

Introduction

A classical type pelvis III resection involves the entire symphysis pubis, superior pubic rami and ischium. The acetabulum and pelvic brim are preserved. Type III hemipelvectomy encompasses resection of the ischio-pubic region area sparing the acetabulum. Reconstruction is not necessary. Functional outcome in these patients is good as the hip joint is maintained. Patients often return to functional activities as there is no loss of pelvic bony continuity between the acetabulum and sacrum.

Surgical Anatomy

The anterior pelvis brim consists of the symphysis pubis, superior pubic rami, and inferior pubic rami where both meet the medial acetabulum and ischium.

Important structures to be evaluated for osseous margin:

- Symphysis pubis as fibrocartilaginous structures are good as tumour barriers. This is important for partial or total resection of the anterior brim structures
- Superior and inferior pubic rami marrow extension for bony margin. Extension to the acetabulum and ischium needs to be evaluated prior to surgery, as different surgical approaches and reconstructions are required.

W. F. N. B. W. Ismail (✉)
Prince Court Medical Center, Kuala Lumpur, Malaysia

Orthopaedic Oncology Reconstructive Unit, Universiti Sains Malaysia, Kubang Kerian, Kelantan, Malaysia

A. Puri, W. F. N. B. W. Ismail (eds.), *Atlas of Orthopedic Oncology Volume 1*,
https://doi.org/10.1007/978-981-95-8958-6_19

Major vessels and nerve

- The femoral vessels and nerve cross the superior pubic rami below the inguinal ligament and are closely held to the bone by the femoral fascia.
- The obturator nerve and vessels enter the obturator fossae from the medial brim of the acetabulum to supply the adductor muscle of the thigh. Tumour extending to this obturator foreman requires sacrificing the nerve and subsequent adductor weakness.

The urethra passes closely below the symphysis pubis and is at risk during surgical procedures and needs to be protected. The urinary bladder is occasionally infiltrated by huge intrapelvic tumour and needs to be evaluated for oncological resection and bladder reconstruction.

Assessment

There are no definite anatomical boundaries for Type III resection. Tumours can grow intrapelvic and push the bladder without infiltration. The space of Retzius is a potential area for mobilisation of the bladder in posterior tumour extension. Areas can be pushed or directly infiltrated by anterior pelvic tumours, and this is an important part of the assessment to achieve oncological clearance.

- Symphysis pubis joint
- Lateral osseous extension of superior and inferior pubic rami
- Femoral neurovascular structures
- Abdominal wall insertion of rectus abdominis muscle
- Pectineus muscle
- Urinary bladder
- Urethra

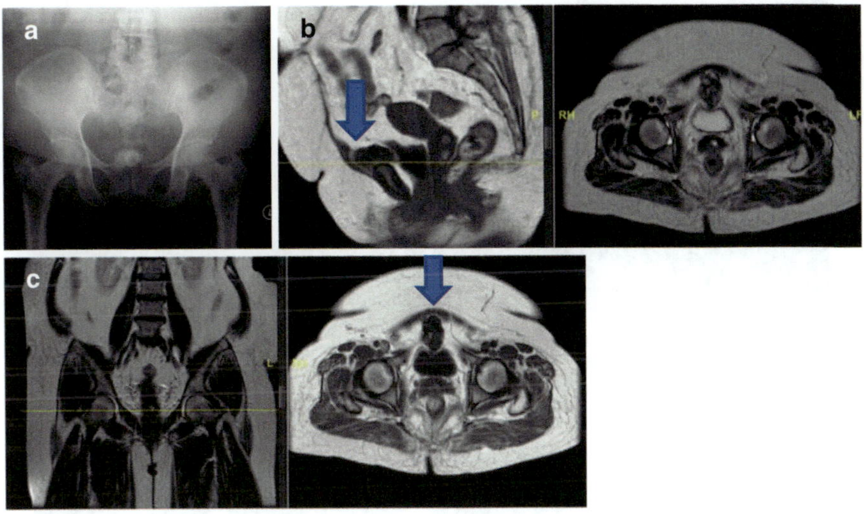

A 60-year-old lady presented with rapidly growing suprapubic mass. Radiograph revealed pedunculated bony mass at the symphysis pubis. The MRI showed a well-circumscribed lesion that was confined to the symphysis pubis and pushed the bladder. No evidence of involvement of local structures (Fig. 1a–c).

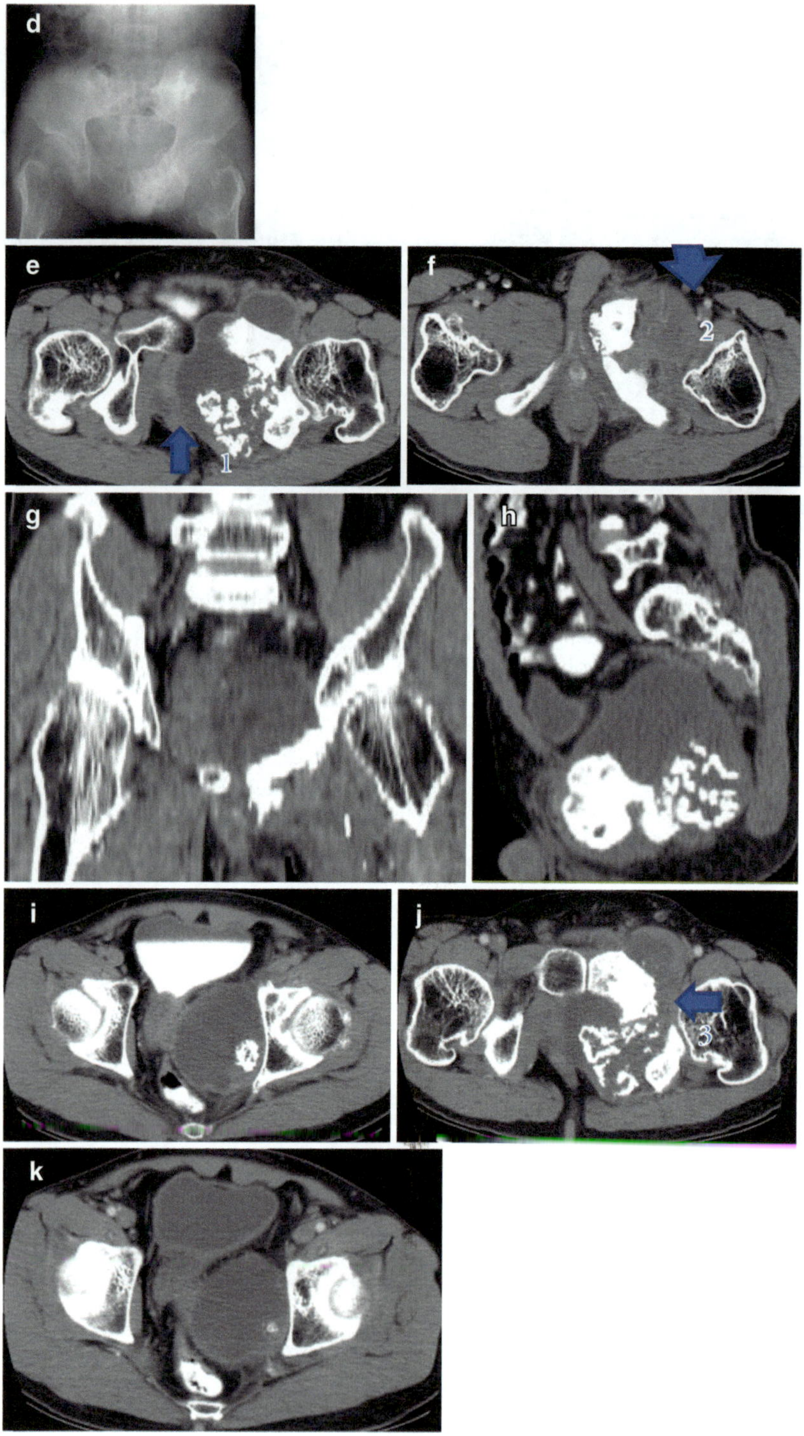
d
e
1
f
2
g
h
i
j
3
k

1. Crus penis—corpus spongiosum
2. Femoral vessels pushed by the tumour
3. Acetabulum involvement

Secondary chondrosarcoma in the superior pubic rami. The lesion arose from the superior pubic rami and extended to the acetabulum and inferior pubic rami to the ischium. The intrapelvic extension pushed the bladder and infiltrated the crura and corpus cavernosum of the penis. In view of extensive involvement, we decided for external hemipelvectomy (Fig. 1 d–k).

Surgical Steps

- Anterior ilioinguinal approach is planned for a retroperitoneal approach to the iliac vessels, femoral nerve exploration and mobilisation of the iliopsoas tendon laterally for visualisation of the medial pelvic wall
- The rectus femoris insertion is cut over the superior pubic rami with muscle margin to expose the space of Retzius for manipulation of the anterior bladder
- 3-window approach for mobilisation of vital structures anterior to the superior pubic rami
  - Iliopsoas tendon retracted laterally together with the femoral nerve
  - Middle mobile femoral vessels
  - Spermatic cord/broad ligament medially
- Perineal extension of the incision is used in large pubic lesions that will expose
  - Adductor origin—detached with good cuff of tissue margin
  - Entire inferior pubic rami to the ischium
  - Ischiorectal fossa
- The bladder neck is mobilised below the symphysis pubis from the inner and outer pelvis prior to osteotomy. Hohmann Muller bone spike lever or malleable retractor is used to protect the urethra and prevent injury.
- Lateral osteotomy based on osseous margin and usually includes part of the obturator membrane structure, including the obturator artery and nerve
- External iliac-obturator anastomosis 'corona mortise' should be identified and ligated prior to these procedure.

Abdominal wall defect must be reconstructed with Prolene mesh to prevent abdominal content hernia

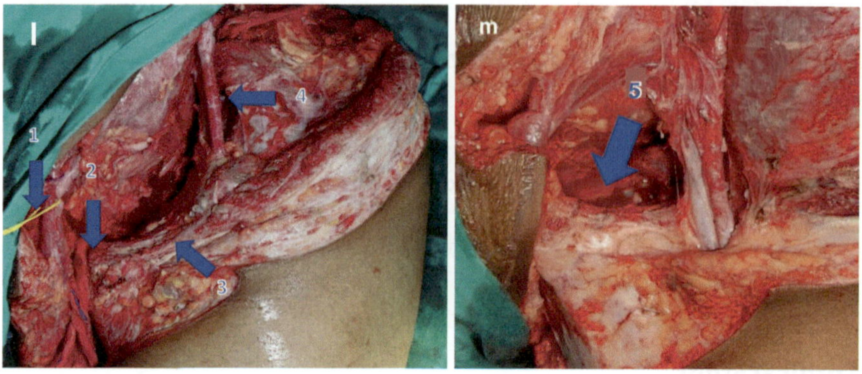

Overview ilioinguinal approach and major anatomical structures (Fig. 11, m)

1. Spermatic cord
2. Symphysis pubis—roller gauze passed through below symphysis pubis
3. Superior pubic rami
4. Iliac vessels
5. Bladder

Chondrosarcoma Symphysis Pubis

Chondrosarcoma at the superior pubic rami and symphysis pubis with posterior extension to the Retzius space with a clear plane with the bladder. The entire symphysis pubis and part of the ischium are removed to achieve good oncological margin (Fig. 2a–c).

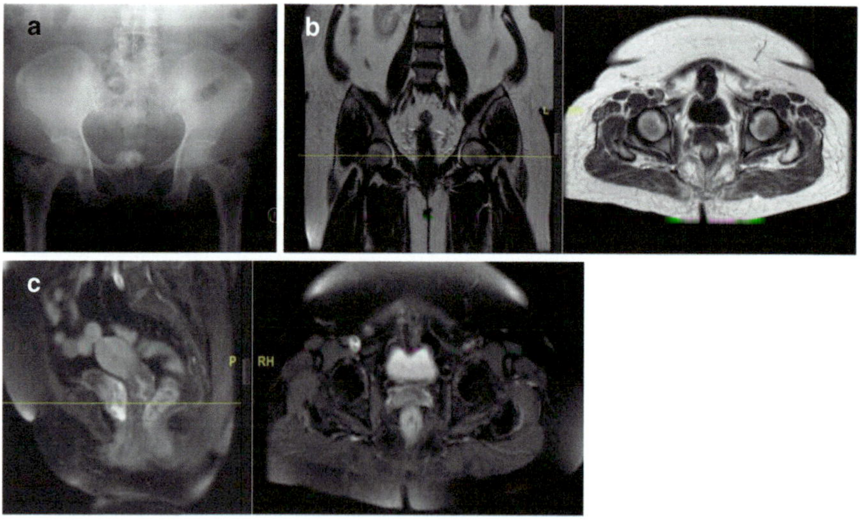

The external oblique aponeurosis is exposed by elevating the subcutaneous tissue. Broad ligament is identified laterally over cribriform opening, and the inguinal ligament is elevated. Both lateral borders of the rectus abdominis are identified and elevated, then transacted with cuff of muscle from the superior border of tumour. The retropubic space of Retzius is developed by pushing the bladder posteriorly, protected for superior pubic rami osteotomy. The adductor attachment for the inferior pubic rami is clear for inferior pubic rami osteotomy. The bladder must be protected before the pubic rami osteotomy to prevent injury (Fig. 2d–k).

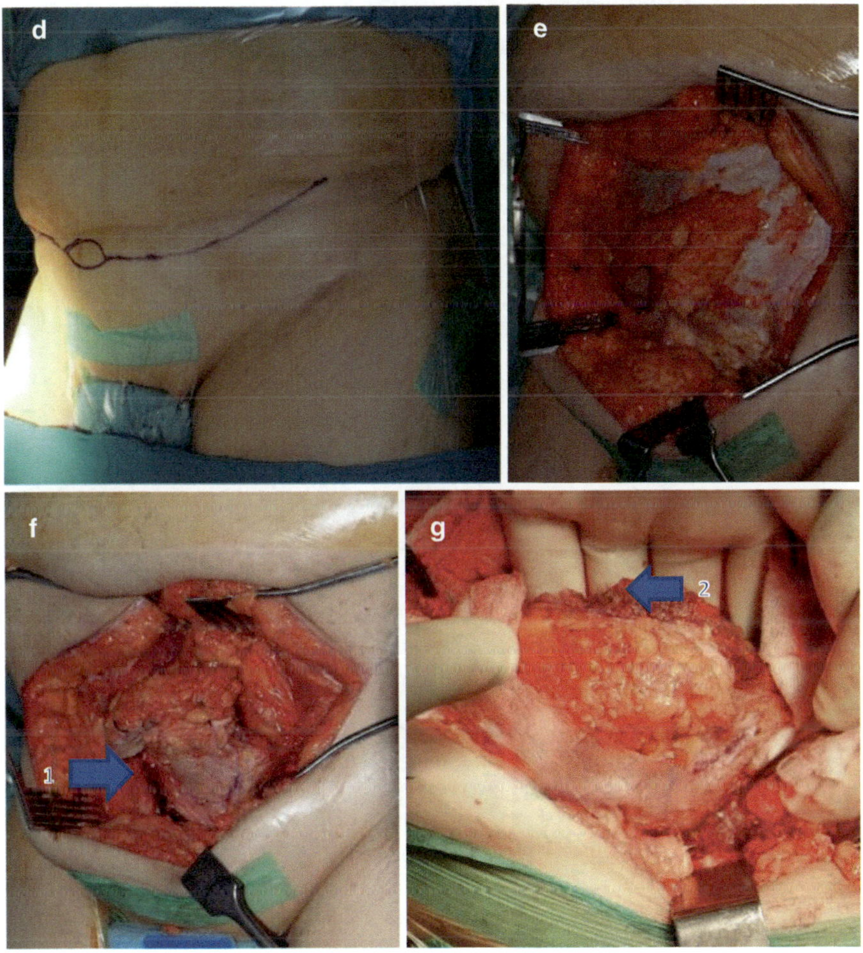

1. Lateral border of the rectus
2. The finger protects the bladder for superior pubic rami osteotomy
3. Superior pubic rami—acetabulum junction

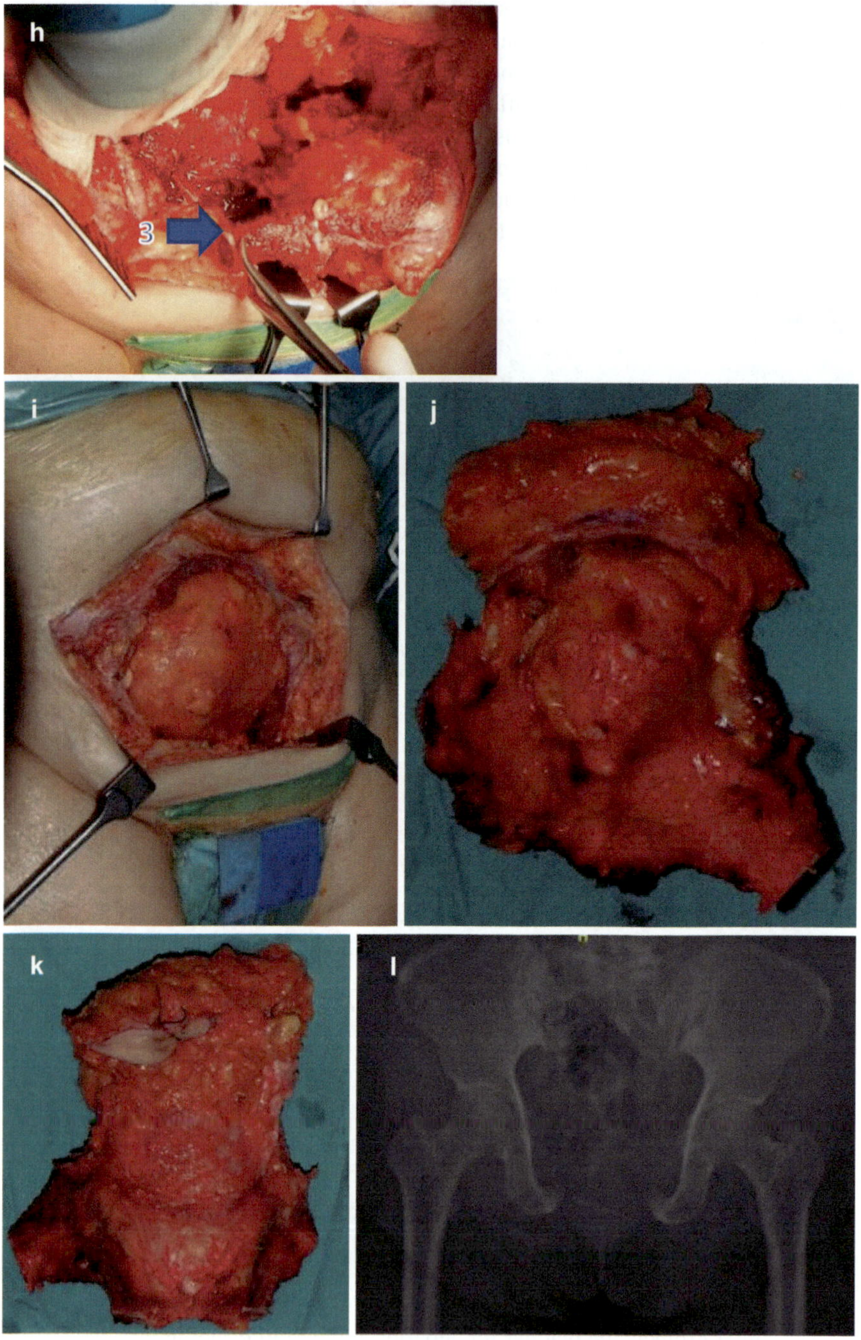

Complete resection of symphysis pubis with bilateral superior pubic rami (Fig. 2l)

Partial Type III Resection

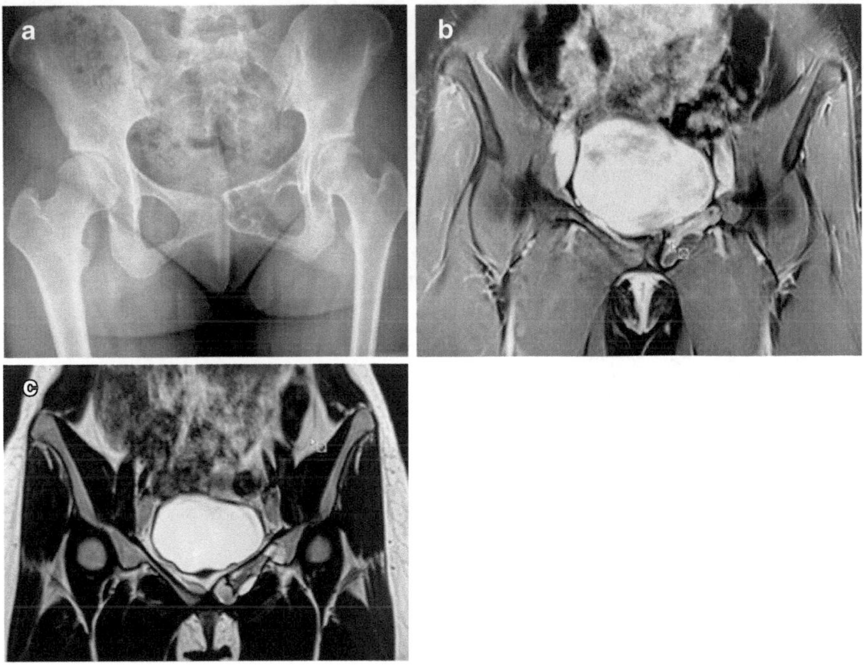

Case of aneurysmal bone cyst not responding to ethyl bloc injection presented with painful recurrence and fracture. The lateral margin planned was medial acetabulum rim and ischium junction (Fig. 3a–c).

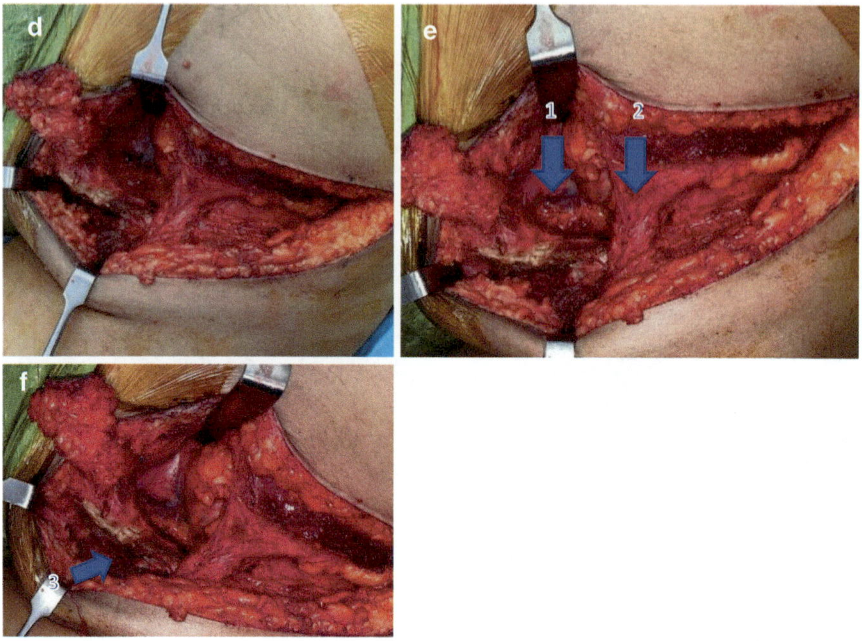

1. Space of Retzius 'Bladder wall'
2. External iliac vessels
3. Adductor muscle origin

The inner pelvis was secured by mobilising the bladder wall from both the pubic rami and symphysis pubis. Attachment of common adductor muscle was detached from the obturator membrane and inferior pubic rami to the ischium border. Mobilisation of the femoral vessels from the superior pubic rami to medial acetabulum region (Fig. 3d–f).

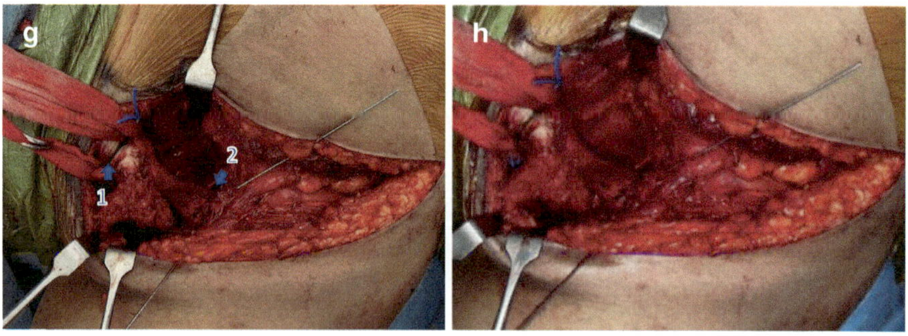

The symphysis pubis, protected by rolled gauze, passed above the bladder neck. The medial wall acetabulum and pubis-ischium border were marked with K-wire for lateral osteotomy. (Fig. 3g–k).

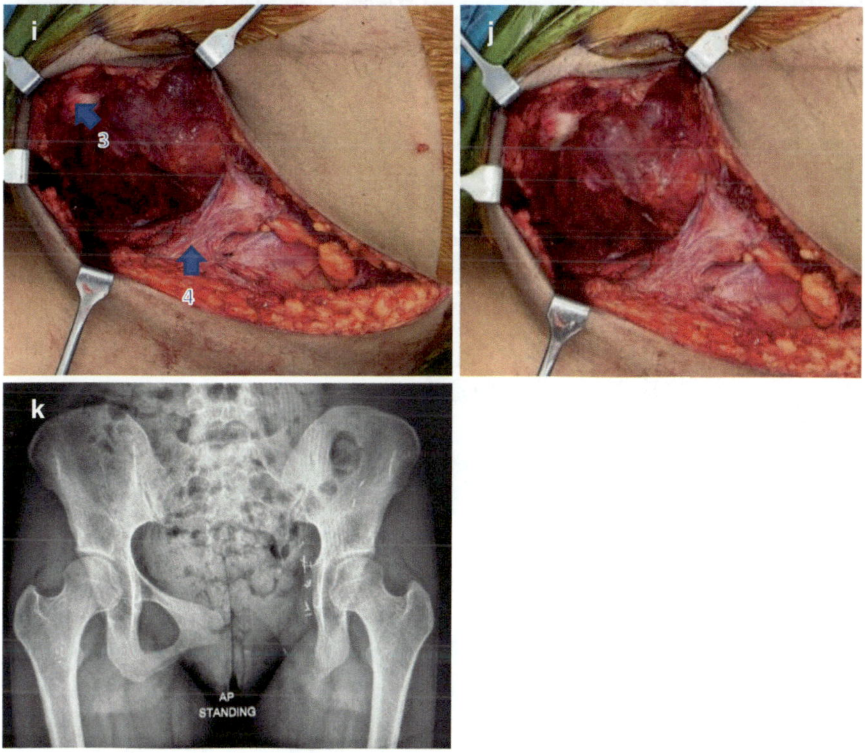

1. Symphysis pubis—roller gauze
2. Medial wall acetabulum
3. Remnant of symphysis pubis
4. External iliac vessels

Extensive Chondrosarcoma Type III with Intrapelvic Extension

Large chondrosarcoma arising from the superior pubic rami that grew posteriorly and suspicion of infiltration of the anterior bladder wall. The inner table of the medial acetabulum was spared, and main neurovascular structures were not involved (Fig. 4a–f).

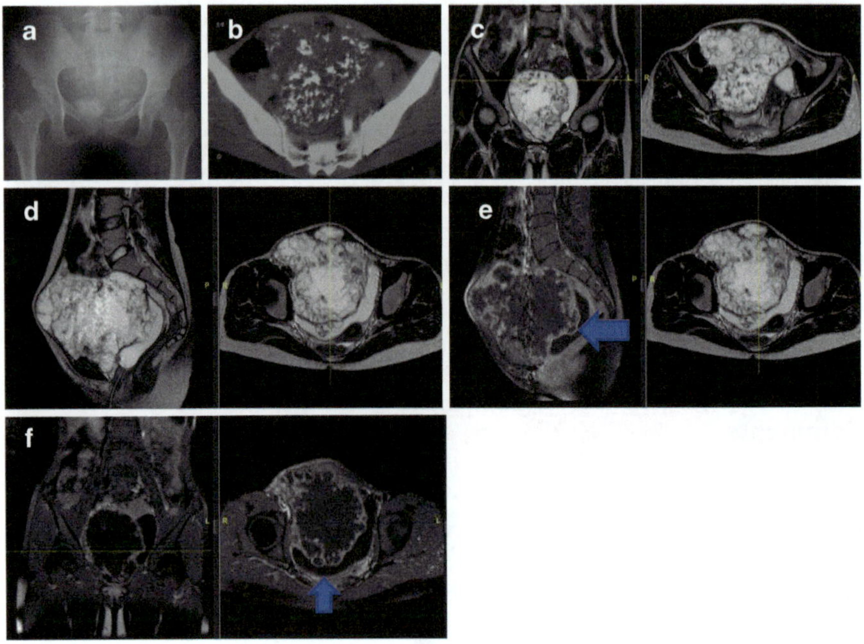

Arrow—Bladder wall infiltration

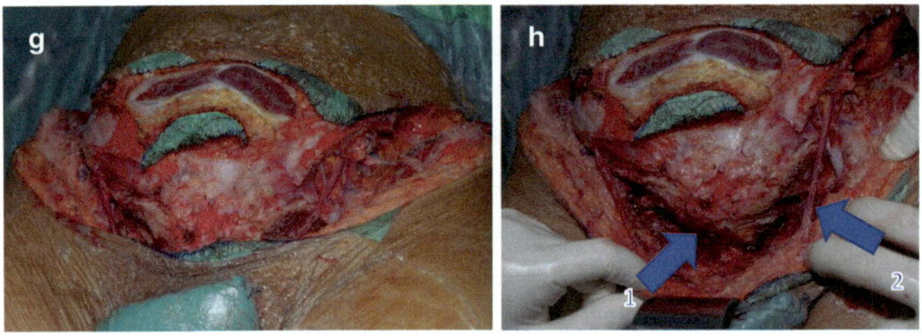

1. Common origin of the adductor compartment thigh
2. Broad ligament

The initial approach is through elevation of the inguinal ligament to reach the retroperitoneal space and lateralmost part of the superior pubic rami over the medial wall of acetabulum. The adductor origin over the superior and inferior pubic rami was detached, and the lateral border of the pubic rami was identified superficially for the bony cut. Each broad ligament was preserved from the superficial inguinal ring. Spermatic cord is crucial to maintain in male patients, especially in young patients (Fig. 4g, h).

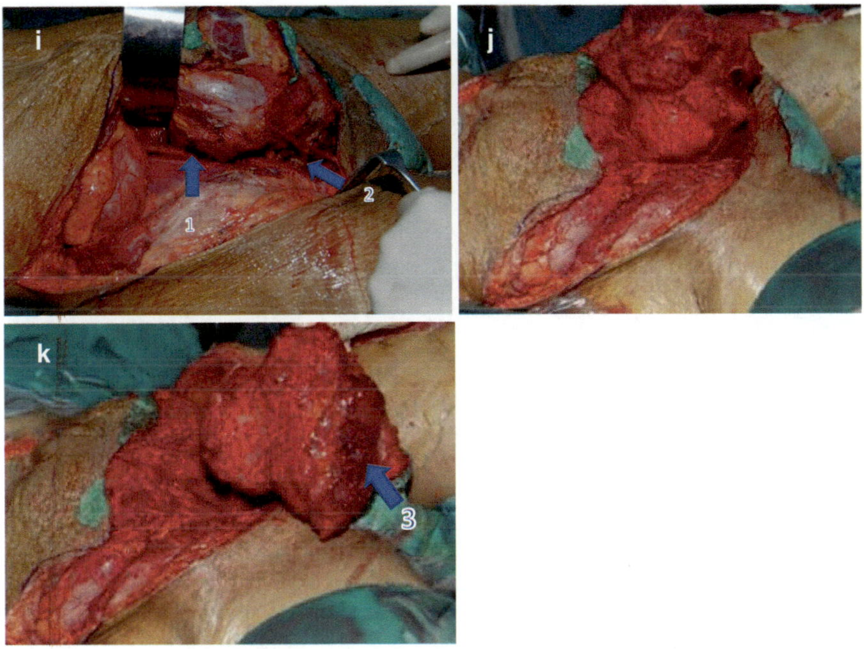

1. External iliac vessels
2. Intended osteotomy of superior pubic rami at the medial acetabulum
3. Four-corner osteotomies for mobilisation of the anterior pelvic brim

Exploration and identification of the external iliac vessels and medial wall of the acetabulum are important prior to osteotomy. Once the lateral border of the superior and inferior pubic rami oncological border is identified, both sides can be safely osteotomised and the entire tumour can be lifted up from its inferior border. Superior border of the tumour, mainly the three layers of anterior abdominal muscle, mainly rectus abdominis at the centre, can be detached and the peritoneum maintained intact (Fig. 4i–k). The bladder's involvement is identified, and resection based on oncological margin is best done with a urologist (Fig. 4l–q).

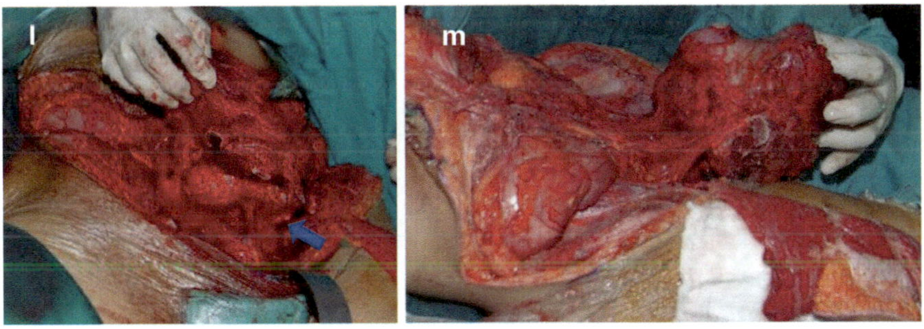

Mobilisation of tumour mass from the bladder neck and urethra, and resection of the anterior bladder wall together with the mass.

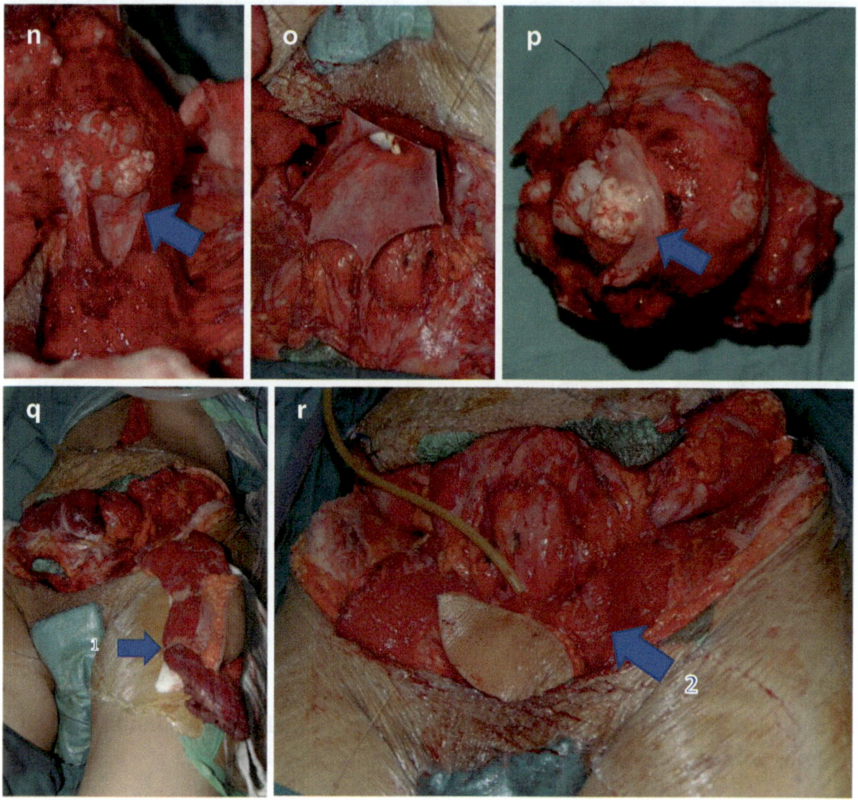

1. Vertical rectus abdominis flap (VRAM) mobilisation prior to complete tumour resection to maintain inferior epigastric vessel supply
2. Sling of the VRAM to cover anterior defect

Large tumour with anticipated soft tissue defect following resection is best covered with good soft tissue flap. Rectus abdominis muscle with inferior epigastric supply is an option that provides anterior cover and slings to prevent post-surgical incisional hernia. Function is good as pelvis acetabulum continuity is maintained (Fig. 4q–s).

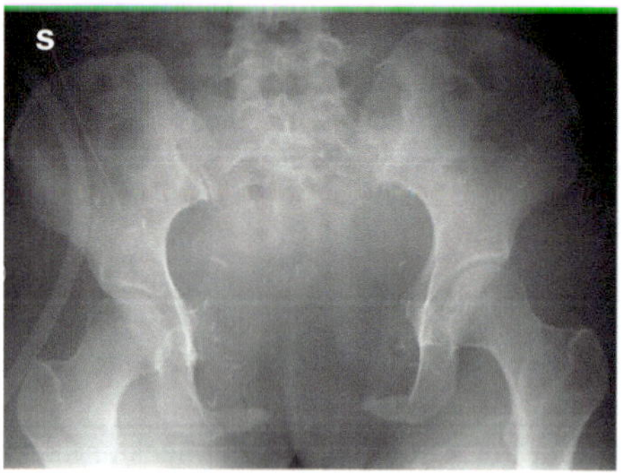

Sarcoma Anterior Abdominal Wall with Symphysis Pubis Infiltration

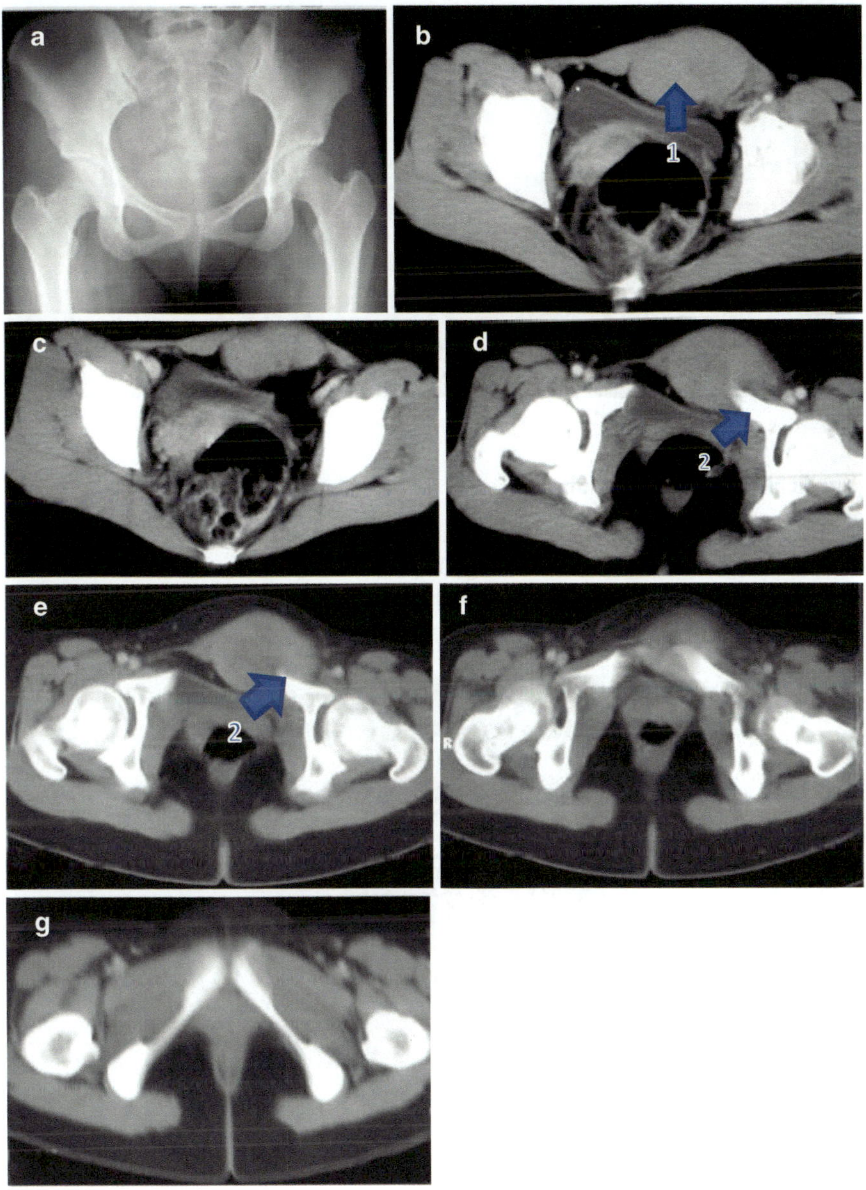

1. Rectus abdominis and anterior abdominal wall
2. Superior pubic rami involvement

The rectus abdominis and left lateral 3-layer abdominal wall involved with inferior extension to the superior pubic rami and symphysis pubis. The inferior pubic rami is spared for pelvic continuity. The peritoneum and intraabdominal content were not breached (Fig. 5a–g).

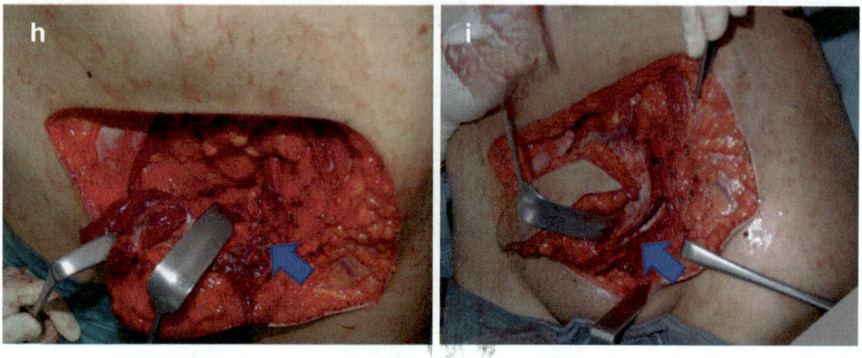

Surgical technique (Fig. 5h–j)

1. External iliac vessels after lateral wall abdomen and rectus abdominis muscle with the tumour mobilised, leaving the peritoneum intact
2. Superior pubic rami exposed from below for osteotomy

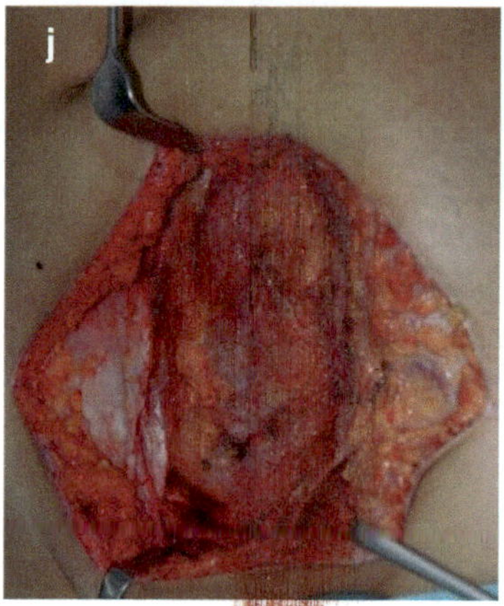

Acknowledgement The author thanks Professor Wan Azman Wan Sulaiman from the plastic reconstructive unit and Dr Mohamed Ashraf Mohamed Daud from urology unit, department of surgery at Universiti Sains Malaysia for their contributions and team member for managing the patients.

Suggested Reading

1. Mavrogenis AF, Papadopoulos D, Tsantes AG, Angelini A, Papagelopoulos PJ, Ruggieri P. Reconstruction vs. no reconstruction for pelvic resections. In: Surgery for pelvic bone tumour. Springer Nature; 2021. p. 165–83.
2. Aratani A, Chan CM, Parker Gibbs C, Scarborough M. Principles of pelvic surgery. In: Surgery for pelvic bone tumour. Springer Nature; 2021. p. 113–22.
3. Du X, Wei H, Zhang B, Gao S, Li Z, Yao W. The pedicled sartorius flap and mesh (PSM) technique vs no reconstruction in repairing the defect after type III pelvic bone tumor resection: a retrospective study. World J Surg Oncol. 2023;21(1):14.
4. Conrad Ill EU, Weisstein J, Lisle J, Stemheim A, Malawer MM. Overview on pelvic resections: surgical considerations and classifications. In: Operative technique in orthopaedic surgical oncology. Lippincott Williams &: Wilkins, A Wolters Kluwer; 2012. p. 161–79.
5. Karim SM, Colman MW, Lozano-Calderón SA, Raskin KA, Schwab JH, Hornicek FJ. What are the functional results and complications from allograft reconstruction after partial hemipelvectomy of the pubis? Clin Orthop Relat Res. 2015;473:1442–8.
6. Krieg AH, Lenze U, Gaston MS, Hefti F. The outcome of pelvic reconstruction with non-vascularised fibular grafts after resection of bone tumours. J Bone Joint Surg Br. 2010;92(11):1568–73.
7. Peter FM. Choong general considerations pelvis. In: Master techniques in orthopaedic surgery orthopaedic oncology and complex reconstruction. Lippincott Williams & Wilkins, A Wolters Kluwer; 2011. p. 3–13.
8. Puchner SE, Funovics PT, Böhler C, Kaider A, Stihsen C, Hobusch GM, Panotopoulos J, Windhager R. Oncological and surgical outcome after treatment of pelvic sarcomas. PLoS One. 2017;12(2):e0172203.

Hemipelvis Resection Type I, II & III

Wan Faisham Nu'man Bin Wan Ismail

Resection of the entire hemipelvis is an uncommon procedure. It is mainly done in extensive marrow infiltration of Ewing's sarcoma, though it may also be needed in other malignant tumours. The sacroiliac joint and symphysis pubis are used as the anatomical bony boundaries for oncological clearance. Understanding oncological boundaries of the entire pelvis and careful evaluation of preoperative MRI staging is mandatory to achieve local clearance. Neo-adjuvant treatment with chemotherapy and local adjuvant radiotherapy further improves the chances for local control.

The main challenge after resection is achieving stable pelvis and hip function for ambulation as well as good long-term outcomes.

Surgical Anatomy and Assessment

Refer to a combination of surgical anatomy and margin in the previous topics of pelvic resection and external hemipelvectomy.

W. F. N. B. W. Ismail (✉)
Prince Court Medical Center, Kuala Lumpur, Malaysia

Orthopaedic Oncology Reconstructive Unit, Universiti Sains Malaysia, Kubang Kerian, Kelantan, Malaysia

A. Puri, W. F. N. B. W. Ismail (eds.), *Atlas of Orthopedic Oncology Volume 1*,
https://doi.org/10.1007/978-981-95-8958-6_20

Ewing's Sarcoma of the Entire Pelvis

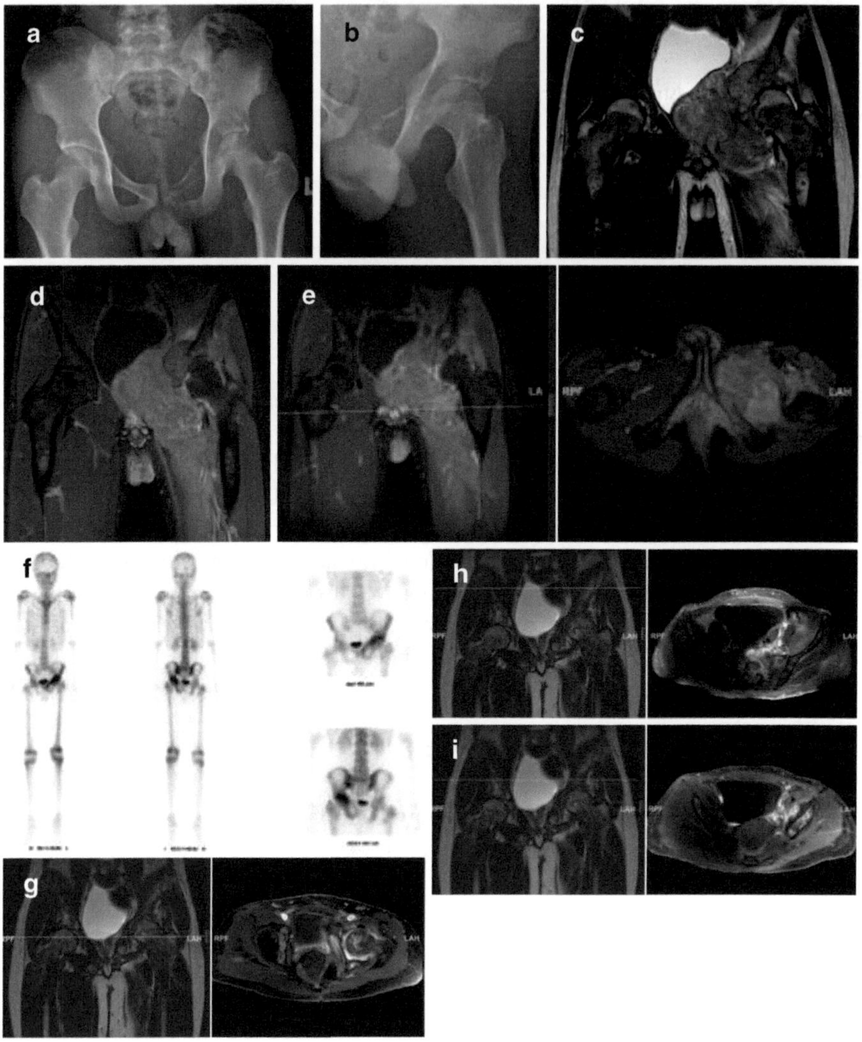

A case of Ewing's sarcoma of the peri acetabulum with marrow infiltration superior to the ilium with soft tissue extension to the iliacus muscle, obturator internus and adductor attachment to the pubic rami. Post chemotherapy MRI showed good response with resolution of soft tissue extension. The gluteus muscle was not involved (Fig. 1a–i).

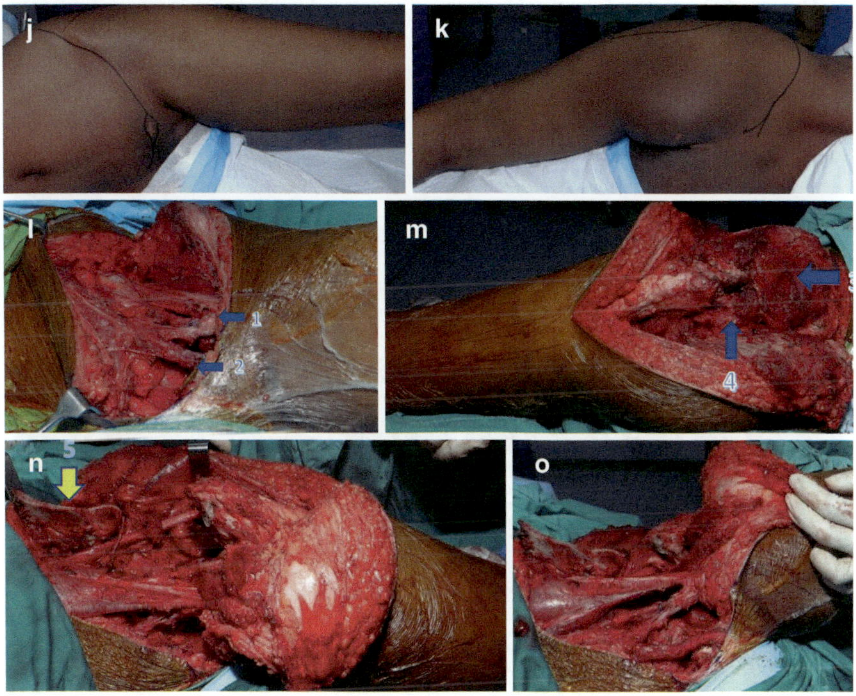

1. Mobilisation of the external iliac vessels and femoral nerve together with the psoas muscle
2. Spermatic cord
3. Gluteus medius was kept as a margin
4. Mobilisation of the sciatic nerve to the greater sciatic foreman
5. Remaining ilium

An extended ilioinguinal approach was used for mobilisation of the external iliac vessels, psoas muscle with femoral nerve and spermatic cord. The abdominal muscle was mobilised to the symphysis pubis for medial osteotomy. The adductor origin at the pubic rami and obturator ligament were detached with good cuff of tissue for margin (Fig. 1j–o).

The gluteus maximus was mobilised by detaching the femoral attachment for exploration of the sciatic nerve at the greater sciatic foreman. The gluteus medius and minimus were kept as the margin and the hamstring origin were detached from the ischium. The sacrospinous and sacrotuberus ligament were detached from the pelvis for complete mobilisation of the hemipelvis.

Options for reconstruction after resection of the entire pelvis with small segment of ilium:

- Custom 3D printing prosthesis
- Allograft
- Recycled bone
  - extracorporeal radiotherapy
  - cryotherapy with liquid nitrogen

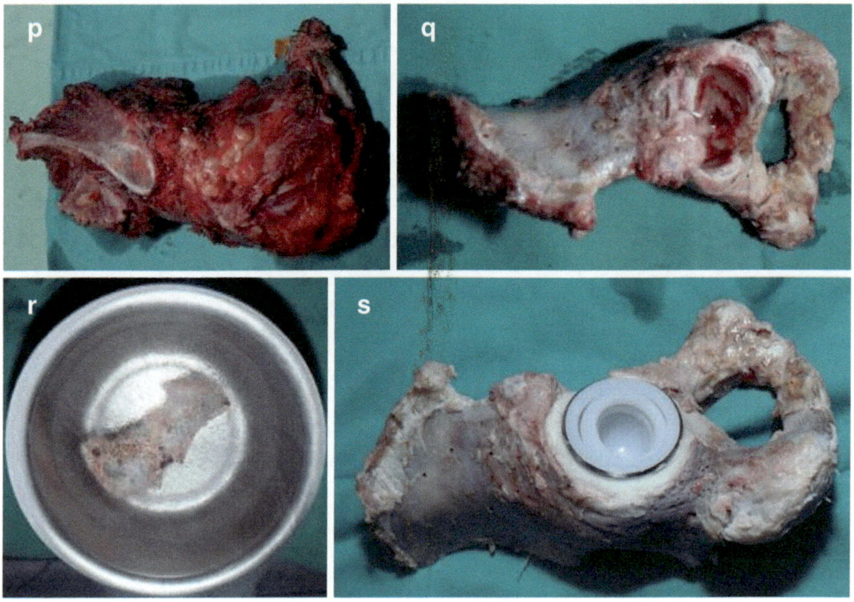

- Cemented capture cup inserted prior to reimplantation

Preparation for cryotherapy involves removal of the soft tissue tumour component. Cryotherapy using liquid nitrogen requires thawing and preparation for total hip replacement. We used a constraint cup acetabular reconstruction as the soft tissues and abductor muscle which act as dynamic hip stabilizers were removed as an oncological margin (Fig. 1p–s).

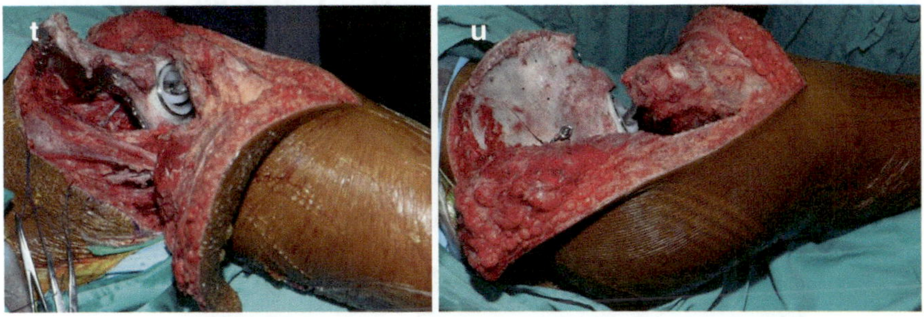

Final reconstruction was stabilized with plates and screws for stabilisation of the entire pelvic ring (Fig. 1t–v).

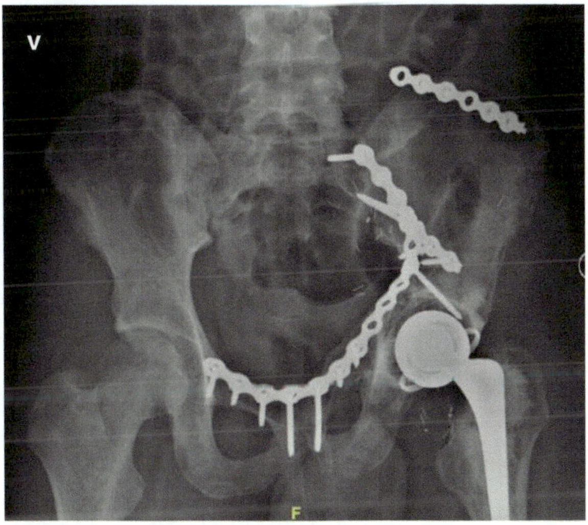

Solitary Metastases Adenocarcinoma Hemipelvis 'Ilium and Acetabulum'

A case of solitary metastases of low-grade adenocarcinoma originating from the mandibular with history of hip pain and limping. Local MRI showed an intraosseous destructive lesion of the acetabulum that extended to the entire ilium. The pubic rami and ischium were not involved (Fig. 2a–g).

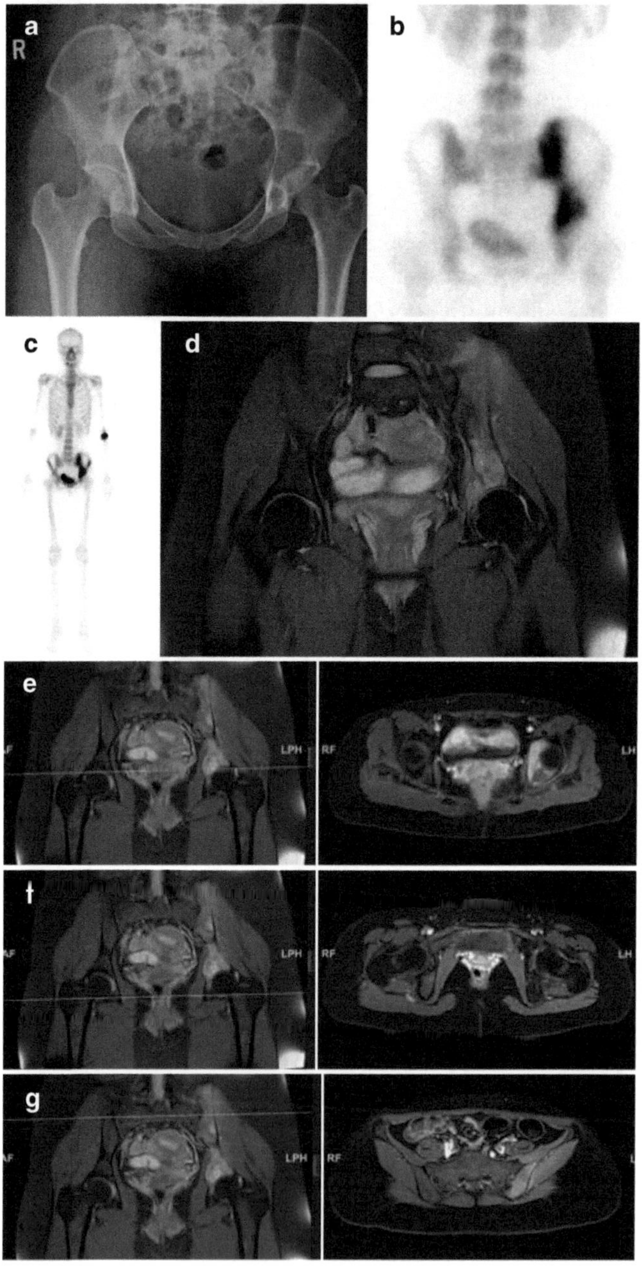

The tumour was resected with superior margin at the sacroiliac joint and inferior margin at superior pubic rami and upper ischium. The surrounding soft tissues were cleared after resection prior to cryotherapy (Fig. 2h–m).

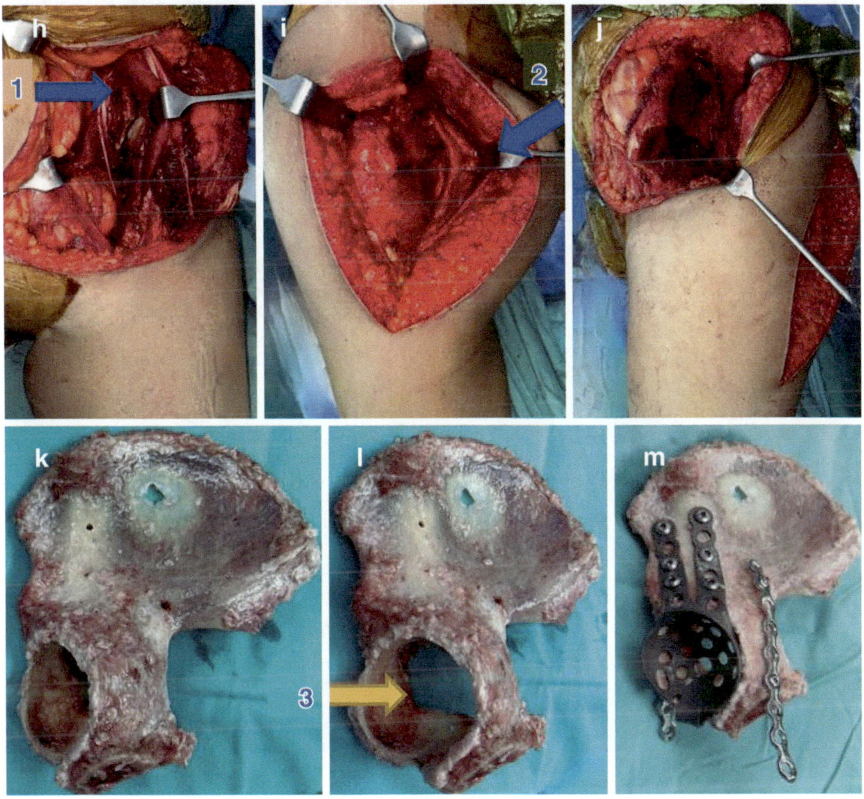

1. Sacroiliac joint for superior margin
2. Mobilisation of the sciatic nerve for ischium osteotomy
3. Medial acetabulum defect

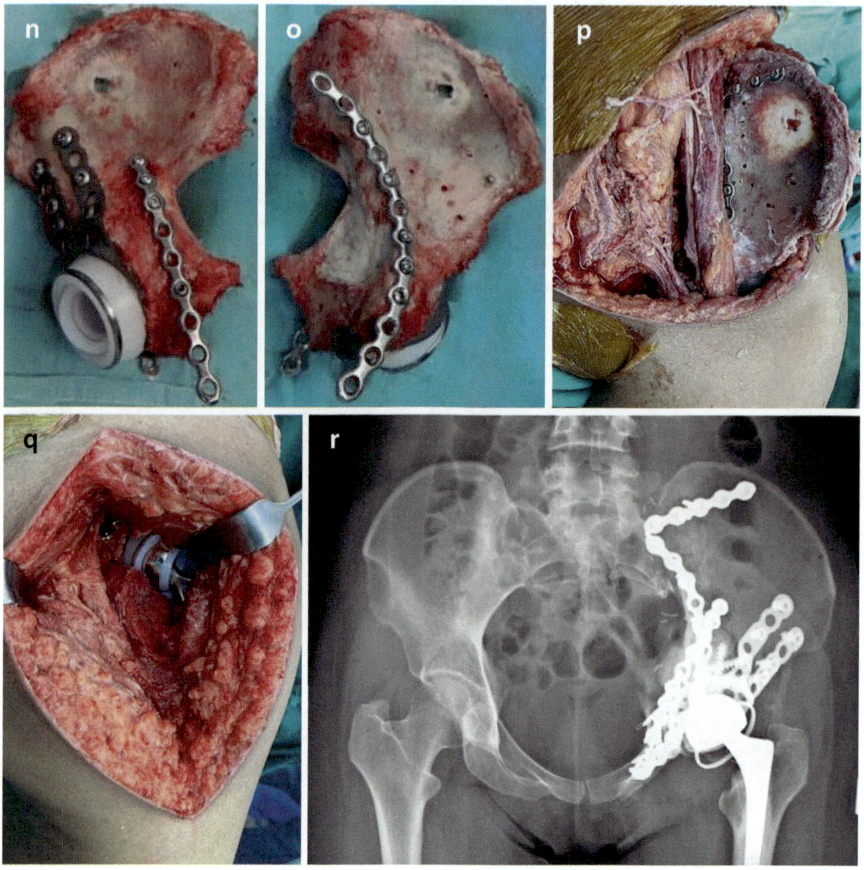

The bone defect was reconstructed with cemented cages and a constrained cup and finally reattached using an anterior plate to the remnant of the sacral ala and superior pubic rami. The sacroiliac joint construct was reinforced by a 90/90 plate to the sacral ala. Posteriorly, the acetabulum column was stabilized to the remnant of the ischium for completion of ring stability (Fig. 2n–r).

Chondrosarcoma with Ischio Femoral Fusion

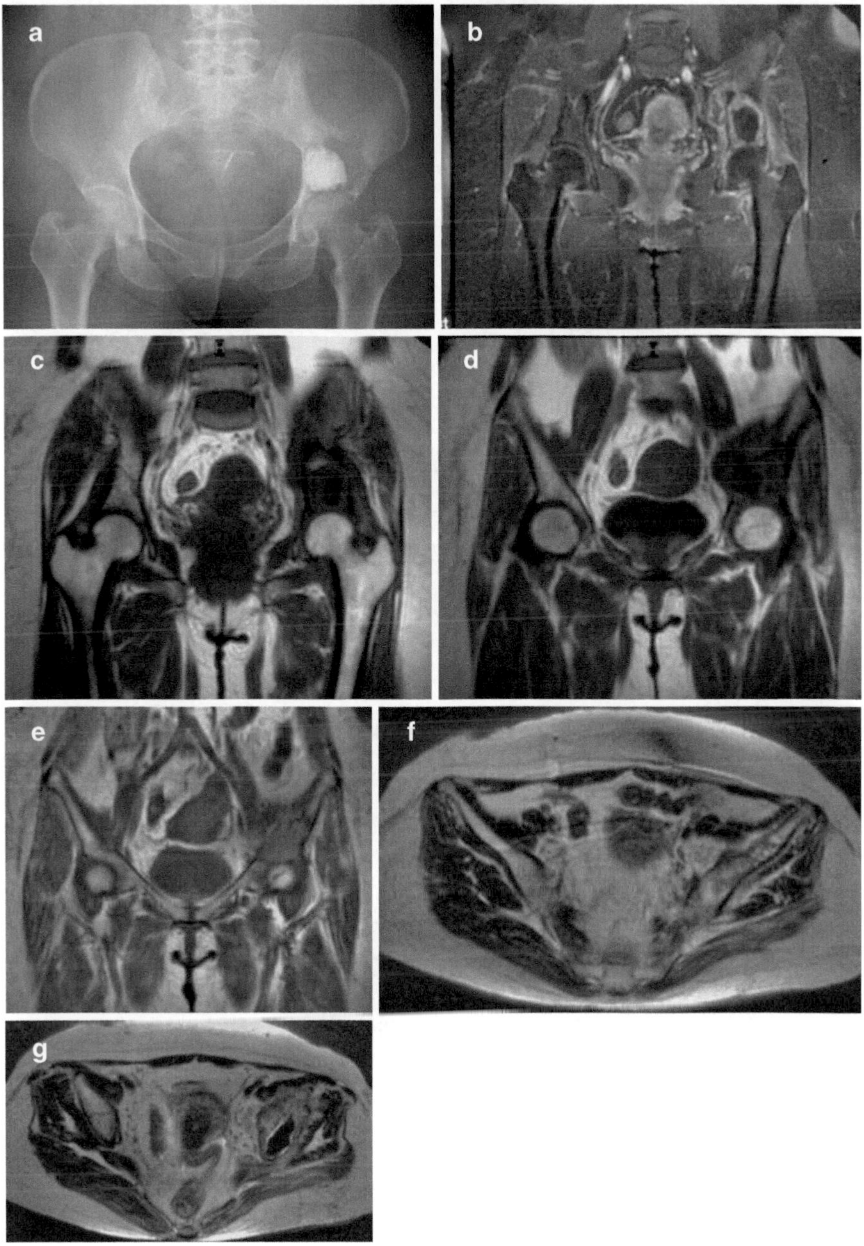

A 45-year-old lady with history of chondrosarcoma initially treated with curettage and bone substitute, through a posterior approach, had recurrence. The disease extended to the entire ilium and acetabulum. The pubic rami were spared (Fig. 3a–g).

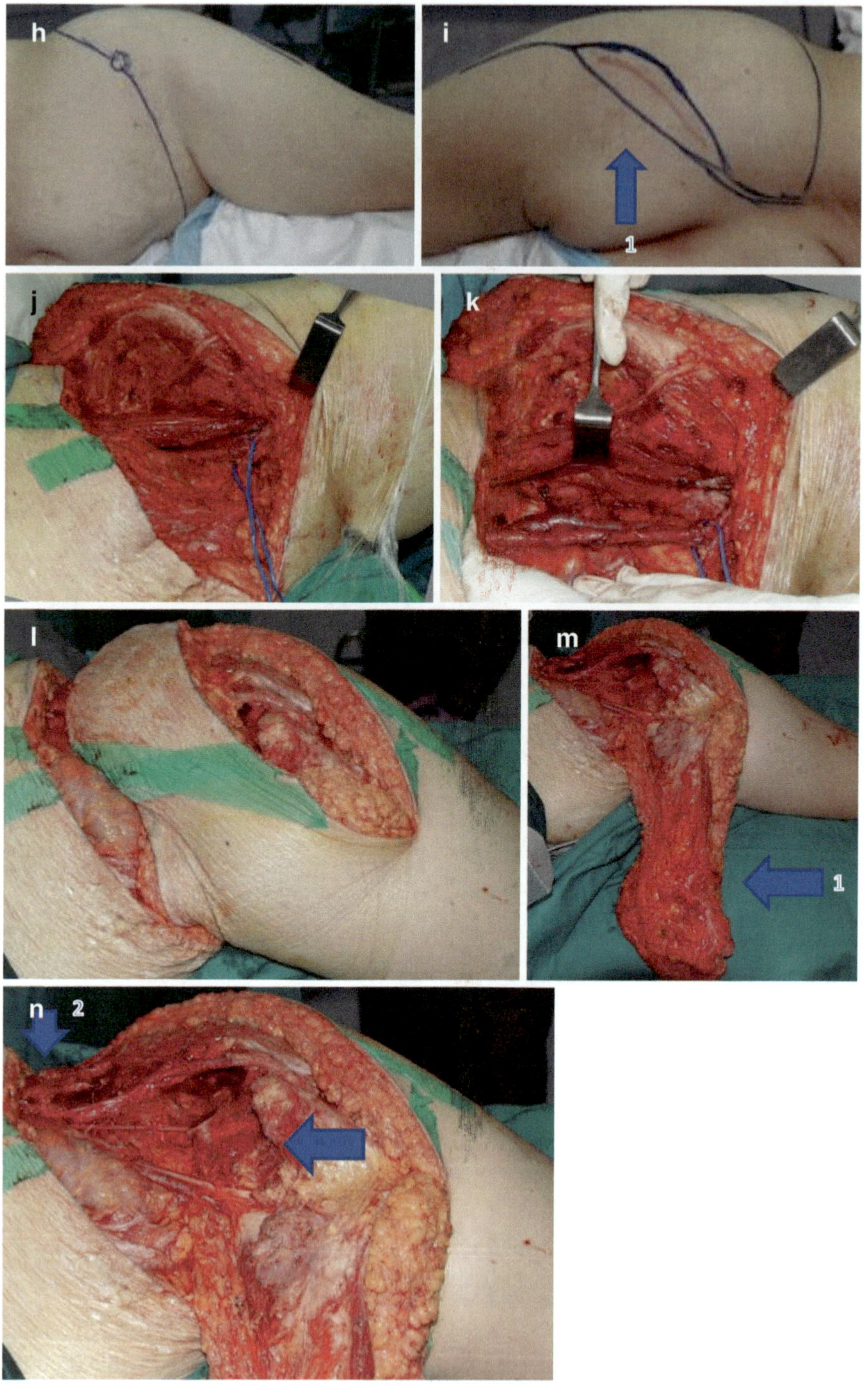
h
i
1
j
k
l
m
1
n
2

1. Extensive mobilisation of the flap from the previous surgery (Fig. 3h–m)
2. Resection at the sacroiliac joint and inferior border acetabulum (Fig. 3n)

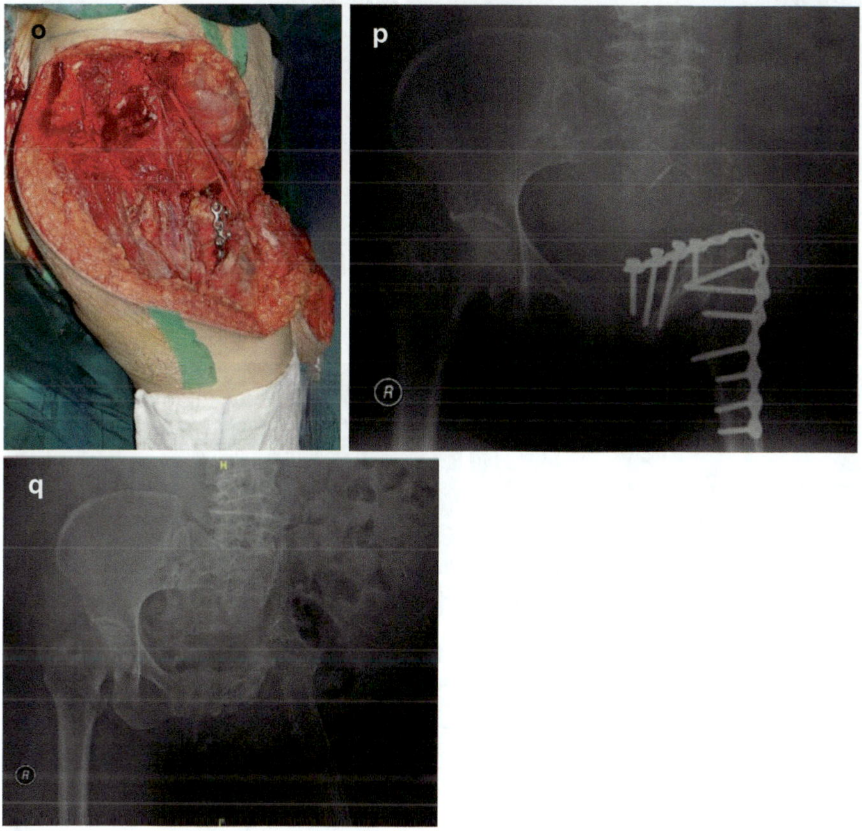

Ischio-femoral fusion was achieved and stabilized with a pre-contoured plate and screws; however, it was removed after three years due to non-union and loosening of the screws. Patient ambulated with a tripod walking stick pain-free with 2 cm shortening (Fig. 3o–q).

Entire (Type I–III) Hemipelvis Resection with Extracorporeal Radiation and Implantation

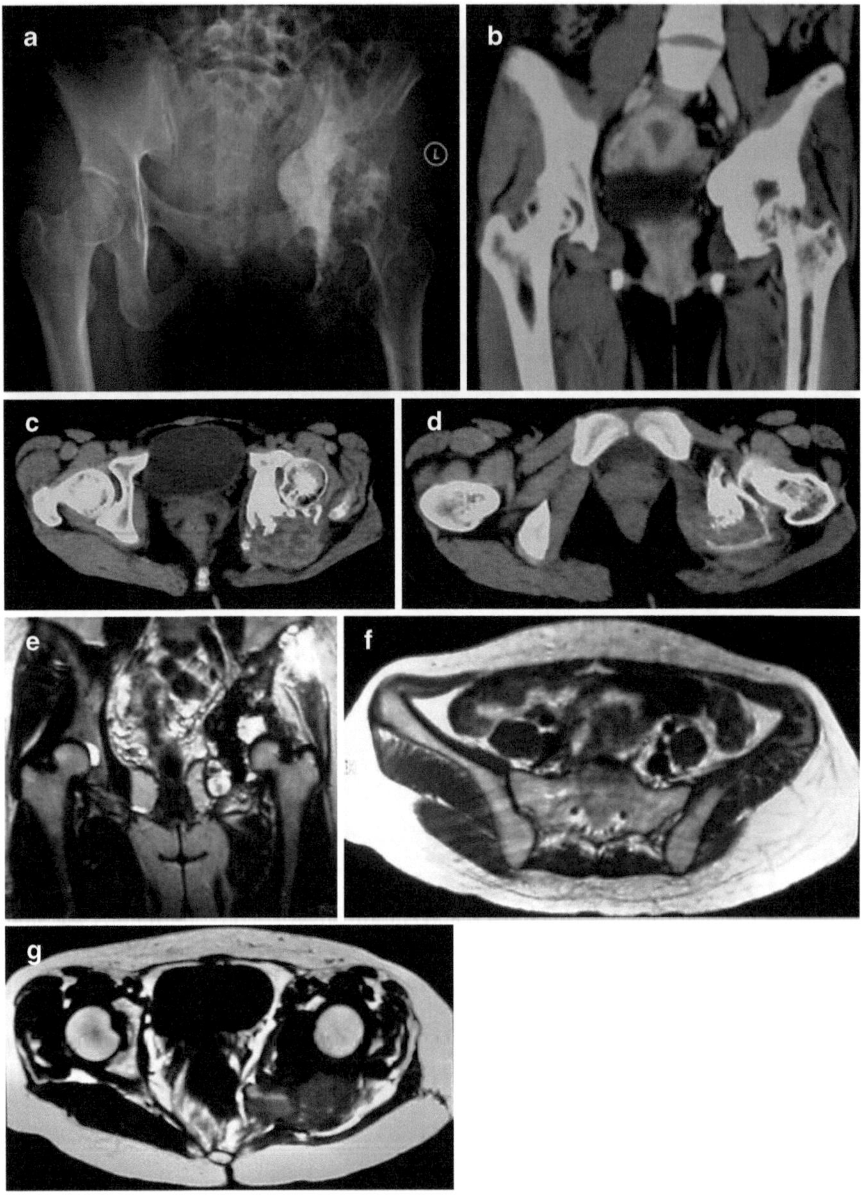

A case of osteosarcoma peri-acetabulum with good response to chemotherapy. The tumour extended mainly to the posterior column of the acetabulum and ischium. The marrow infiltration involved the iliac brim and did not cross the sacroiliac joint. The greater sciatic foramen was clear, and the sciatic nerve was free from tumour extension (Fig. 4a–g).

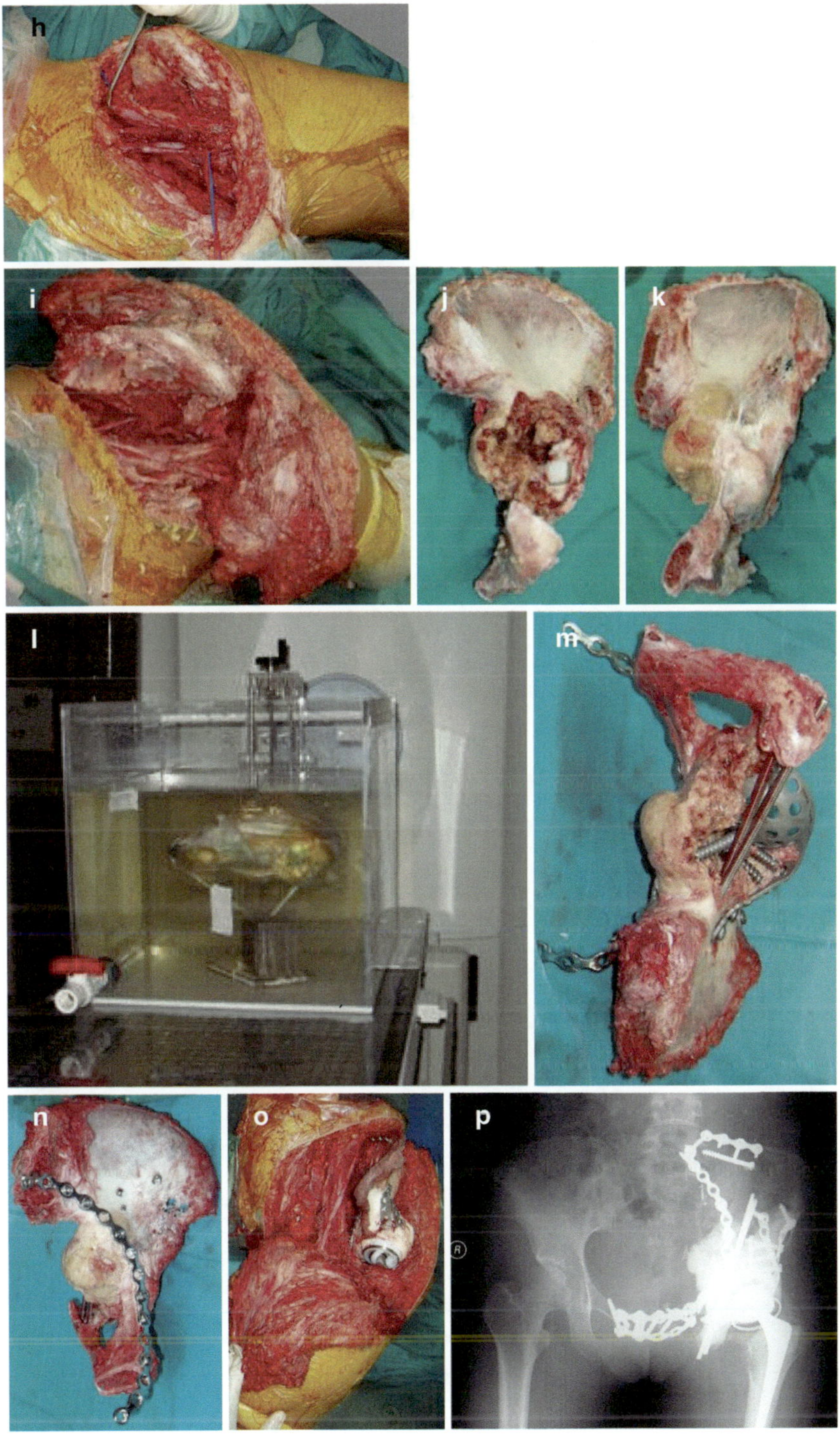
h
i
j
k
l
m
n
o
p

Hemipelvis resection with the iliacus muscle, gluteus medius, obturator internus and all short rotator muscles as muscle margin was achieved. The hamstring origin to the ischium was also removed for oncological margin. The soft tissue component and tumour infiltration to the bone were cleared from the resected hemipelvis after excision prior to radiation. Radiation of 60 Gy was delivered as a single fraction (Fig. 4h–l).

Pre-contoured pelvic plate, gap II cage and multiple threaded pins were applied on the final specimen prior to cemented hip replacement. Stability of the hip was provided by a constrained acetabulum liner as static and dynamic hip stabilizers, which were excised as margin (Fig. 4m–p).

Entire (Type I–III) Hemipelvis Resection with High Hip Centre Reconstruction

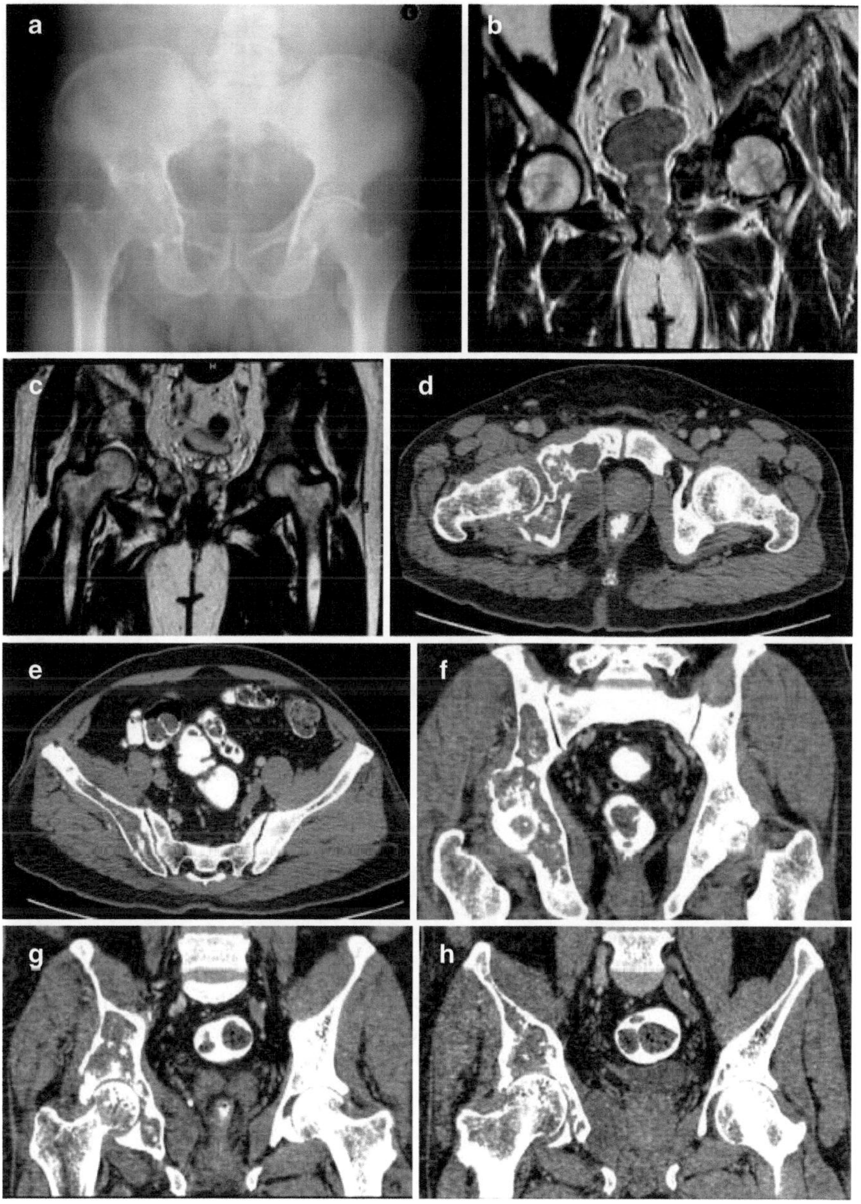

A case of chondrosarcoma where the entire hemipelvis (Fig. 5a–h) underwent complete hemipelvis resection. The hip joint was created by inserting a cone prosthesis into the S1 & L5. The stability was reinforced by purse string of a Dacron graft to the cup and the femoral head. The segment length was built up with a proximal femur replacement to achieve correct limb length. The anterolateral rotational thigh flap was performed as a primary soft tissue reconstruction to minimise wound breakdown and flexibility of closure (Fig. 5i–m).

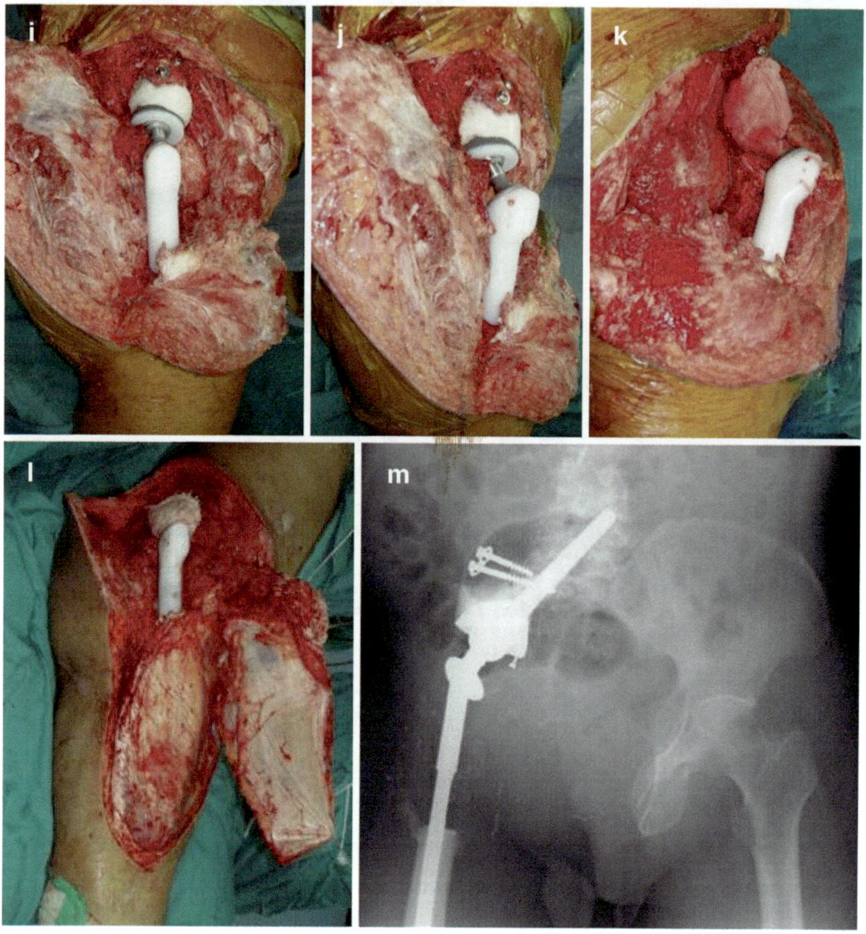

A case of chondrosarcoma where the entire hemipelvis (Fig. 5n–q) underwent resection and reconstruction with cages and mesh wire, which was hooked over S1 remnant of the sacral alar. The limb length was built up by proximal femur endoprosthesis (Fig. 5r–t).

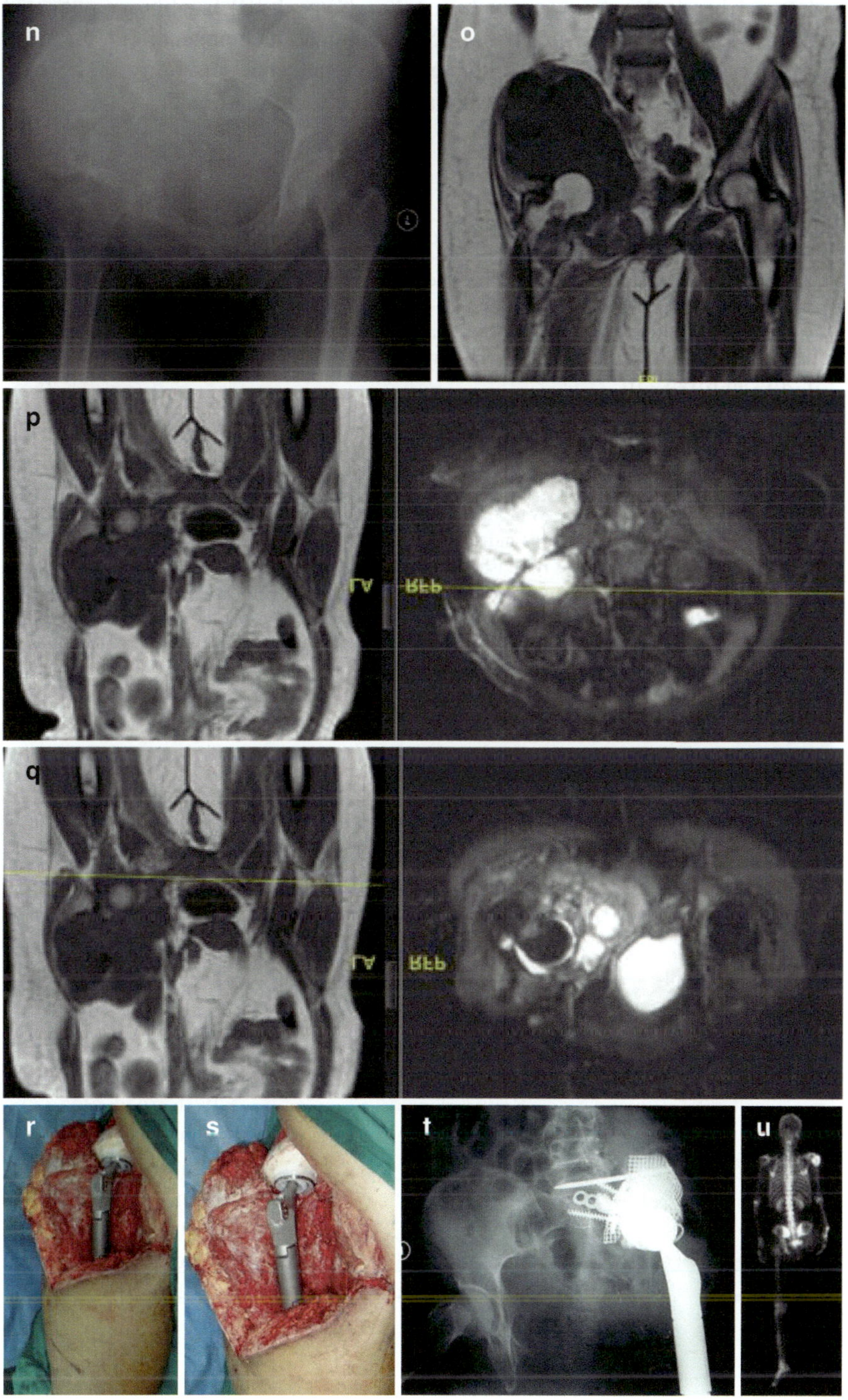
n
o
p
q
r
s
t
u

Internal hemipelvectomy entire hemipelvis (Type I–III) is often complicated with chronic pain and poor function. Reconstruction to the remnant of the S1 & L5 to provide stability is associated with higher hip joint centre, disability and chronic pain. Both patients ended up with external hemipelvectomy (Fig. 5u).

Suggested Reading

1. He F, Zhang W, Shen Y, Pei Y, Bao Q, Wen J, Chuanzhen H, Qiu S. Effects of resection margins on local recurrence of osteosarcoma in extremity and pelvis: systematic review and meta-analysis. Int J Surg. 2016;36:283e292.
2. Wafa H, Grimer RJ, Jeys L, Abudu AT, Carter SR, Tillman RM. The use of extracorporeally irradiated autografts in pelvic reconstruction following tumour resection. Bone Joint J. 2014;96-B:1404–10.
3. Lee JS, Kelly CM, Edmund K. Bartlett management of pelvic sarcoma. Eur J Surg Oncol. 2022;48:2299e2307.
4. Puri A, Gulia A, Pruthi M. Outcome of surgical resection of pelvic osteosarcoma. Indian J Orthop. 2014;48:273–8.
5. Qu H, Li D, Tang S, Zang J, Wang Y, Guo W. Pelvic reconstruction following resection of tumour involving the whole ilium and acetabulum. J Bone Oncol. 2019;16:100234.
6. Fujiwara T, Ogura K, Christ A, Bartelstein M, Kenan S, Fabbri N, Heale J. Periacetabular reconstruction following limb-salvage surgery for pelvic sarcomas. J Bone Oncol. 2021;31:100396.
7. Fujiwara T, Rincon MRM, Sambri A, Tsuda Y, Clark R, Stevenson J, Parry MC, Grimer RJ, Jeys L. Limb-salvage reconstruction following resection of pelvic bone sarcomas involving the acetabulum. Bone Joint J. 2021;103-B(4):795–803.

Pseudoarthrosis of Hip Joint (Meshplasty) After Periacetabular Resection

Ajay Puri, Rudra Pratap Singh, and Ashwin Prajapati

Introduction

Reconstruction after periacetabular resection ranges from conventional implants to custom-made 3D-printed implants to biological options like sterilized reimplanted tumor bone. Pseudarthrosis is yet another option. Reconstructing the bone defect with a polypropylene mesh (Prolene TM Mesh, Johnson & Johnson, Ethicon division, Aurangabad, India) (meshplasty) results in a stable construct after significant fibrosis, and this provides a durable, cost-effective, and mobile long-term reconstruction option with minimal complications.

Surgical Anatomy

- Enneking and Dunham classified pelvic resections into three broad categories: type 1—iliac resection, type 2—periacetabular resection, and type 3—resection of pubis and ischium. Reconstruction is necessary after periacetabular resection to create stability for subsequent ambulation.
- Preserving the gluteus maximus muscle along with the skin flap and preserving the inferior gluteal vessels whenever feasible helps decrease wound-related complications.
- The continuity of the psoas muscle to its femoral attachment helps in postoperative stability.
- Visualizing the greater sciatic notch from both, the outer brim and inner brim is the key to safeguarding the sciatic nerve and its nerve roots in pelvis resection.
- Bony landmarks like ASIS (anterior superior iliac spine), AIIS (anterior inferior iliac spine), ischial tuberosity, pubic symphysis, superior and inferior pubic

A. Puri (✉) · R. P. Singh · A. Prajapati
Department of Surgical Oncology, Tata Memorial Centre, Mumbai, Maharashtra, India

A. Puri, W. F. N. B. W. Ismail (eds.), *Atlas of Orthopedic Oncology Volume 1*,
https://doi.org/10.1007/978-981-95-8958-6_21

ramus, SI joint, and sacral foramen are used as reference points to plan the three-dimensional multiplanar cuts.
- Severing the ligaments, i.e., iliolumbar, sacrospinous, and sacrotuberous, is a necessary prerequisite to mobilize the specimen after bony osteotomy.
- The femoral head is anchored to the residual pelvis after resection (sacrum or ilium) depending on the extent of resection.
- If ischial tuberosity with pubic rami is preserved, pseudarthrosis can be achieved with them so that subsequent shortening is minimized.

Assessment

An MRI assessment of pelvis with bilateral hips includes:

- Evaluating the extraosseous soft tissue component and its relation to visceral structures like bladder, urethra, ureter, bowel, spermatic cord/ adnexa, etc., sciatic nerve and its nerve roots, femoral neurovascular bundle, and involvement of gluteal muscles.
- Evaluating the extent of intraosseous extent of the disease to decide bony cuts.
- Evaluating the presence of intraarticular disease and extent, if any, across the sacroiliac joint.

Surgical Steps

Position Floppy lateral position with the involved side up and the arm resting on a support. Side supports applied above the level of umbilicus to facilitate free tilting of pelvis on either side. All bony prominences are padded adequately.

Resection
- Resection involves dissection of the tumor with standard oncological margins and preservation of vital structures, i.e., femoral neurovascular bundle, sciatic nerve and its nerve roots, psoas major muscle, and visceral organs.
- Preserving as much hip joint capsule as possible helps anchor the mesh during meshplasty.
- Precise three-dimensional bony cuts are taken based on preoperative planning, and necessary ligaments are cut to deliver the specimen out.
- Navigation is a useful tool in guiding the bony cuts.

Reconstruction with Meshplasty
- In isolated type 3 and type 1 resections, hip joint reconstruction is not necessary. For periacetabular resections, meshplasty is done to anchor the proximal femur/ prosthesis to the remaining part of the pelvis.

- A 15 × 15 cm or 30 × 30 cm commercially available polypropylene mesh (Prolene TM Johnson & Johnson, Ethicon division, Aurangabad, India) is soaked in vancomycin-infused saline while resection is ongoing (Fig. 1a).

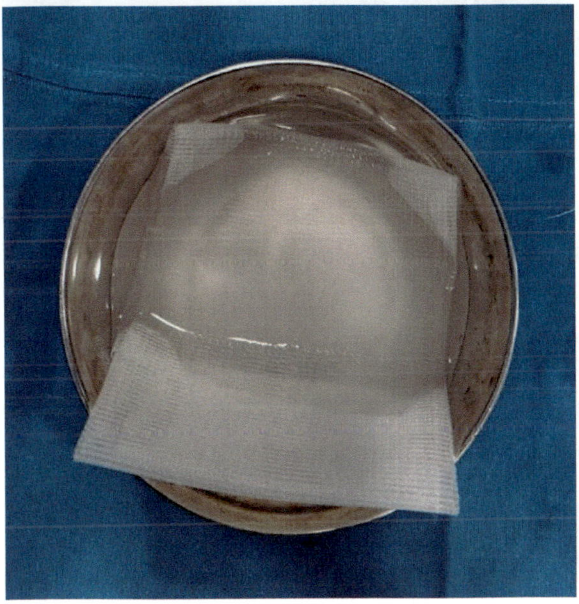

- After resection is completed, the mesh is folded on itself, and the loose ends are sutured with No. 1 Vicryl TM (Johnson & Johnson) to form a double-layered rectangular sheet.
- Depending on the area to be stabilized, one of the longer sides of the rectangle is anchored circumferentially to the femur neck with the help of four to six sutures passed through bone or remnent joint capsule using No: 2 Ethibond Excel TM (nonabsorbable, braided, polyester suture manufactured by Johnson & Johnson Ltd., Ethicon division, Chihuahua 32575 Mexico), a polyester braided nonabsorbable material.
- The other end is fixed to the remaining bone of the pelvis in various patterns shown in the cases below.
- Remaining muscles and tendons can be anchored to the mesh.
- The concept is to provide a scaffold on which fibroblastic tissue ingrows to form a biological pseudoarthrosis, which provides stability by preventing proximal and medial migration of the femur while retaining mobility of the head of the femur.

Case 1: Type 1 + Type 2 + Partial 3 Internal Hemipelvectomy and Meshplasty Reconstruction

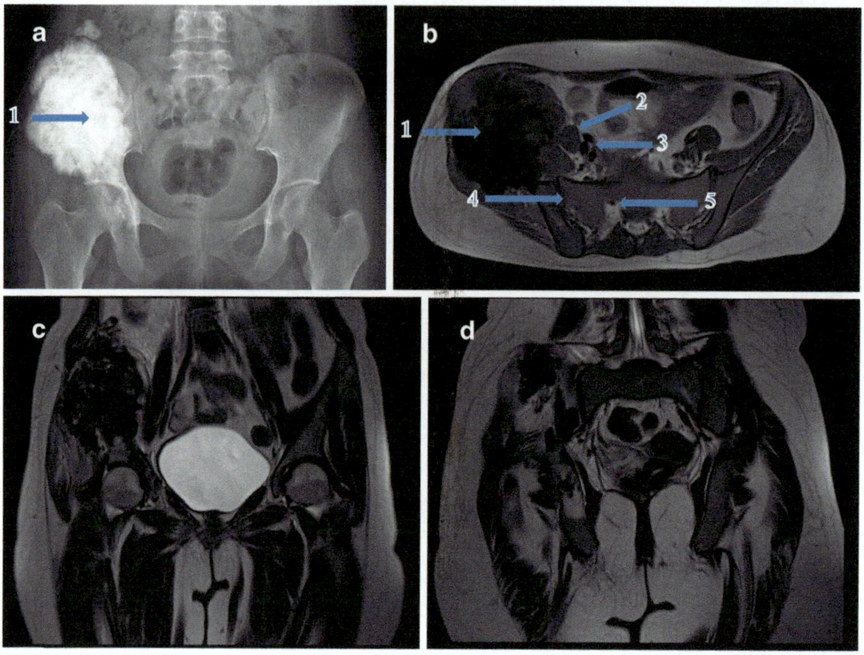

1. Tumor
2. Psoas muscle
3. External iliac vessels
4. Sacroiliac joint
5. S1 Nerve root

Osteosarcoma of ilium involving anterior and posterior columns. Sacroiliac and hip joints are not involved. External iliac vessels, the femoral nerve, and sciatic nerve roots are uninvolved by the tumor (Fig. 2a–d).

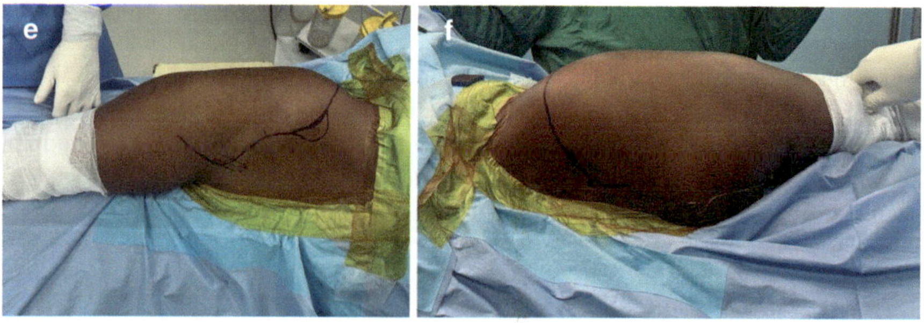

A single incision is taken from PSIS to ASIS, extending along the inguinal ligament, and curving distally and laterally in the thigh from a mid-inguinal point (islanding the biopsy scar) (Fig. 2e, f). A type 1 + 2 internal hemipelvectomy is performed with three osteotomies through superior pubic ramus, through ischium, and through sacrum just medial to SI joint (Fig. 2g–i).

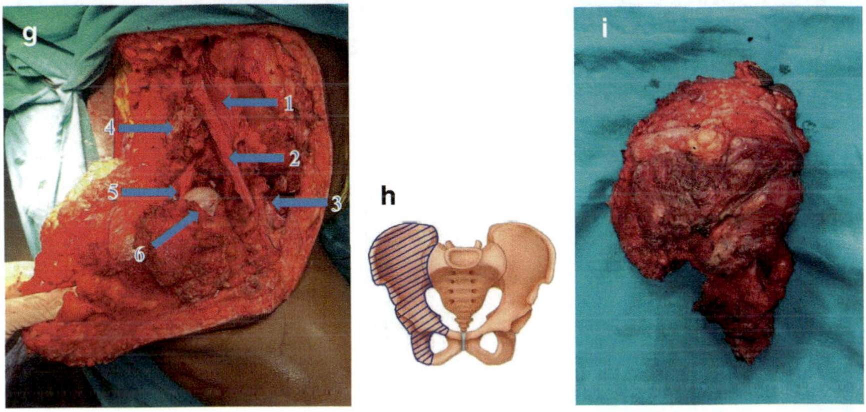

1. Psoas muscle
2. Femoral nerve
3. Femoral vessels
4. Sacral ala
5. Sciatic nerve
6. Femur head and capsule

Mesh reconstruction is planned between the proximal femur and sacral ala. A 15 × 15 Prolene mesh is folded on itself and secured with No. 1 Vicryl sutures to form a sleeve. The broader end of the sleeve is fixed circumferentially to remaining hip joint capsule with No 2 Ethibond sutures. Drill holes are made in sacral ala. With limb in neutral rotation and without undue tension on soft tissue, proximal end of the sleeve is secured to sacral ala with Ethibond sutures (Fig. 2j–m).

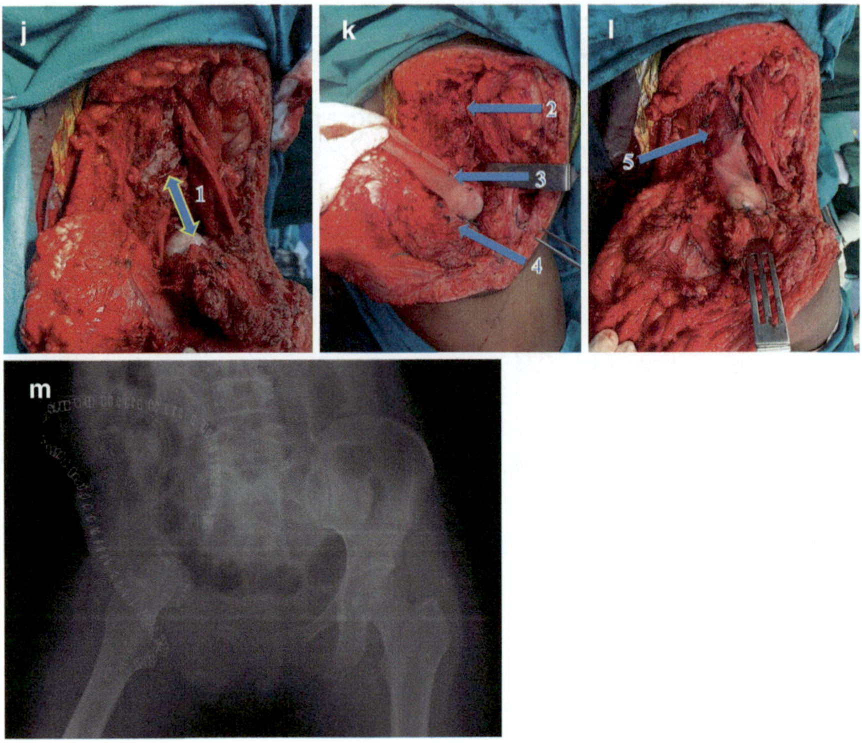

1. Bone defect for reconstruction.
2. Sacrum ala.
3. Prolene mesh folded and secured with Vicryl sutures.
4. Mesh sutured to hip joint capsule.
5. Mesh sutured to sacral ala.

Case 2: Type 1 + Type 2 + Type 4 + Partial 3 Internal Hemipelvectomy and Meshplasty

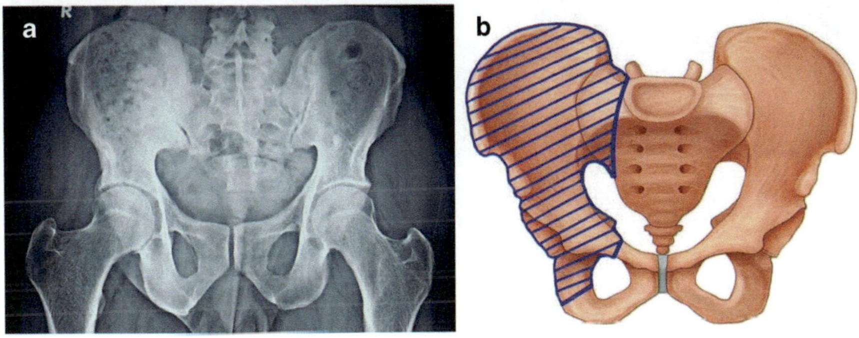

Chondrosarcoma of right hemipelvis requiring resection of sacral ala along with ilium and periacetabular area. Extended resection of sacrum along with SI joint is classified as type 4 resections (Fig. 3a, b).

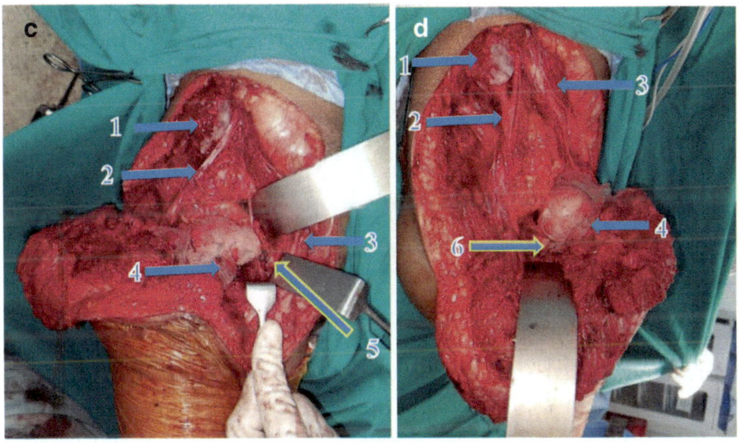

1. Sacral cut.
2. Sciatic nerve.
3. Psoas muscle and femoral nerve.
4. Mesh sutured to hip joint capsule.
5. Superior pubic ramus cut end, mesh sutures to it.
6. Ischium cut end mesh sutured to it.

After type 4 resection in which remaining bone stock of sacrum is not adequate for mesh attachment, mesh is sutured to the hip capsule and its ends are secured to osteotomized ends of superior and inferior pubic ramus or ischial tuberosity if it is available (Fig. 3c–e).

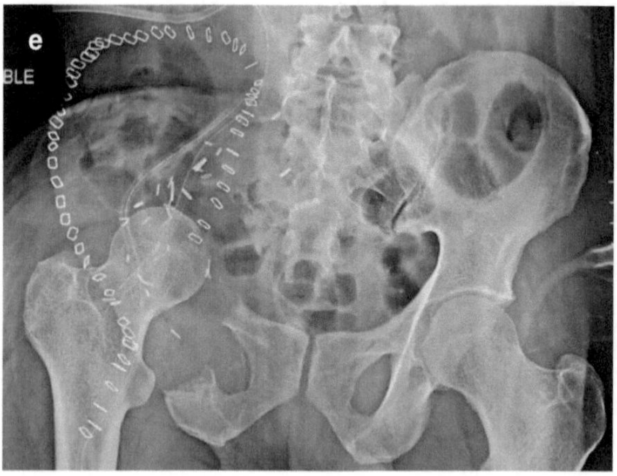

Case 3: Type 1 + Partial 2 Internal Hemipelvectomy and Meshplasty

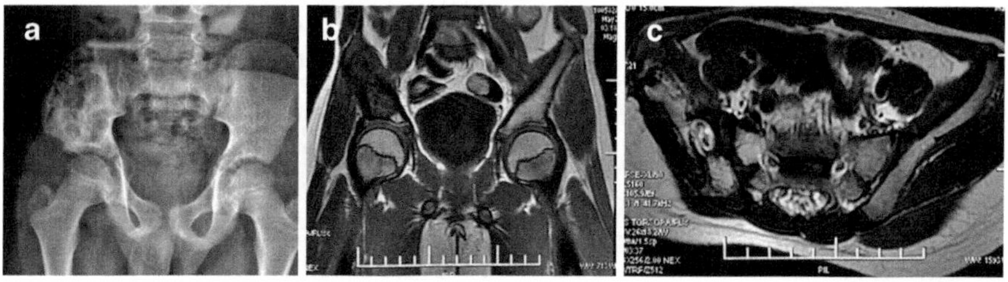

Ewing's sarcoma of ilium in a young child involving the acetabular roof. Sacroiliac and hip joints are uninvolved. External iliac vessels, femoral nerve and sciatic nerve roots are preserved (Fig. 4a–c). A type 1 + Partial 2 internal hemipelvectomy is performed by performing 2 osteotomies through triradiate cartilage and another through sacrum medial to SI joint. Ligamentum teres attachment to femur head is preserved (Fig. 4d–g).

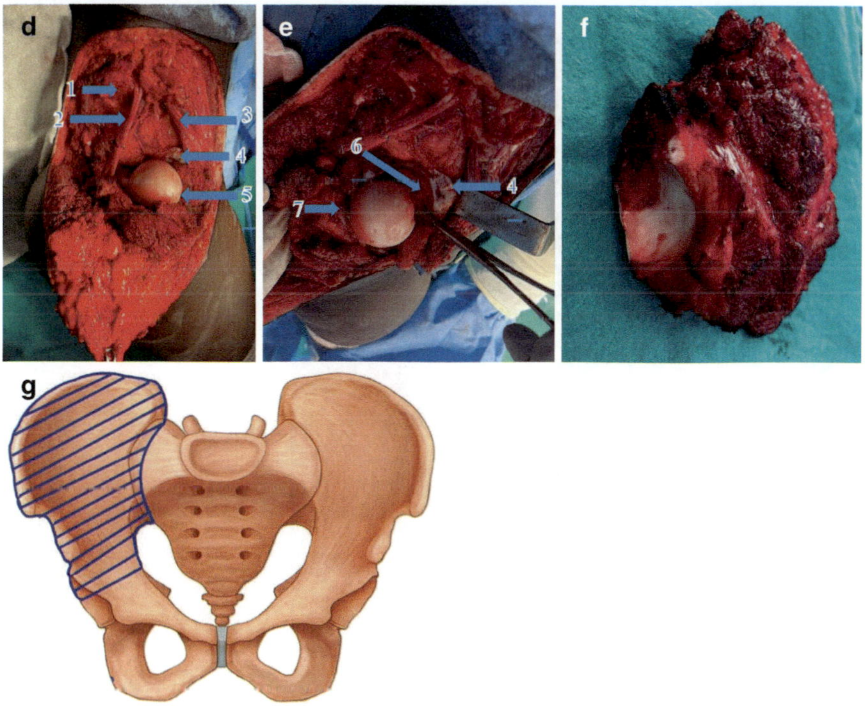

1. Sacral ala
2. Sciatic nerve
3. Psoas muscle and femoral nerve
4. Osteotomy through triradiate cartilage
5. Femur head
6. Ligamentum teres
7. Hip joint capsule

Mesh reconstruction is planned to reconstruct the deficient acetabular roof. A piece of Prolene mesh is folded on itself and secured with No. 1 Vicryl sutures to form a rectangular piece. The lateral end is fixed to remaining hip joint capsule with

Ethibond sutures. Drill holes are made in medial wall of acetabulum and columns. With limb in neutral rotation, medial end of the mesh is attached to remaining acetabulum with Ethibond sutures, forming a hood over the femur head (Fig. 4h).

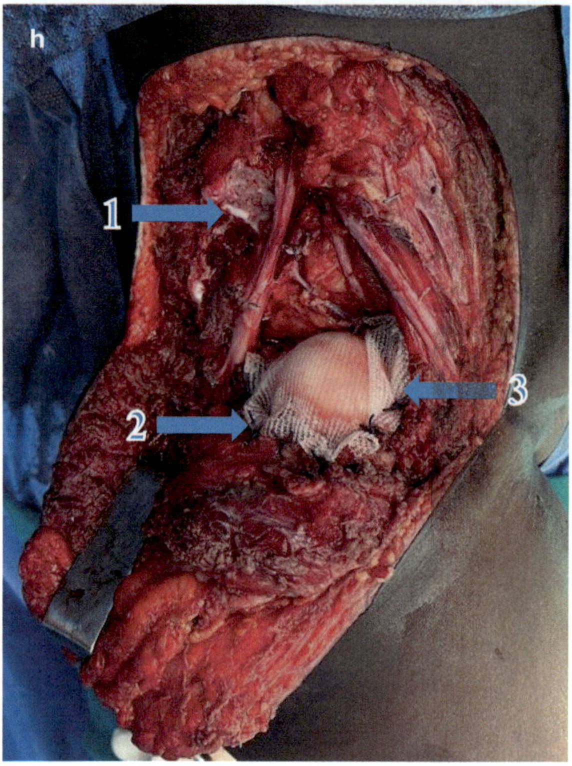

1. Sacrum ala.
2. Mesh sutured to hip joint capsule.
3. Mesh sutured to remaining acetabulum.

Case 4: Type 3 + Partial Type 2 Internal Hemipelvectomy and Meshplasty

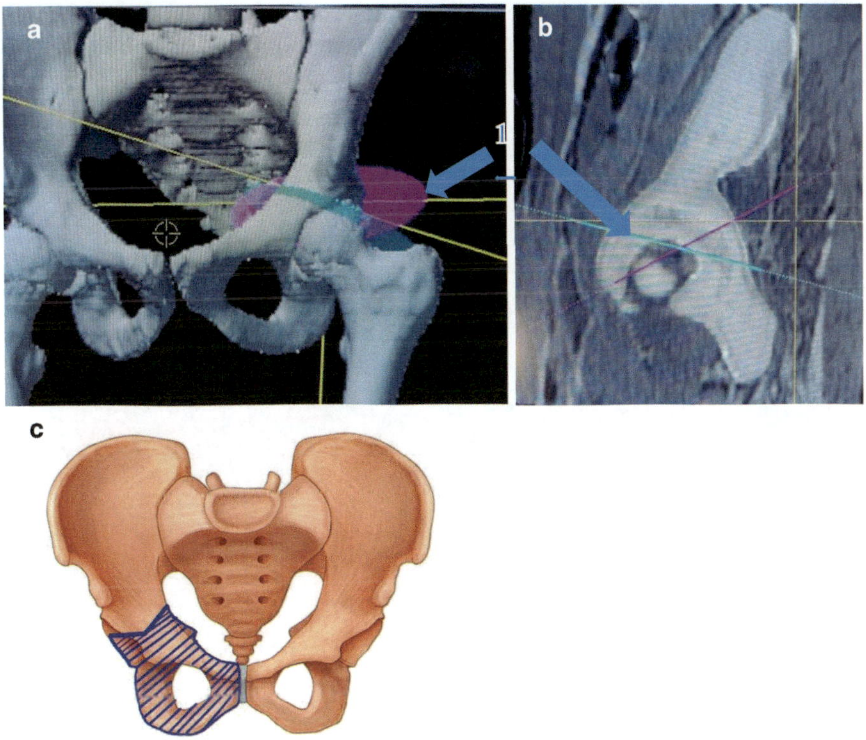

1. Planes of acetabular cuts

Ewing's sarcoma of ischium and pubis involving the lower half of the acetabulum. A broad "V" shaped cut is planned and executed with navigation guidance, preserving a part of acetabular dome. Specimen is detached from symphysis and delivered out (Fig. 5a–c).

A burr hole is made in the ilium above the acetabular dome where the bone stock is good. A rectangular piece of mesh is passed through this hole. Broad ends of the mesh are sutured on either side to the hip joint capsule with the femur head reduced to remaining acetabulum and limb kept in neutral rotation. This prevents superior-inferior and mediolateral translation of the head, thereby preventing limb shortening (Fig. 5d, e).

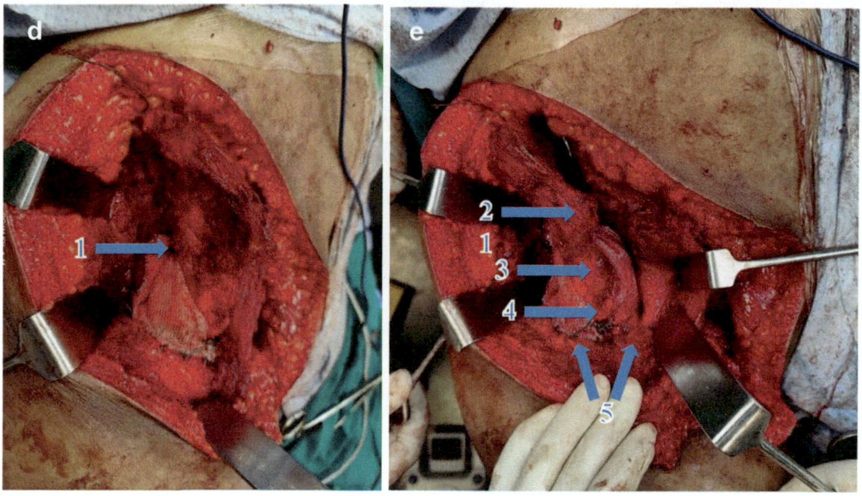

1. Burr hole in Ilium
2. ASIS
3. AIIS
4. Acetabular dome
5. Hip joint capsule

Case 5: Type 3 + Type 2 Internal Hemipelvectomy with Extra-Articular Hip Resection and Meshplasty

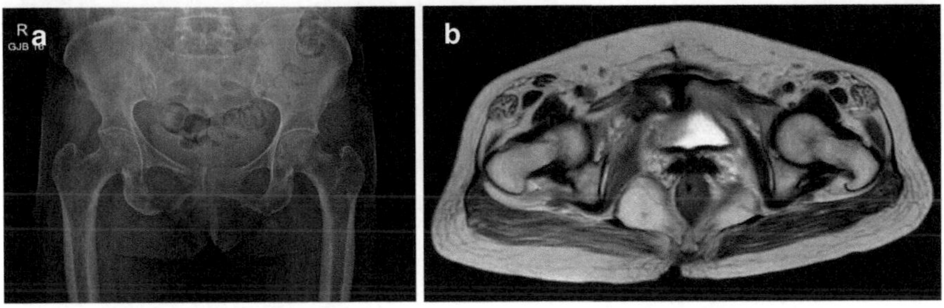

High-grade bony sarcoma of ischium and pubis involving the acetabulum and hip joint (Fig. 6a, b). Pelvic osteotomies are performed through the symphysis and through the greater sciatic notch. Hip joint is excised along with the specimen by doing a femoral osteotomy (Fig. 6c, d).

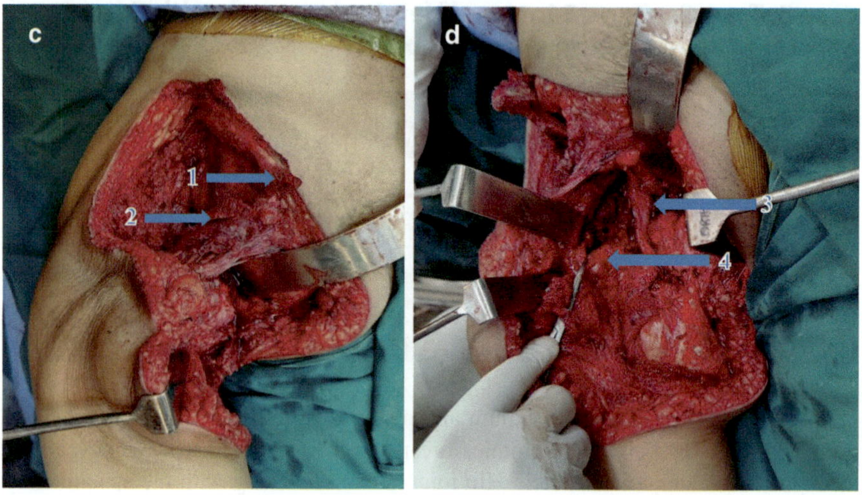

1. ASIS
2. Osteotomy through greater sciatic notch
3. Psoas muscle and femoral neurovascular bundle
4. Femoral osteotomy

Hole is made in the ilium with a high-speed burr where the bone stock is good. A 15 × 15 mesh is the passed through this hole and tied with a knot on itself. Femoral defect is reconstructed with a cemented endoprosthesis. Mesh is then wrapped around endoprosthesis and secured with Ethibond sutures. Abductor (gluteus medius and minimus) muscles are then reattached to the mesh (Fig. 6e–k).

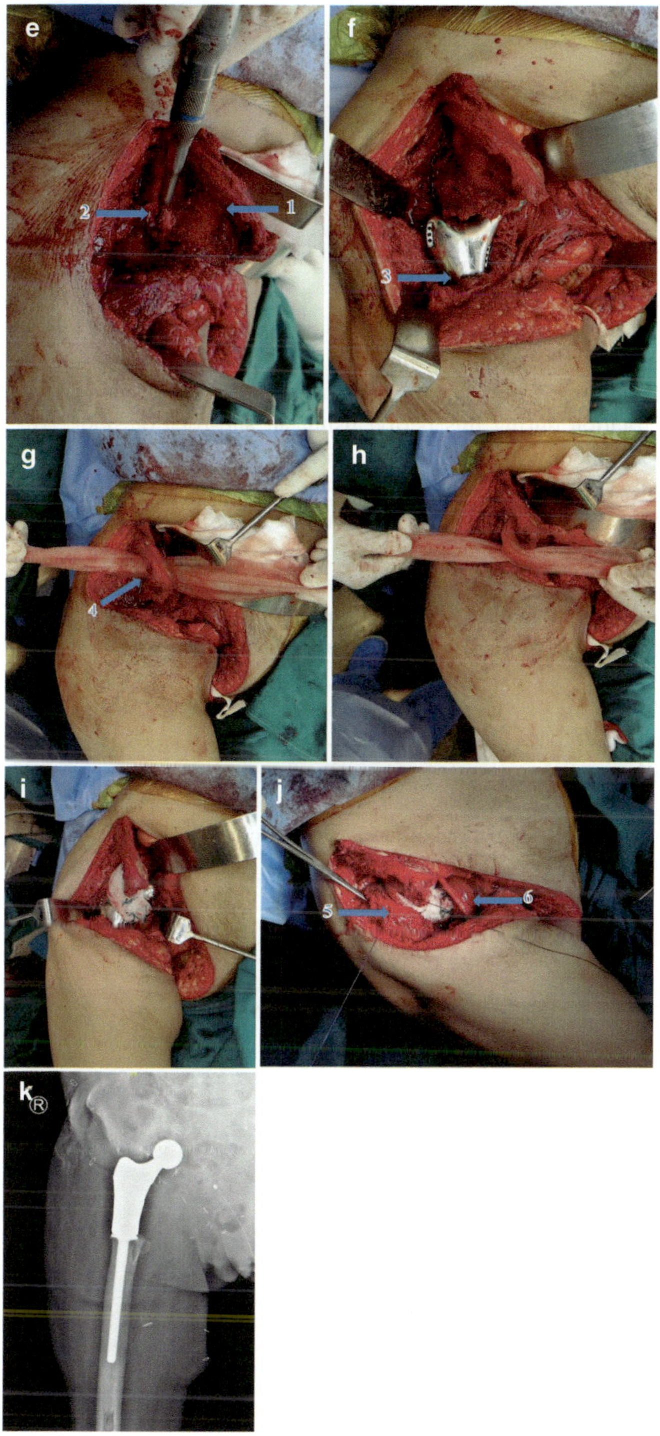
e
2
1
f
3
g
4
h
i
j
5
6
k

1. Ilium
2. Burr hole
3. Endoprosthesis
4. Mesh passed through burr hole
5. Abductors sutured to mesh
6. Psoas muscle and femoral nerve

Rehabilitation

The patient is kept on bed rest for 6 weeks after surgery. Change of posture and sitting is permitted. In bed mobilization, pelvic lifts, core strengthening exercises, static quadriceps, and hamstring exercises are encouraged. Care is taken to maintain the limb in neutral rotation during this period using an anti-rotation boot. After 6 weeks, the patient is gradually started on partial weight bearing with walking aids. The patient is gradually shifted to full weight bearing without support. SLR (straight leg raising) and abductor strengthening are encouraged during the latter part of the rehabilitation period.

Depending on the extent of resection and individual patient rehabilitation and ability, patients ultimately ambulate without walking aids or with a walking stick. Shoe lifts to compensate for shortening aid in better ambulation and improving the gait.

Suggested Reading

1. Enneking WF, Dunham WK. Resection and reconstruction for primary neoplasms involving the innominate bone. J Bone Joint Surg - Series A. 1978;60 A(6):731–46.
2. Hillmann A, Hoffman C, Gosheger G, Rödl R, Winkelmann W, Ozaki T. Tumors of the pelvis: complications after reconstruction. Arch Orthop Trauma Surg. 2003;123(7):340–4.
3. Puri A, Gulia A, Pruthi M. Outcome of surgical resection of pelvic osteosarcoma. Indian J Orthop. 2014;48(3):273–8.

Computer-Assisted Tumor Surgery (CATS) in Orthopedic Oncology: Computer Navigation and 3D Printing

Kwok Chuen Wong

Learning Objectives

- Computer-Assisted Tumor Surgery (CATS) enables surgeons to meticulously plan and replicate surgeries by mitigating surgical errors. It may translate into better oncological and functional results.
- Computer navigation and 3D printing technology are the two assistive precision tools for CATS that integrate 3D preoperative surgical planning and utilize precision tools for intraoperative implementation.
- Two cases are illustrated with practical steps to utilize the technology in orthopedic oncology surgery.

Introduction

Inaccurate bone sarcoma resection may result in positive margins with compromised oncological results or the sacrifice of more normal bone than oncologically necessary, thus adversely affecting limb function after reconstruction.

Computer-Assisted Tumor Surgery (CATS) enables surgeons to meticulously plan and replicate the surgical plans by mitigating surgical errors.

The integration of CATS into orthopedic oncology is driven by its capacity to fuse preoperative CT and MRI imaging, which offers a three-dimensional roadmap for surgeons. This is particularly crucial in technically demanding resections, such as those regions with complex anatomy and nearby vital neurovascular structures in

K. C. Wong (✉)
Orthopaedic Oncology, Department of Orthopaedics and Traumatology, Prince of Wales Hospital, The Chinese University of Hong Kong, Hong Kong SAR, China
e-mail: skcwong@cuhk.edu.hk

A. Puri, W. F. N. B. W. Ismail (eds.), *Atlas of Orthopedic Oncology Volume 1*,
https://doi.org/10.1007/978-981-95-8958-6_22

the pelvis and sacrum. CATS facilitates joint-preserving surgeries and allows for more sophisticated reconstructions with better host bone matching to custom-designed prostheses or allografts, enhancing patient limbs' functional outcomes.

CATS Workflow

The clinical CATS workflow for orthopedic oncology surgery involves integrating 3D preoperative surgical planning and utilizing precision tools for intraoperative implementation (Fig. 1).

Preoperative Planning

- Virtual bone resections are simulated in 3D bone-tumor models generated from CT-MRI image fusion and MRI-based tumor mapping. Surgeons choose their familiar and available tools (navigation or 3D printed resection guides) for the surgery.
- Navigation may be better for sarcoma surgery in complex regions like the pelvis or sacrum, where real-time image feedback helps in surgical anatomy. 3D-printed resection guides facilitate geometric bone resections and reconstruction with custom implants but are limited by design and manufacturing lead time and the availability of engineers' support.

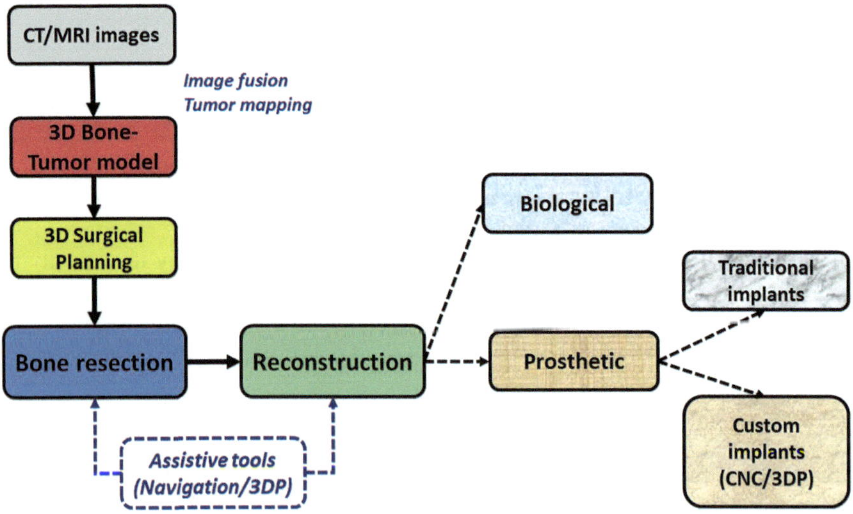

Fig. 1 Shows the CATS workflow. 3DP 3D printing (as a type of additive manufacturing), CNC Computer Numeric Control (as a type of subtractive manufacturing)

Intraoperative Implementation

For navigation, a learning curve is associated with performing an accurate image-to-patient registration, and a reliable navigated saw is not available. 3D-printed guides are intuitive to use without attention shift, but the correct guide placement as planned may be difficult, particularly with bone sarcoma having a big extraosseous component.

3D Printing

Additive manufacturing, also known as 3D printing, involves constructing a 3D physical object from a digital model by depositing material like plastic or metal in successive layers. It has the advantages of flexible designs and porous lattices for better osseointegration.

The design of a 3D-printed patient-specific resection guide (PSG) requires surgical considerations, which include the surgical approach, the amount of exposed bone footprints for stable and correct guide placement, the width of the osteotomy platform, K-wire holes to stabilize the guide, and a handle to connect two osteotomy platforms for long bone resections.

The 3D-printed patient-specific implants (PSI) should

- Match the patient's bony anatomy and the bone defect created after tumor resections
- Achieve the initial primary bone stability using extracortical flanges and multiple screw fixation
- Have porous lattices at the bone-implant junctions to enhance secondary osseointegration to the host bones for implant longevity.

A close collaboration between surgeons and engineers is crucial to producing 3D-printed guides and implants that meet surgical and manufacturing needs.

Case 1 (Computer Navigation)

A 25-year-old man had Ewing sarcoma involving the left posterior iliac crest and sacroiliac joint (Fig. 2a). Systemic staging showed no distant metastases. He received preoperative chemotherapy with a good clinical and radiological response (Fig. 2b).

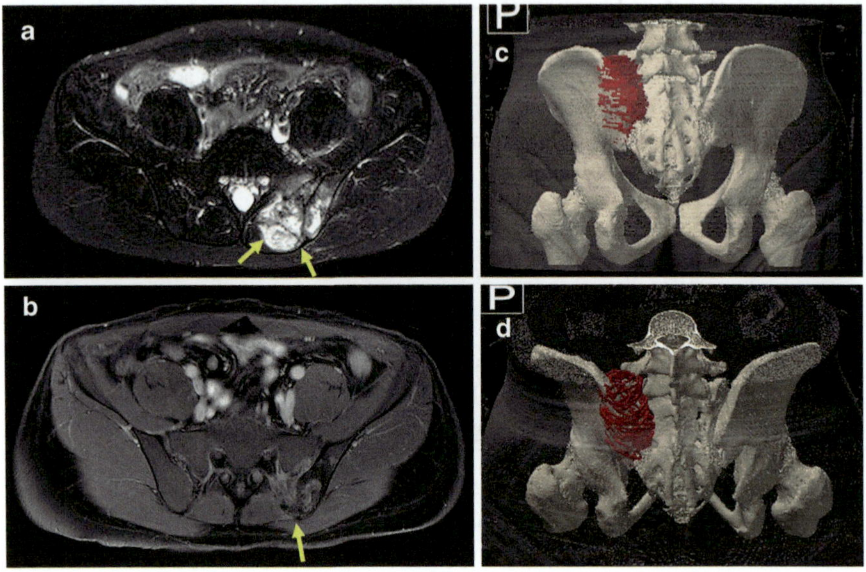

Fig. 2 (**a**) The axial view of a T2-weighted MRI of the pelvis in a 25-year-old man shows Ewing sarcoma at the left posterior iliac crest with an extraosseous tumor component (yellow arrow) extending to the paraspinal muscle region. (**b**) The patient responded well to the neoadjuvant chemotherapy, as significant tumor shrinkage (yellow arrow) was noted on the axial view of T1-weighted MRI with fat suppression and less contrast enhancement. (**c**) and (**d**) show the 3D-bone tumor model for resection planning in the navigation software

Preoperative Navigation Planning

- DICOM images of the CT pelvis and post-chemotherapy MRI pelvis were imported into the navigation system (OrthoMap 3D, Stryker). CT and MRI images were co-registered, and the tumor was mapped on the MRI images. 3D bone-tumor model (Fig. 2c, d) was generated.
- By studying the co-registered CT-MRI image dataset and the 3D model, the surgeon defined resection planes around the sarcoma based on the surgical approach, the tumor extent, and nearby vital structures (Fig. 3a–d).
- Four bone surface points were selected and marked on the CT images for intraoperative image-to-patient registration (Fig. 3e, f).

Intraoperative Navigation

- The patient lay in a prone position. A curvilinear skin incision was made along the iliac crest and the lateral aspect of the left sacrum (Fig. 4a).
- The Gluteal Maximus, Gluteal Medius, Iliocostalis Lumborum, Longissimus Thoracis, and Multifidus muscles, except the portions covering the sarcoma, were mobilized to expose the planned osteotomies (Fig. 4b).

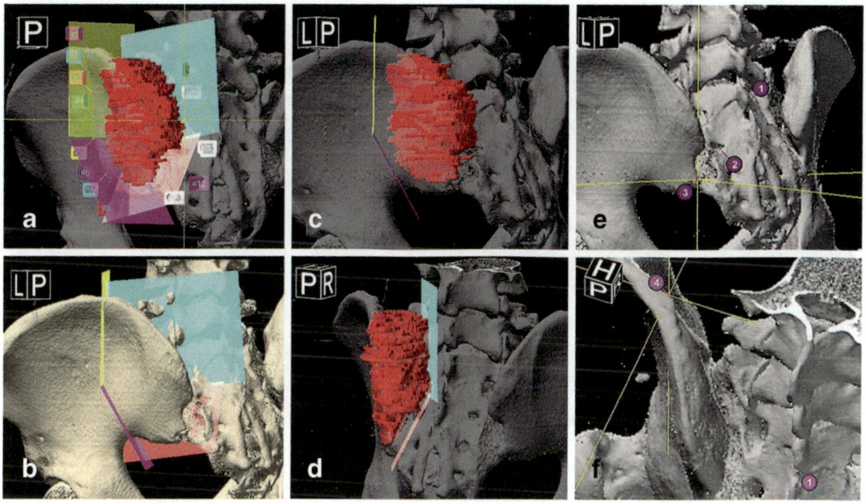

Fig. 3 (**a–d**) Shows the intended multiplanar resections around the sarcoma (red) at the posterior ilium and sacral ala bone in the navigation software. (**e**) and (**f**) show that four bony surface points were selected on the 3D pelvic bone model for the subsequent intraoperative image-to-patient registration

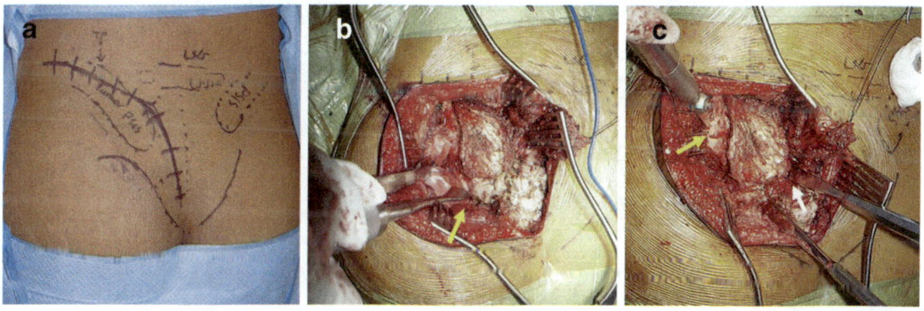

Fig. 4 (**a**) Skin markings of the anatomical landmarks and the surgical incision for the patient with Ewing sarcoma at the left posterior iliac crest. (**b**) Surgical exposure of the bone sarcoma after mobilizing gluteal and paraspinal muscles, exposing the intended osteotomy sites. A retractor was placed at the greater sciatic notch (yellow arrow) to protect the superior gluteal vessels and the sciatic nerve before performing the osteotomies. (**c**) After the image-to-patient registration, the osteotomy sites were marked by diathermy or Kirschner wires (yellow arrow) under the navigation assistance. The bone resection was completed by an oscillating saw (yellow arrow) and osteotomes (white arrow) at the marked osteotomies

- A patient navigation tracker was placed at the right posterior iliac crest. A navigation probe was calibrated with the navigation system. The image-to-patient registration was first performed by matching the four paired-point bony surface points (Fig. 5). The registration accuracy was improved by surface matching (Fig. 6). The navigation probe touching the exposed bone surface further verified the registration. Surgeons trust and rely on virtual images to execute their 3D

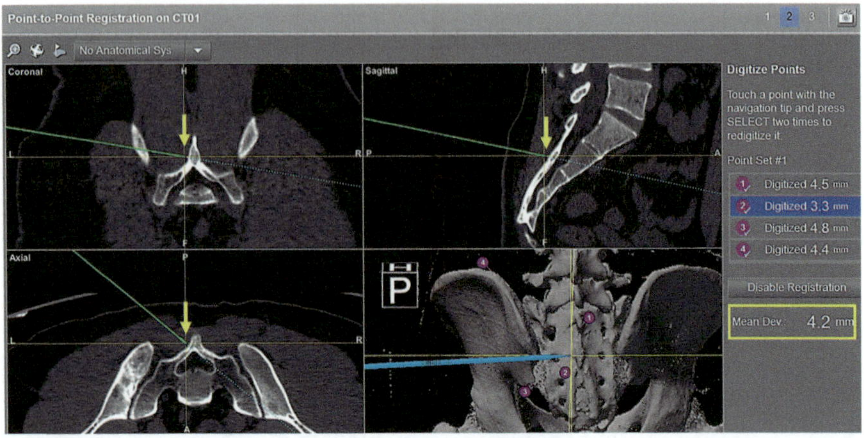

Fig. 5 The navigation display shows the mean deviation error was 4.2 mm (yellow rectangle) after the paired-point image-to-patient registration. When the tip of the navigation probe touched the bone surface to verify the registration accuracy, the virtual tip of the navigation probe (green line) was offset from the bone surface (yellow arrows)

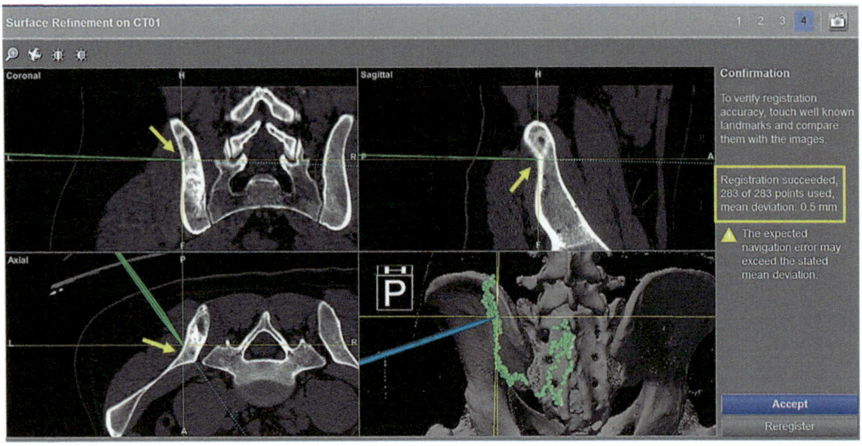

Fig. 6 The navigation display shows the mean deviation error was 0.5 mm (yellow rectangle) after surface matching. The green dots represented the 283 bone surface points collected near the intended osteotomies. The surface points formed a 3D surface cloud that matched the patients' respective CT bone models. The registration was accurate as the virtual tip of the navigation probe precisely tracked the bone surface (yellow arrows)

surgical plans only if the patient's operative anatomy matches their preoperative images and the operated bones can be physically tracked by the navigation system.

- With the real-time feedback of preoperative CT images, the locations and orientations of the planned osteotomies were identified using the navigation probe (Figs. 7 and 8), which were marked by diathermy or Kirschner wires.

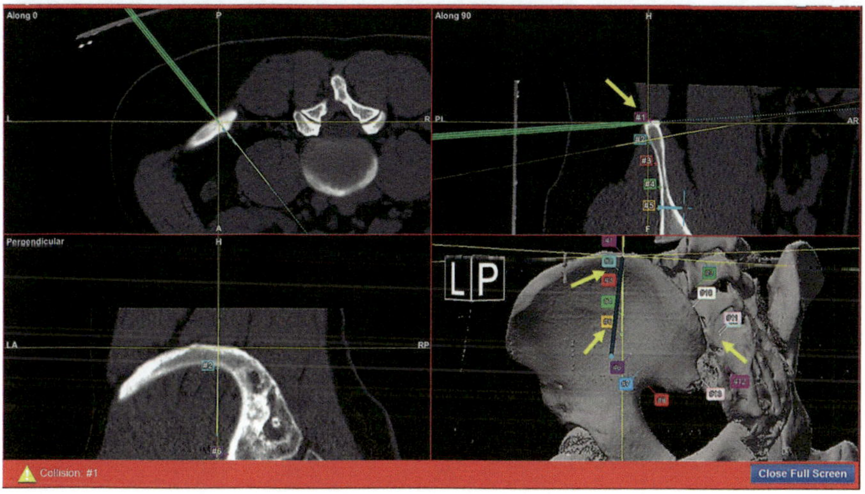

Fig. 7 The navigation display shows the tip of the navigation probe (green line), which identified the intended osteotomy sites (yellow arrows) under navigation assistance

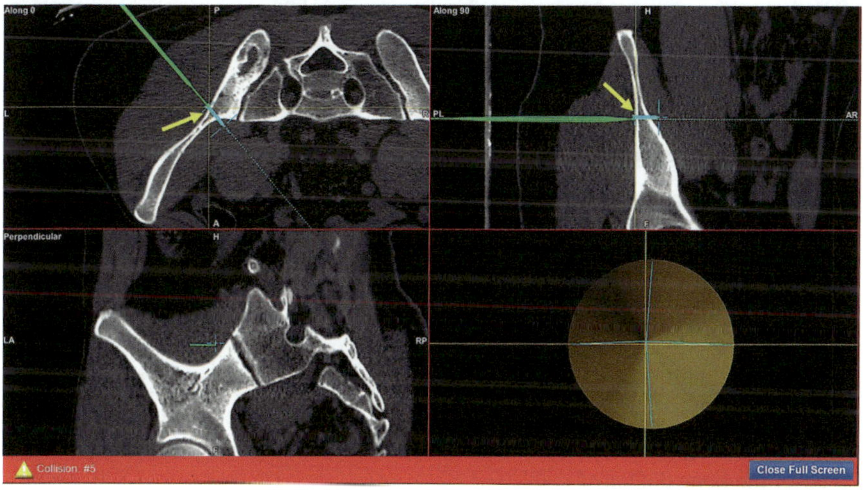

Fig. 8 The navigation display shows the tip of the navigation probe (green line) matched to the virtual screw (yellow arrow) that was planned along the osteotomy plane. A Kirschner wire was inserted along the trajectory of the virtual screw, and osteotomy could be performed along the orientation of multiple Kirschner wires

- The osteotomies were performed using an oscillating saw and osteotomies along the orientations of K-wires and the navigation probe (Fig. 4c). After resection, the resection margin at the remaining sacrum bone was verified using the navigation probe, confirming the negative bone margin (Fig. 9a, b).

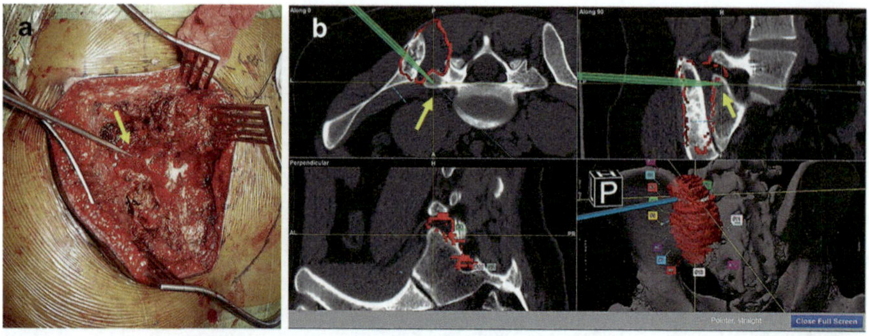

Fig. 9 (**a**) After bone sarcoma resection, the negative resection margin could be verified by placing the tip of the navigation probe (yellow arrow) on the resected bone surface. (**b**) The navigation display shows that the tip of the navigation probe (green line) was outside the tumor edge (yellow arrow), confirming the negative resection margin intraoperatively

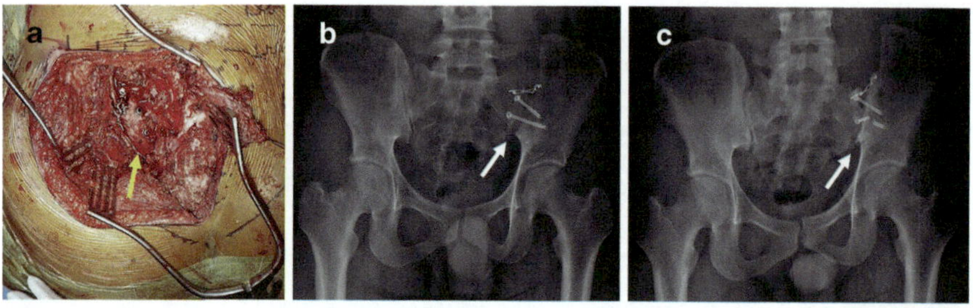

Fig. 10 (**a**) Shows an iliac crest bone graft (yellow arrow) filled up the bone defect at the sacroiliac joint and secured by titanium screws and wires. The plain radiograph of the pelvis 2 weeks after surgery (**b**) and 5 years after surgery (**c**) shows partial bone healing with fibrous union (white arrow) and upward migration of the left hemipelvis

- A cortico-cancellous bone graft was harvested from the left iliac crest and was placed to bridge the bone gap between the remaining left iliac crest and left sacral ala (Fig. 10a). The gluteal muscle and paraspinal muscle were repaired to cover the bone defect.

Postoperative Outcome

- The histology of the tumor specimen showed a negative resection margin with 100% chemonecrosis.
- He completed his postoperative chemotherapy without external radiotherapy.
- The patient had partial weight-bearing walking with aids for 4 weeks after his wound was well.

- He enjoyed normal leg function without evidence of sarcoma recurrence 5 years after surgery. The plain radiograph of the pelvis showed a fibrous union at the left sacroiliac region with some upward migration of the left hemipelvis, hinging at the pubic symphysis (Fig. 10b, c).

Case 2 (3D-Printed, Patient-Specific Guides and Pelvic Implant)

A 48-year-old man complained of a painful left hip with swelling and stiffness. He had a left pelvic stage III giant cell tumor of bone involving pubic rami and acetabulum (Fig. 11a). The expansile extraosseous component extended to the adductor component and posterior acetabulum (Fig. 11b–d). The patient received 6 months of denosumab for pain relief and tumor consolidation before undergoing PII & III resection (with the assistance of a 3D-printed PSG) and reconstruction with a 3D-printed pelvic implant and a Duo Mobility hip arthroplasty.

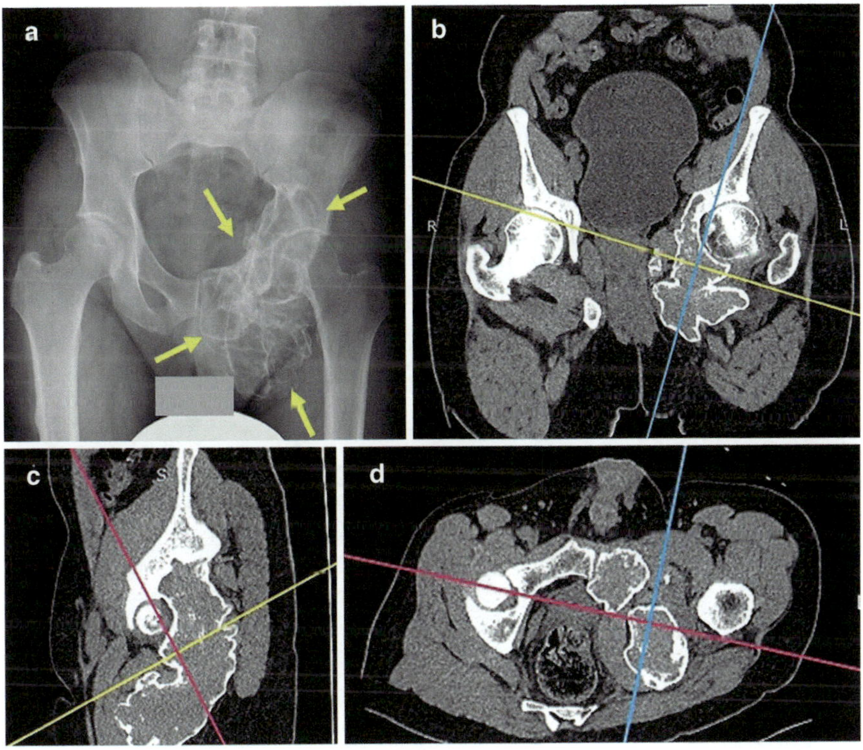

Fig. 11 (a) A plain radiograph of the pelvis shows a left pelvic giant cell tumor (yellow arrows) after denosumab treatment in a 48-year-old man. The coronal (b), sagittal (c), and axial (d) views of the reformatted CT pelvis show the extent of the tumor involving the left superior and inferior pubic rami and posterior acetabular column

Preoperative Planning

- DICOM images of the CT pelvis (slice thickness of 0.625 mm) were imported into the medical engineering software (MIMICS, version 16, Materialise, Belgium). After mapping the tumor on the CT images, the 3D bone-tumor model was generated for surgical planning.
- By studying the reformatted views of CT images and the 3D model, the surgeon defined the multiplanar resections at the ilium (Fig. 12a, b) via the anterolateral direction, thereby maximally preserving the normal host bone at the anterior inferior iliac spine with its muscle attachment and also the remaining ilium and sacroiliac joint for better load transfer of the implant reconstruction.
- The engineer designed a PSG to replicate the surgeon-defined bone resections. The guide was positioned on the outer surface of the ilium at the intended resection planes, with its footprint wrapping around the inferior part of the anterior inferior iliac spine and greater sciatic notch (Fig. 12c).
- The engineer further designed a pelvic PSI that matched the planes of intended bone resections (Fig. 13a, b). The hip center of the PSI was the same as the opposite normal side. It did not connect to the pubic rami, as inaccurate iliac osteotomies may result in implant mismatch, and more extensive revision is required if the whole construct fails. The primary fixation of the implant was achieved by the extracortical flanges and multiple screw fixation (Fig. 13c), while the secondary osseointegration for implant longevity was enhanced by porous lattices coated with calcium sulfate at the implant-bone interface (Fig. 13d).

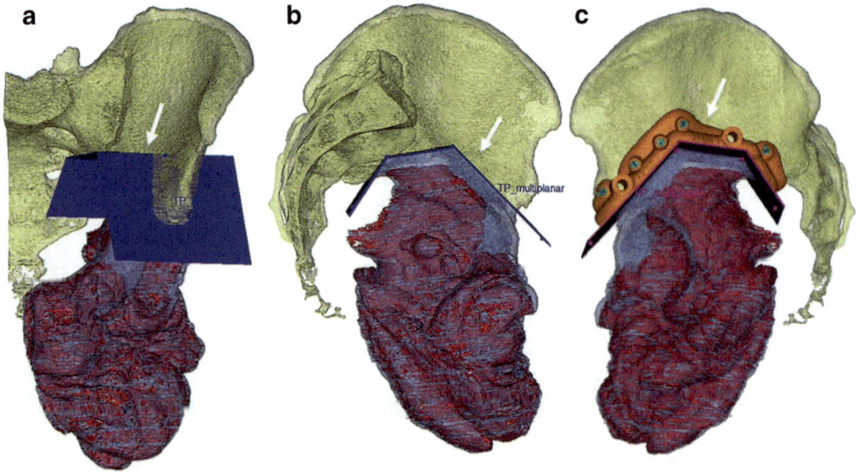

Fig. 12 The surgeon defined the resection planes (white arrows) at the left ilium in the 3D virtual bone-tumor models (**a**, **b**). (**c**) The engineer designed a patient-specific resection guide (white arrow) on the outer table of the left ilium that matched the surgeon-defined resection planes. A few 3.2 mm pins were used to secure the guide to the bone after its correct placement on the bone surface

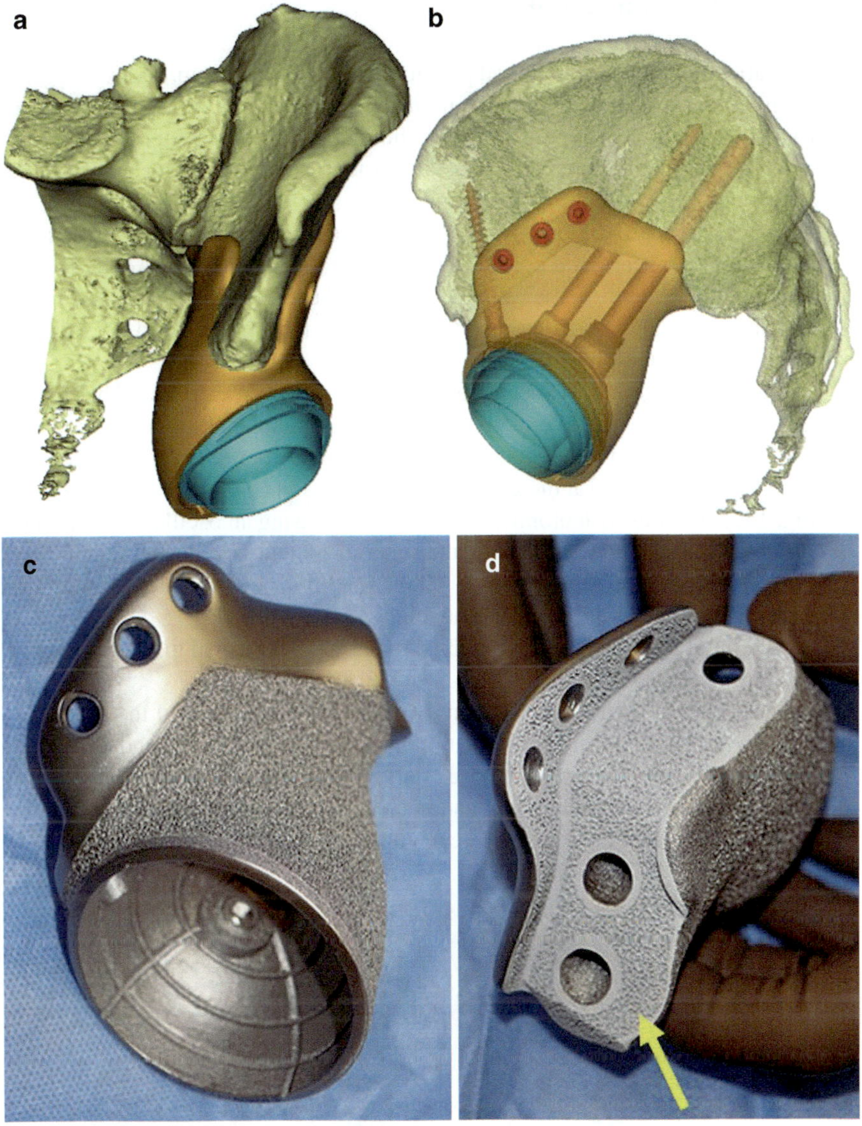

Fig. 13 An implant engineer designed a patient-specific pelvic implant (**a**, **b**) that matched the bone defect after bone resection. Extracortical flanges and multiple screws achieved the primary stability of the implant. (**c**, **d**) show the 3D-printed patient-specific implant with porous lattice and calcium sulfate coating (yellow arrow) for better soft tissue healing and secondary osseointegration

Intraoperative Implementation

- The patient lay in a floppy lateral position with the left side up.
- A utilitarian surgical approach was used. The transverse skin incision was made from the proximal adductor and the ilioinguinal to the posterior iliac crest regions. The anterolateral skin incision started from the anterior superior iliac spine to the level of the proximal femur.
- The three surgical windows—the iliopsoas muscle, the femoral neurovascular bundle, and the spermatic cord—were identified and protected. Adductor muscles were detached from the calcified tumor at the pubic rami (Fig. 14a).
- The gluteal muscles were detached from the outer table of the ilium to expose the intended iliac osteotomy sites (Fig. 14b).
- The femoral head was dislocated after releasing the hip capsules. The femoral neck was osteotomized to expose the posterior acetabular column.
- The PSG was placed and secured with fixation pins after its footprint fitted well to the bone surface and at the greater sciatic notch and anterior inferior iliac spine (Fig. 14c). The iliac osteotomies were performed using an oscillating saw on the cutting platform of the PSG, while the superior gluteal vessels and sciatic nerve were protected at the greater sciatic notch. The tumor was resected en bloc after releasing the remaining soft tissue attachment.
- A 3D-printed drill guide was assembled to the PSG to predrill the screw tracts of iliac screws (Fig. 15a).
- The pelvic PSI was fixed to the ilium with multiple screws, and the hip arthroplasty with Duo Mobility articulation was performed in a standard fashion (Fig. 15b). Passive hip movement was stable on table examination. All remaining pelvic-hip muscles were repaired and reattached meticulously to restore the suspensory soft tissue balance of the new hip joint (Fig. 15c).

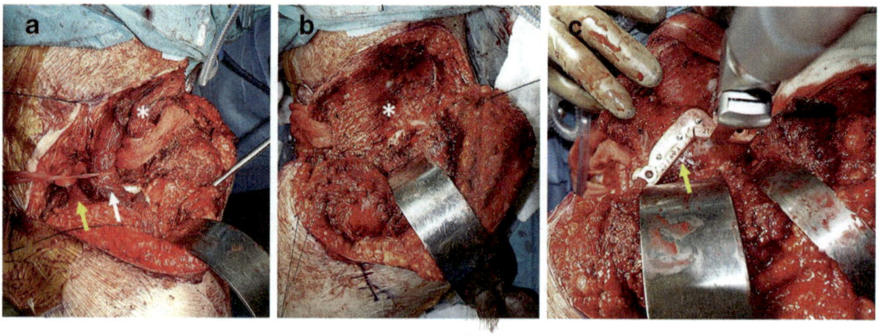

Fig. 14 (**a**) Shows the ilioinguinal approach to expose the ilium (*), iliopsoas muscle (white arrow), and femoral neurovascular bundle (yellow arrow). (**b**) Shows the outer table of the left ilium (*) to expose the intended iliac osteotomy site after the gluteal muscle detached and retracted distally. (**c**) The osteotomy was performed with an oscillating saw along an orientation guided by the patient-specific resection guide (yellow arrow)

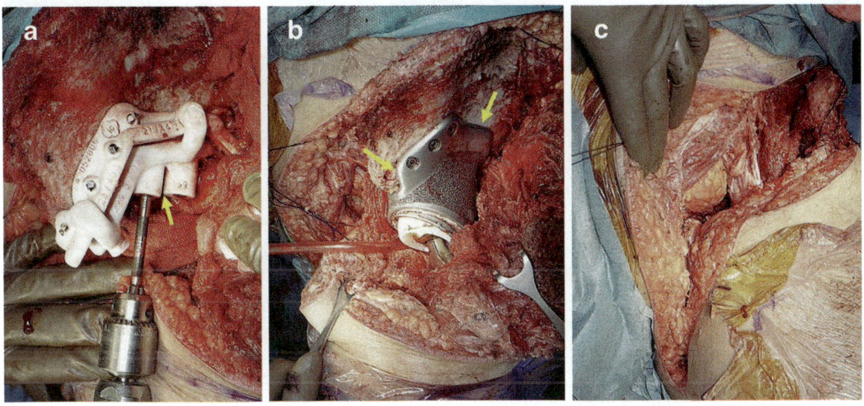

Fig. 15 (**a**) The patient-specific drill guide (yellow arrow) was placed at the bone defect by connecting to the resection guide after bone tumor resection. The posterior iliac bone was predrilled with the predetermined screw diameter and length via the drill guide. (**b**) The patient-specific implant matched well with the ilium (yellow arrows). A duo mobility cup with traditional hip replacement was performed. (**c**) All remaining pelvic-hip soft tissue was meticulously repaired to restore the suspensory muscle function of the hip joint

Postoperative Outcome

- The patient started mobilization after the wound was well.
- He wore a hip-knee-ankle-foot orthosis for 3 months while standing and walking. The orthosis protected the soft tissue reconstruction and controlled the leg alignment.
- He had partial-weight-bearing walking for 6 weeks after surgery and then walked as tolerated.
- The histology of the tumor specimen confirmed the giant cell tumor of bone with the denosumab effect.
- At 3 years after surgery, he did not have pain, and there was no evidence of local tumor recurrence. A plain radiograph of the pelvis showed no implant loosening (Fig. 16a). He could achieve hip flexion from 0 to 90° (Fig. 16b). He could walk unaided for a short distance with a mild Trendelenburg gait due to some weakness of his abductor muscles (Fig. 16c). He needed a walking stick for outdoor and long-distance walks.

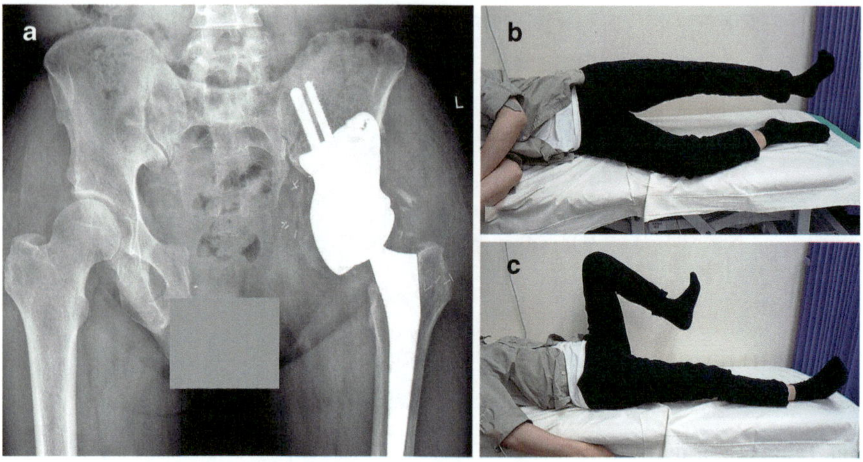

Fig. 16 Shows the patient's plain radiograph of the pelvis (**a**), his hip abduction (**b**), and flexion (**c**) 3 years after surgery

Summary

- The advent of CATS technology enables tumor surgeons to 3D plan and precisely replicate surgical plans that may translate into better oncological and functional results.
- Close collaboration and teamwork between surgeons and engineers are crucial to the success of CATS.
- Surgeons should embrace the CATS technology and select the best tools for their tumor patients.
- A long-term follow-up with more patients from various tumor centers is required to determine the clinical efficacy of the CATS.

Suggested Reading

1. Wong KC. 3D-printed patient-specific applications in orthopedics. Orthop Res Rev. 2016;14(8):57–66.
2. Wong KC, Kumta SM. Use of computer navigation in orthopedic oncology. Curr Surg Rep. 2014;2(4):47.
3. Wong KC, Scheinemann P. Additive manufactured metallic implants for orthopaedic applications. Sci China-Mater. 2018;61:440–54.
4. Wong KC, Sze LKY, Kumta SM. Complex joint-preserving bone tumor resection and reconstruction using computer navigation and 3D-printed patient-specific guides: a technical note of three cases. J Orthop Translat. 2021;29:152–62.

Tips and Tricks in Allograft Reconstructions

Domenico Andrea Campanacci, Roberto Scanferla,
Maurizio Scorianz, Francesco Muratori,
and Guido Scoccianti

Allograft Prosthesis Composite (APC) of the Proximal Femur

Introduction

Proximal femur is one of the most common sites of primary bone tumors. After proximal femur resection, allograft-prosthesis composites (APC) and modular prostheses represent the most frequently used reconstructive options. The advantages of APC reconstruction over endoprosthesis include biological attachment of gluteal and iliopsoas tendons, improving stability, function recovery, and gait, restoration of bone stock, and load-sharing properties of the allograft if union occurs. In particular, restoration of bone stock is very helpful in young patients who are likely to require further surgeries. Nonetheless, proximal femur reconstruction in growing children poses several challenges. Cementless prosthetic stem fixation in an immature bone may induce stress shielding, while cemented implants pose concerns related to the bone loss during subsequent revision surgery.

Proximal femur APCs have been described with two different assemblies: long stem prosthesis cemented into the allograft, bypassing the osteotomy line and achieving fixation in healthy bone with or without cement, and short stem prosthesis cemented into the allograft and fixed with a compression plate to the femoral diaphysis.

D. A. Campanacci (✉) · R. Scanferla · M. Scorianz · F. Muratori · G. Scoccianti
Orthopaedic Oncology Unit, Careggi University Hospital, Florence, Italy
e-mail: domenicoandrea.campanacci@unifi.it

A. Puri, W. F. N. B. W. Ismail (eds.), *Atlas of Orthopedic Oncology Volume 1*,
https://doi.org/10.1007/978-981-95-8958-6_23

Surgical Anatomy

The proximal femur is characterized by several tendinous insertions and an intra-capsular location of the femoral head and neck. The anatomical structures potentially involved in proximal femur tumors include:

- Joint space and capsule: intra-articular tumor extension is quite rare and usually occurs after a pathologic fracture. In this case an extra-articular resection should be planned.
- Hip abductor (gluteal) tendons, inserted on the greater trochanter. These tendons should be preserved for subsequent reattachment to the graft. If infiltrated by the tumor and resected, an endoprosthetic reconstruction should be considered.
- Gluteus maximus: the tendinous insertion on femoral linea aspera is detached for a variable amount according to tumor extension.
- Ilio-psoas tendon, inserted on the lesser trochanter. The tendon stump should be preserved for its reattachment to the graft, improving hip flexion and balancing.
- Vastus lateralis and medialis, inserted on proximal femur meta-diaphysis. The muscles are usually partially resected, leaving their fibers to cover the tumor, according to tumoral extension, and no reconstruction is needed.
- Adductor muscles insert on the medial femoral diaphysis. They are usually detached at a safe distance from the tumor and no reconstruction is needed.
- Common/superficial femoral artery: if infiltrated by the tumor, a vascular bypass, or a hip disarticulation should be considered.

Assessment

Proximal femur resection and reconstruction with APC requires the availability of a well-functioning bone banking facility; furthermore, there are some religious concerns related to the use of human allografts in different countries. Finally, in children, the small size of the residual femur and acetabulum requires small hip stems and head prostheses.

Important assessments to be done before resection include:

- Femoral deformity, through preoperative whole femur X-rays.
- Tumor extension, through a contrast-enhanced MRI of the entire femur and hemipelvis. This reconstructive option is contraindicated in case of abductor muscle and/or acetabular tumor involvement.
- Common/superficial femoral artery. The tumor involvement of the common/superficial femoral artery contraindicates the reconstruction with an APC due to the high risks of subsequent complications.

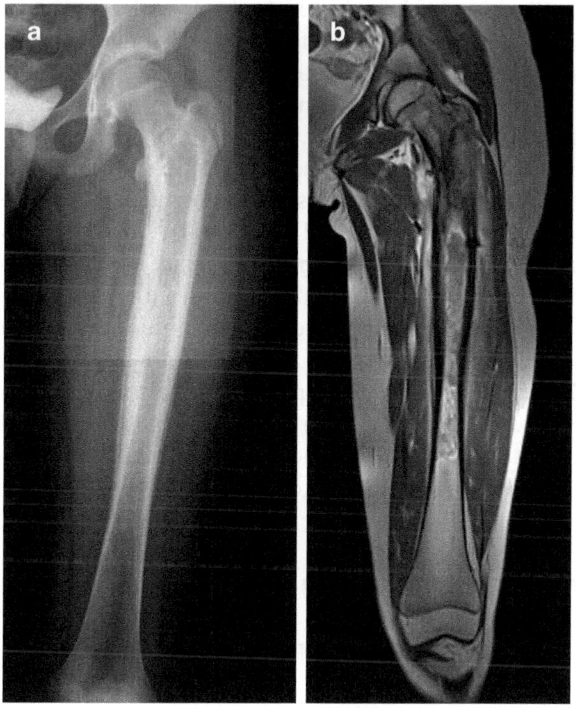

These figures show an Ewing' sarcoma of the left proximal femur in a 12-year-old female. Contrast-enhanced MRI shows the tumor involvement of the proximal femur, without extraosseous mass nor articular invasion (Fig. 1a, b).

Surgical Steps

Proximal Femur Resection Surgical Steps

- Lateral approach to the proximal femur, with patient in supine or lateral position
- Detachment of the hip abductor tendons from the greater trochanter, taking care to mark the tendon stump.
- Detachment of vastus lateralis, intermedius, and medialis from proximal femur metadiaphysis; the proximal fibers of these muscles are usually resected along with the tumor, leaving a layer of healthy tissue surrounding the specimen. The amount of muscular resection is decided case by case, according to tumor extension.
- Posteriorly, gluteus maximus insertion on the femur is resected, paying attention to the sciatic nerve, which lies nearby (a useful tip is to put finger behind the tendon when cutting it). With the lower limb in internal rotation, the external rotator muscles (piriformis, superior and inferior gemellus, obturator internus and externus, and quadratus femoris) are sectioned.

- After freeing the lateral side of the femur, diaphyseal osteotomy is performed at a distance from the tip of the greater trochanter determined by preoperative planning, according to the extension of the tumor as assessed by MRI. A specimen from the distal medullary canal is sent for frozen section to have confirmation of oncological margin at the osteotomy.
- Once the osteotomy is performed, the proximal femur can be abducted, making it easier to detach the adductor muscle, paying attention to possible bleeding from branches of the deep femoral artery and vein. The iliopsoas tendon is detached from lesser trochanter, taking care to mark its tendon stump. During the detachment of medial structures from proximal femur, it's mandatory to locate and protect the common femoral artery along its superficial and deep branches (the deep vessels can be sacrificed if required by tumor location and extension).
- Hip capsule incision, marking the capsule. If there is no involvement of the capsule by the tumor, it should be preserved, receiving an inverse T-shaped incision with subsequent resuturing, to enhance stability of the reconstructed joint.
- Section of ligamentum teres and hip dislocation.

Options for Bone Reconstruction

Several reconstructive options have been described after proximal femur resection:

- Massive osteoarticular allografts
- Modular prosthesis
- Allograft-prosthesis composites (APC)
- Recycled autograft-prosthesis composites
- Combination between massive allograft and vascularized growing fibula autograft
- Hip arthrodesis.

Nowadays, APC represents our preferred reconstructive option after proximal femur resection in skeletally immature patients; we also use this reconstructive option in young adults with diagnoses of aggressive benign and low-grade malignant bone tumors.

In adults, we usually prefer APCs with long stem cemented into the allograft and bypassing the osteotomy line, with uncemented fixation on host bone (Fig. 1c, d).

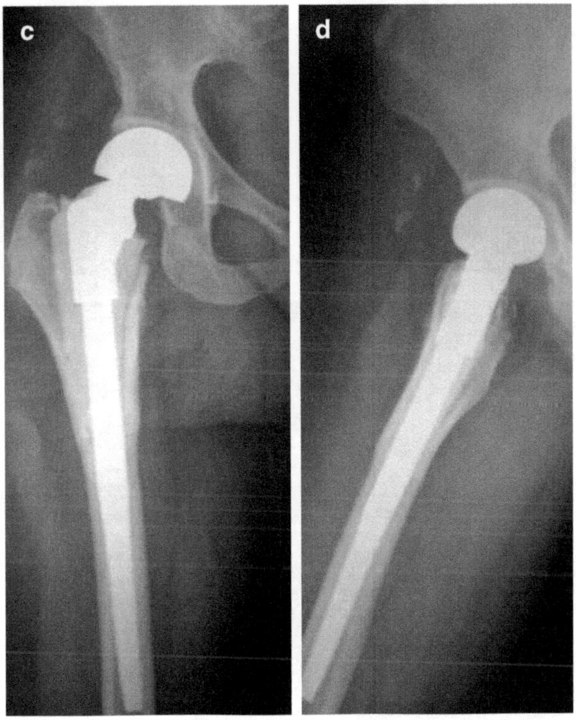

In long proximal femur resection, where it would be difficult to adequately shape the allograft, an APC made by a proximal femur massive allograft combined with a modular cementless proximal femur prosthesis can be used (Fig. 1e–k) This allows an effective abductor and iliopsoas tendons reattachment with no need to adapt a long straight stem to the allograft shaft procurvatum

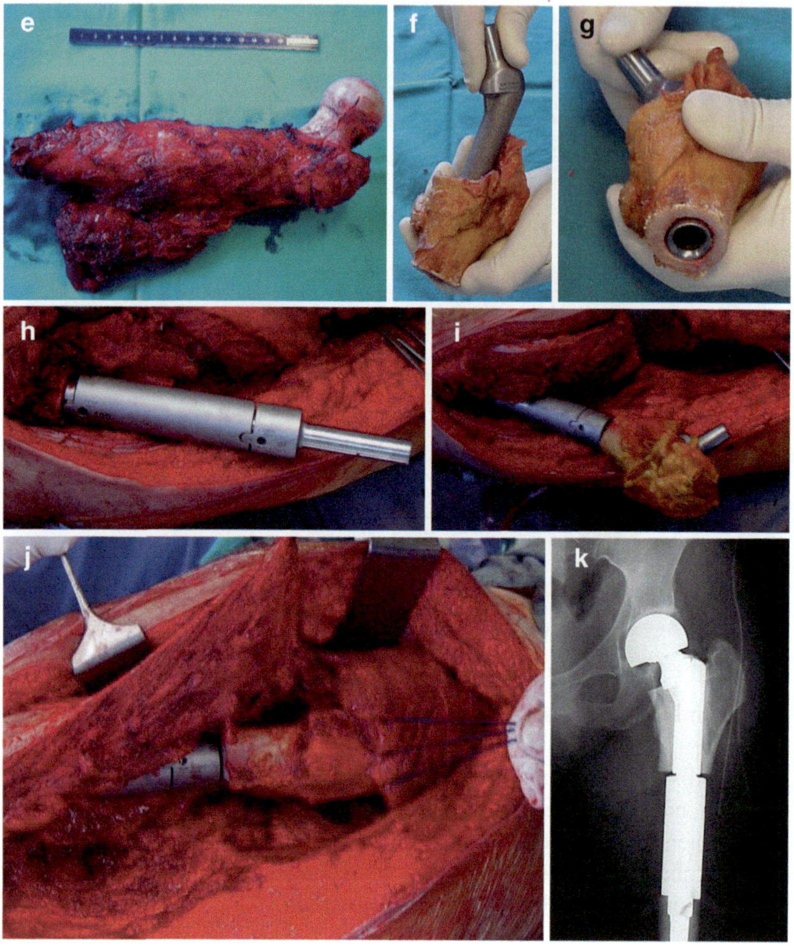

On the contrary, short stem APCs are preferred in proximal femur pediatric reconstructions for the following reasons:

- Long stems hypothetically decrease the risk of allograft fractures, but on the other hand, they transfer loads directly to the healthy immature femoral diaphysis of the child, leading to an increasing risk of stress-shielding that could impair subsequent revisions;
- Lengthening procedures on the residual femur cannot be performed in the presence of a long stem extending into the distal diaphysis;
- Using a short stem APC, the proximal femur bone stock is preserved by allograft replacement, providing a biologic scaffold for future revisions.

Furthermore, in growing patients the residual femoral shaft dimension does not always accept long stems. In growing patients, an APC using compression plates and short stem prosthesis minimally affects the osteotomy site, allowing physiologic load transfer once union has been achieved by periosteal and endosteal callus formation.

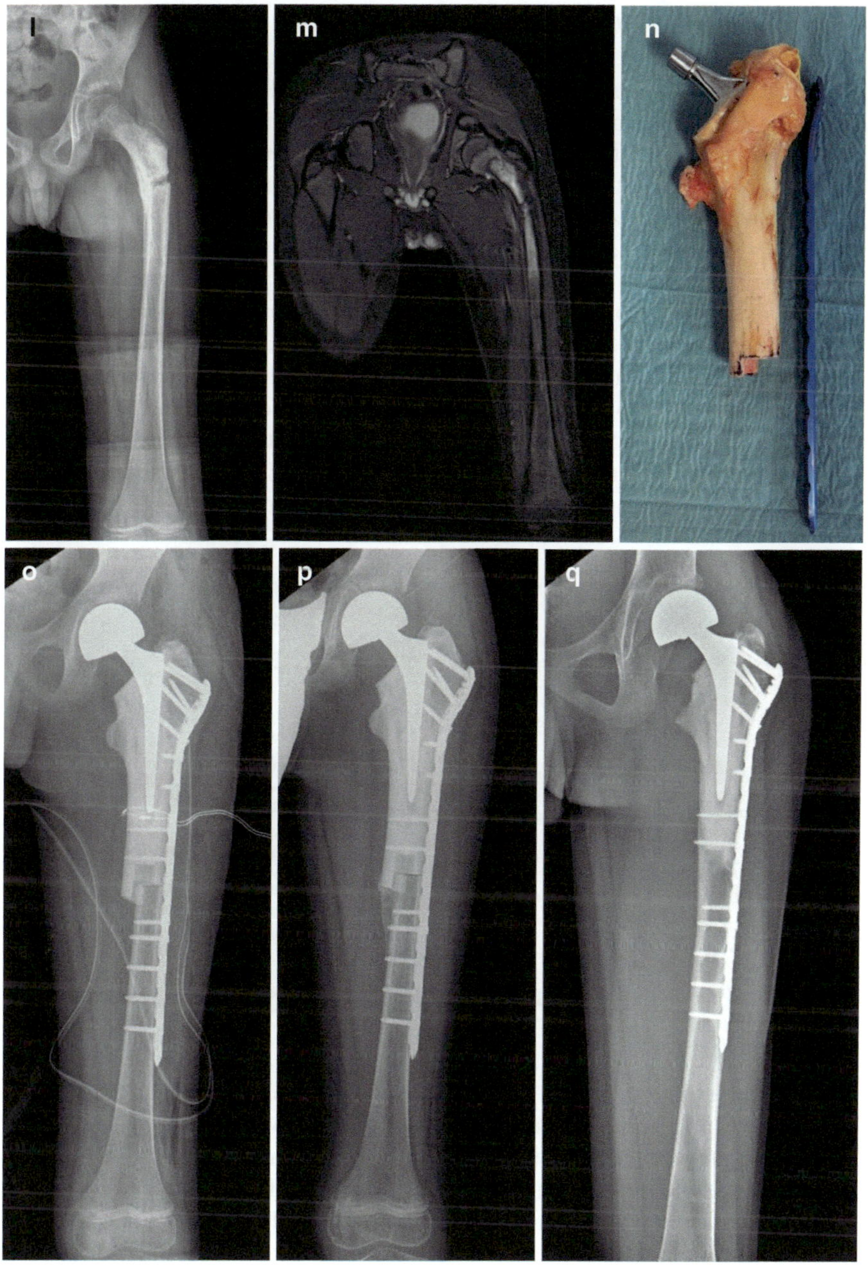

These figures show the case of a proximal femur Ewing's sarcoma in a 9-year-old male, with a pathologic fracture that healed with cast containment after preoperative chemotherapy. The patient underwent intrarticular proximal femur resection and reconstruction with a short stem APC with plate fixation. Few months later the osteotomy healed, and the APC remained in situ 6 years after the index surgery (Fig. 11l–q).

Proximal Femur APC Reconstruction Steps (Fig. 1r–u)

- The proximal femur osteoarticular massive allograft with native tendons is thawed and then shaped according to the length of the defect, resecting the femoral neck and the distal diaphysis. It's mandatory to preserve the abductor and iliopsoas tendon attachments on the graft. A step-cut osteotomy of the graft diaphysis is usually advocated in children to achieve a better matching between graft and host bone, as the allograft is usually larger than the host bone, coming from adult donors.
- After reaming the medullary canal of the graft, the stem of a conventional hip prosthesis is cemented inside the allograft; as mentioned above, we cement a short stem not bypassing the osteotomy line in skeletally immature patients, while we cement a long uncemented stem bypassing the osteotomy line in adults.
- A prosthesis head is then assembled. Usually, a bipolar head is recommended, but in growing patients with small acetabula, a unipolar ceramic head could be required due to the unavailability of very small bipolar heads.

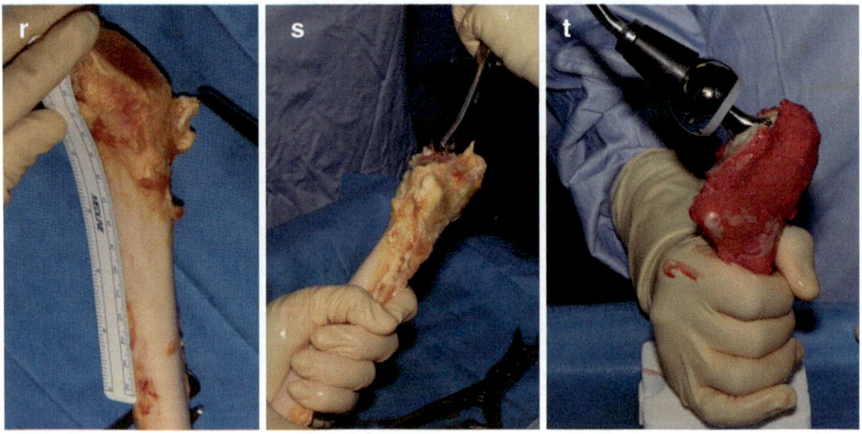

- The entire construct is fixed to the host bone. In children with a short stem APC, a long bridging compression plate and screw fixation is required, using, if possible, a plate extended over the greater trochanter. In adults, the cementless stem protruding from the allograft is inserted press-fit inside the host bone medullary canal after its preparation; a stem at least three times longer than the bone diameter at the osteotomy line is recommended in order to achieve a stable diaphyseal fixation. Cementless stem fixation can be used when at least 4 cm of press-fit fixation is achievable at the isthmus level. In longer resections, modular prostheses or APC with a floating allograft (see Fig 1k) should be considered due to the difficult APC assembly related to the femur procurvatum.
- Finally, once APC has been reduced, the abductors and iliopsoas tendons are reattached to the graft tendons with nonabsorbable sutures.

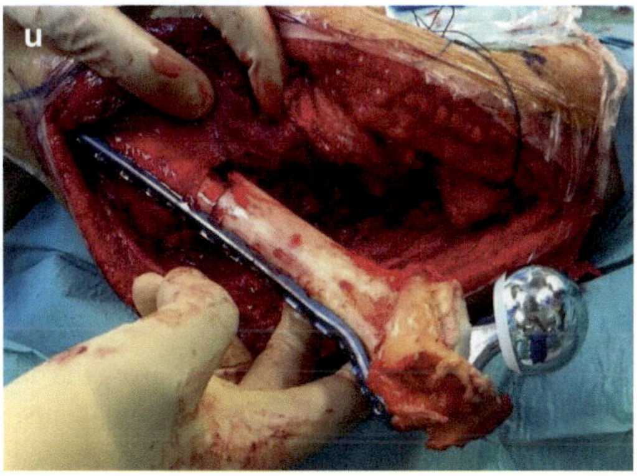

- After surgery, all patients are allowed to walk with two crutches and instructed to do controlled active and passive movements of the hip, knee and ankle. In children, an ischial weight-bearing brace is usually worn. Partial weight-bearing is allowed after initial evidence of callus formation on X-rays; full weight-bearing is given after evidence of osteotomy healing. Time of bone healing at the osteotomy is variable and is usually delayed in case of postoperative chemotherapy.

Allograft-Prosthesis Composite (APC) of the Proximal Tibia

Introduction

The proximal part of the tibia is the second most common location for primary bone tumors, only exceeded by the distal part of the femur, and it is occasionally the site of metastatic disease. Reconstruction of the proximal part of the tibia after surgical resection remains challenging, with different options including the implantation of a metallic endoprosthesis, osteoarticular allograft, or allograft-prosthesis composite (APC). Endoprostheses represent the most widely used technique after proximal tibia resection with the drawback of non-biologic patellar tendon reattachment which may lead to an extension lag. Osteoarticular allograft has the advantage of biologic patellar tendon reconstruction but has been almost completely abandoned, due to frequent mechanical complications and articular surface degeneration. APCs were introduced to merge the advantages of endoprostheses and osteoarticular allografts and to overcome their disadvantages. The use of APC maintains bone stock and provides a more anatomic and biologic reconstruction of the extensor mechanism, decreasing the risk of mechanical complications. Proximal tibia APC can be assembled with a long stem, cemented into the allograft, and implanted with cemented or cementless fixation in the distal tibia, or with a short stem as resurfacing APC, cemented onto the allograft with compression plate fixation of the osteotomy site. The latter option is indicated in pediatric reconstruction in order not to violate the distal femur growth plate. In this case, only the tibial prosthetic component with an ultracongruent polyethylene liner is implanted.

Surgical Anatomy

Proximal tibia is a complex area to be reconstructed due to the regional anatomy and because of a poor soft tissue coverage.

The principal structures that must be considered when performing a resection are:

- Extensor apparatus: Resection of the proximal tibia requires detachment of the patellar tendon from the tibial tuberosity at a variable distance, depending on tumoral extension.
- Capsuloligamentous structures: the disarticulation from the distal femur includes sections of the medial collateral ligament, cruciate ligaments, and joint capsule. APC proximal tibia reconstruction requires a hinged stemmed prosthesis in long stem configuration, while an accurate medial collateral ligament and capsule repair together with the use of an ultra-congruent polyethylene liner is recommended in resurfacing APC.
- Fibular proximal epiphysis: usually a disarticulation of the tibio-fibular joint is performed, unless the involvement of the proximal fibula by the tumor requires an extra-articular resection of the proximal fibula with the tibia.
- Popliteal and tibial neurovascular bundle: the popliteal neurovascular bundle is composed of the tibial nerve and popliteal artery and vein, which distally divides in tibioperoneal trunk vessels; the anterior tibial vessels cross the interosseous membrane extending anteriorly, running beneath the anterior tibial muscle and the extensor hallucis longus and extensor digitorum longus in the anterior compartment of the leg, adjacent to the deep peroneal nerve. The surgical management of the anterior tibial vessels at their anterior crossing is a critical step of the procedure. The possibility of their salvage or the need of their sacrifice must be preoperatively assessed on the basis of extension and location of the tumor; often, the last decision of their management must be adopted intraoperatively. When the need for their sacrifice is evaluated as possible, a preoperative study of the vascular pattern of the limb must be performed (by Angio CT or Doppler ultrasound), to ascertain the adequacy of distal limb perfusion based only on the tibioperoneal trunk vessels.

Assessment of Margins

Achieving wide margins is sometimes a complex issue, due to the anatomy of the site, even in patients who have undergone neoadjuvant therapies. If the lesion is contained inside the tibia without interruption of the cortex, soft tissues can be preserved, and only the biopsy tract is excised.

When the tumor extends outside the tibia, a safe margin must include the surrounding muscles and sometimes the skin, often requiring additional reconstructive procedures, like gastrocnemius rotational flaps or free flaps. Posteriorly, the popliteal muscle is excised with the tumor, representing almost always an adequate anatomical barrier. Anteriorly, the muscles of the anterior compartment are excised according to tumor extension, but medially, in case of tumoral infiltration of the skin, a rotational or free flap may be necessary for soft tissue closure. Laterally, the proximal fibula and the superficial peroneal nerve can be resected in case of tumoral infiltration.

Tibial osteotomy must be performed at 2–3 cm from the distal end of tumoral extension, as assessed by preoperative planning on MRI. A sample from the medullary canal of distal osteotomy is sent for frozen section to assess the quality of diaphyseal margin. The articular cartilage represents a good anatomical barrier, but in case of intra-articular tumor extension or articular pathologic fracture, an extra-articular resection must be considered.

Resection: Surgical Steps

- An anteromedial or anterolateral skin incision can be used, depending on the tumor location and extension. The preoperative biopsy tract is excised with the specimen.
- Section of the patellar tendon is performed.
- From the medial side, after posterior retraction of medial gastrocnemius, exploration and mobilization of the popliteal neurovascular bundle is performed, reaching the origin of anterior tibial vessels, then exposing the tibioperoneal trunk and posterior tibial vessels after section of the tibial insertion of the soleus muscle. Anterior tibial vessels are preserved or ligated and sectioned, according to tumor extension.
- Proximal tibia is surgically isolated, including partial or total sacrifice of muscles of the anterior compartment, if involved by the tumor.
- Distal osteotomy of the tibia and section of the interosseous membrane.
- Medially, section of pes anserinus tendons (sartorius, gracilis, and semitendinosus) and medial collateral ligament and capsule.
- Laterally, disarticulation of the tibiofibular joint and section of the popliteal tendon and lateral capsule.
- After the section of anterior and posterior cruciate ligaments, the resection of the proximal tibia, including the menisci, is completed.

Reconstruction

After proximal tibia resection, several reconstructive options have been reported:

- Megaprosthesis
- Massive osteoarticular allografts
- Recycled autografts
- Allograft-prosthesis composites

- Reconstruction with an osteoarticular allograft has the advantage of preserving bone stock in young patients and allowing a biologic attachment of the patellar tendon to the tendon of the graft. However, in the lower limb, a progressive degeneration of the articular cartilage of the graft is to be expected, eventually leading to subchondral fractures. Therefore, osteoarticular allografts are currently seldom used in the lower limb. Furthermore, allograft reconstruction requires a long period of protected weight bearing until union of the osteotomy.

- A prosthetic reconstruction is technically easier and allows faster functional recovery, with early weight-bearing. However, a limitation of this option is the reconstruction of the extensor apparatus of the knee that requires fixation directly onto the metal parts. To facilitate patellar tendon fixation, mesh augmentation has become popular and commonly used in many centers.
- The use of an APC combines the advantages of an osteoarticular allograft, particularly biologic insertion of the soft tissues and bone stock preservation, with the advantages of a prosthesis, including mechanical stability and long-term durability of joint surface.
- Infection rate after reconstructive surgery of proximal tibia defects is high. Medial gastrocnemius rotational flap is an effective adjunctive procedure to decrease the infection risk in any kind of proximal tibia reconstruction. APCs are often bulkier than modular prostheses, usually requiring a split-thickness skin graft over the flap, and, for this reason, the conditions of superficial soft tissues must be verified before choosing this option.
- APC offers the possibility of a better reconstruction of the extensor apparatus compared to the use of a metallic prosthesis, which requires the reinsertion of the tendon on a metal surface, but evidence of a better long-term functional result is not clearly confirmed by published clinical data.
- The reconstruction is performed with fresh-frozen nonirradiated allografts, which are chosen to match the size of the host bone using radiographs or CT scans.
- The APC is prepared on the back table by cutting off the joint cartilage, reaming the canal, and trimming the bone and soft tissue to the proper size.
- In adults, the use of hinged stemmed prostheses is recommended. In pediatric reconstructions, with the aim to preserve the distal femur growth plate, a resurfacing APC can be implanted, using a short stem proximal tibia prosthetic component cemented into the allograft, which is fixed to distal tibia by a compression plate. An ultra-congruent polyethylene liner is inserted, which is able to provide an adequate anteroposterior stability even in the absence of the cruciate ligaments. No femoral component is implanted, and care must be taken in the accurate suture of medial collateral ligament and joint capsule of the allograft to the host (Fig. 2a–g).
- Fixation of the allograft to the residual tibia of the host can be accomplished by a compression plate in case of short stem resurfacing APC or using a long intramedullary stem, which is always cemented in the graft and can be cemented or inserted press-fit in the host tibia (Fig. 2o–r).
- All cement is removed from the allograft-host bone junction prior to final seating of the allograft.
- The native residual patellar tendon is sutured with multiple interrupted nonabsorbable sutures to the allograft tendon in all patients. The native tendon should overlap the allograft tendon, creating a larger area for the allograft tendon to heal to the native tendon. Care is taken to restore isometry and to maintain the native patellar height.

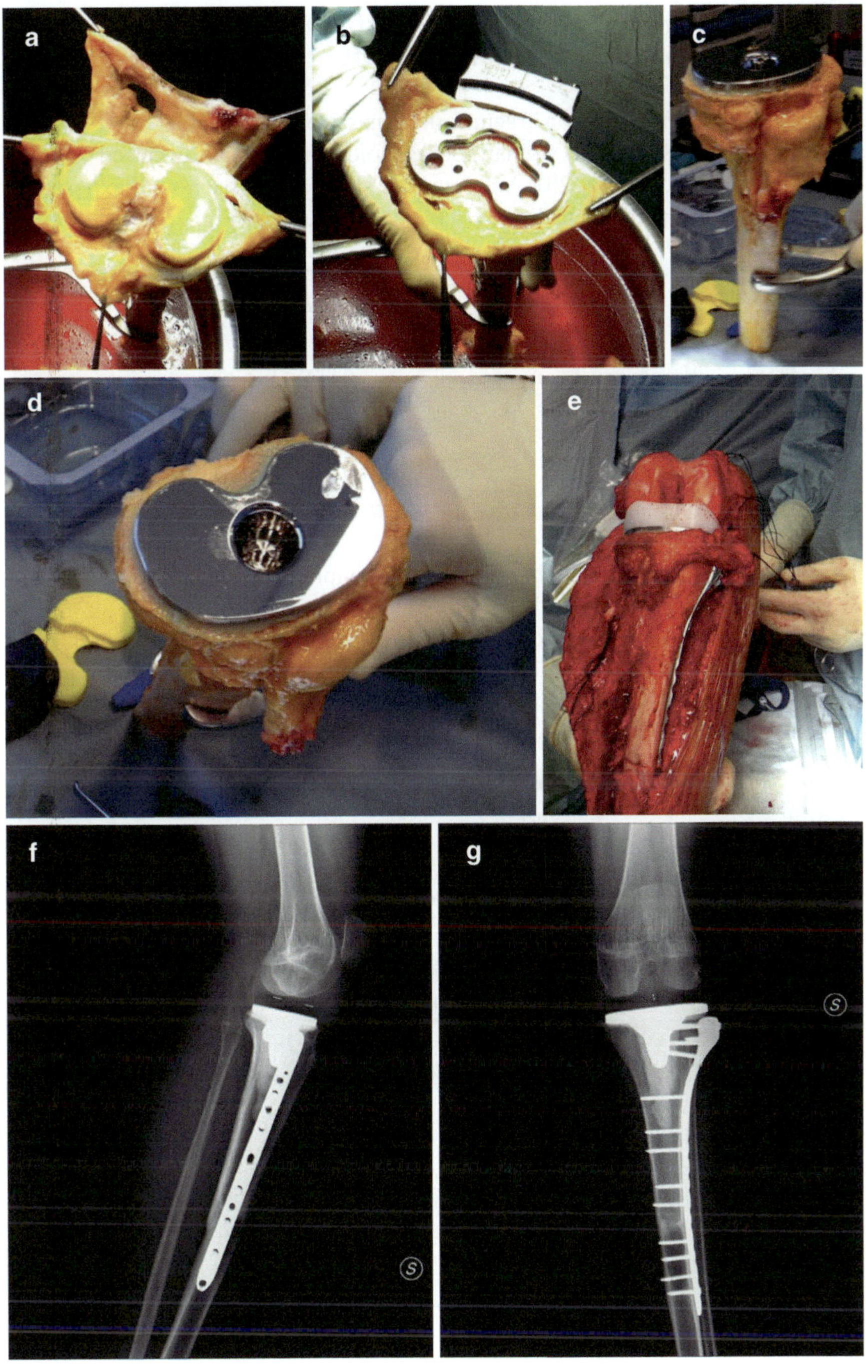
a
b
c
d
e
f
g

Allograft-Prosthesis Composite (APC) After Failure for Fracture of Proximal Tibia Osteoarticular Allograft

X-ray shows the failure for a fracture of a massive osteoarticular tibia allograft implanted in an 18-year-old woman for desmoid tumor, which occurred 15 years after primary surgery (Fig. 2h). Anteromedial surgical approach with exposure of the bone graft and plate. Detachment of the patellar tendon (Fig. 2i).

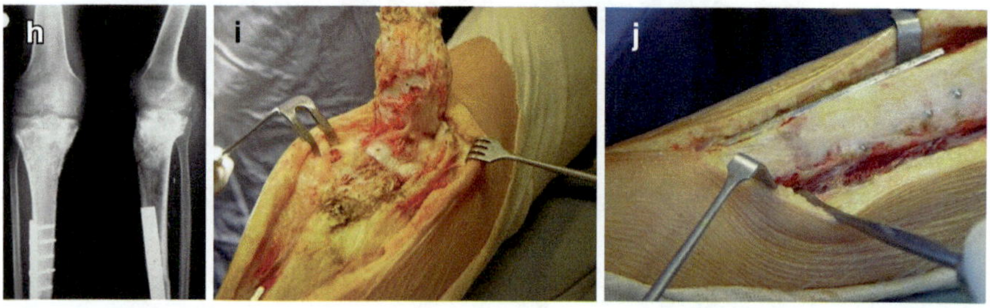

The intraoperative image highlights the complete fusion of the previously implanted allograft (Fig. 2j).

The proximal part of the fractured allograft is resected and the plate is removed. After plate removal, another diaphyseal fracture was detected, running along the screw holes. After allograft removal, the osteotomy section shows a completely necrotic bone after 15 years from implantation (Fig. 2k, l).

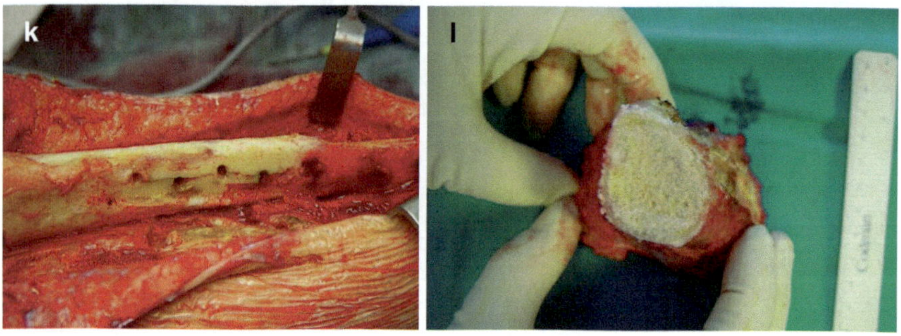

The images show a new allograft with the extensor apparatus necessary for the new reconstruction and the new APC implanted with the suture of the extensor apparatus (Fig. 2m, n).

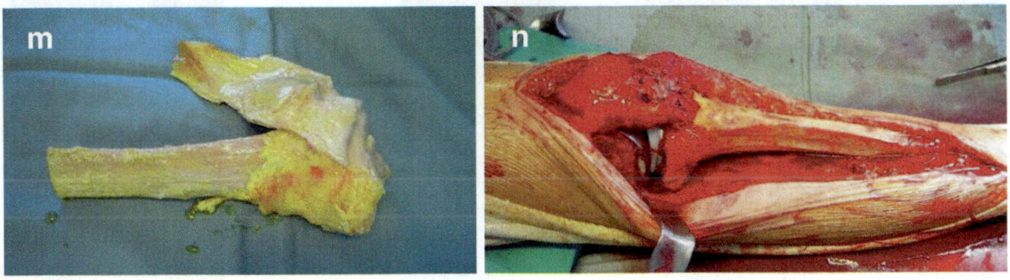

Follow-up radiographs of the APC with rotating-hinged modular prosthesis, with the long stem of the tibial component cemented inside the graft and the host bone and the cementless stem in the femur (Fig. 2o–r).

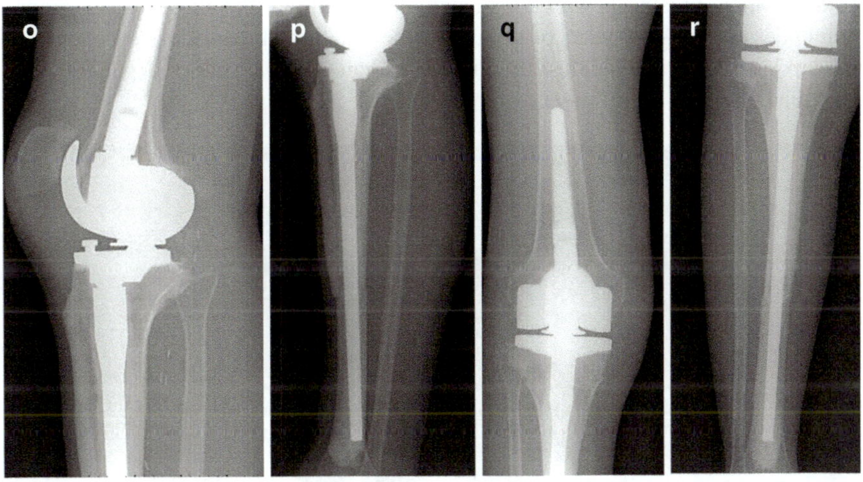

Total Tibia Allograft-Prosthesis Composite (APC) in Chondrosarcoma with Pathological Fracture

Pathological fracture of a high-grade central chondrosarcoma in a 39-year-old man treated elsewhere with an intramedullary nail, spreading the tumor along the entire tibia. The bone scan clearly highlights the dissemination of the tumor along the entire bone segment. Another spot of increased uptake was present in the homolateral proximal femur, which was diagnosed as an enchondroma (Fig. 2s–v).

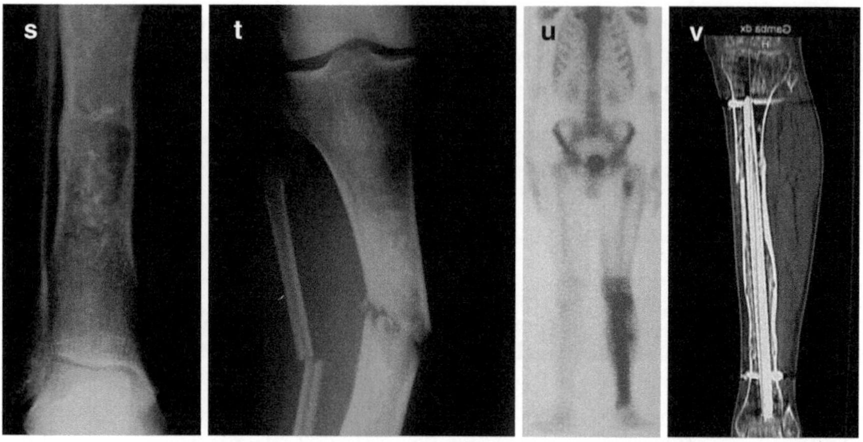

A total tibia resection was performed, reconstructed by a total tibia APC using a rotating hinge prosthesis with a long stem cemented into the allograft and femoral cementless stem. At 15 years of follow-up, the function of the knee is excellent, and the ankle is stable and painless despite the evident articular surface degeneration of the tibial allograft (Fig. 2w–z).

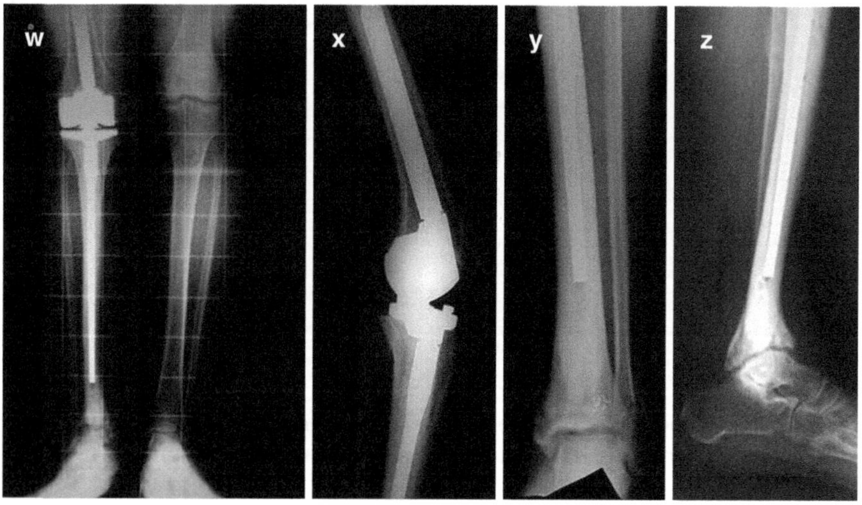

Intercalary Resection of Long Bones and Reconstruction with Massive Allograft and Vascularized Fibula Graft

Introduction

Most of the femoral and tibial tumors involve the meta-epiphysis, requiring an intra-articular resection to obtain adequate surgical margins. Less frequently, when the tumor arises in metadiaphysis, an intercalary resection is feasible with joint preservation. Nowadays, through an accurate imaging-based planning and with the use of intraoperative guides or navigation systems, joint-sparing intercalary resections can be safely performed even in tumors with juxta-articular extension, preserving a small epiphyseal segment with native joint and ligament insertions. After intercalary resection of long bones, several reconstructive options have been reported, such as intercalary prosthesis, massive allografts, bone transport, osteoinductive membrane technique, recycled autografts, and vascularized fibula, combined or not with a massive allograft. Vascularized fibula can be used as ipsilateral pedicle flap or as free flap from contralateral leg. Intercalary vascularized fibula graft (VFG) provides many advantages, such as early union, spontaneous healing potential after fracture, and the ability to hypertrophy under mechanical stress. Capanna et al. in 1993 first described the association between VFG and massive allograft as reconstructive option after intercalary resection for primary bone tumors; the rationale of this technique is represented by the combination of the primary mechanical stability of the allograft and the long-term biological potential of the vascularized fibula.

Surgical Anatomy

The tibia is a subcutaneous bone, with a scarce vascular supply in the lower third. The anatomical structures potentially infiltrated by diaphyseal tumors include.

- Subcutaneous tissue in the anteromedial aspect, sometimes requiring fasciocutaneous flap coverage after tumor excision.
- Tibialis anterior and extensor hallucis longus muscles and tendons are closely related to the bone surface of the tibia diaphysis, along with the anterior tibial vessels and deep peroneal nerve in the lower half. Anterior tibial artery and vein represent the most frequent vessels used for the anastomosis in free VFG reconstruction.
- Tibialis posterior and flexor digitorum longus muscles cover the posterior aspect of the tibia shaft. Posterior tibial nerve and vessels are rarely involved in diaphyseal tumors, and they are usually shielded by the above-mentioned muscles.
- Peroneal vessels are important for the vascular supply of the fibula; a tumor involvement of the fibula and/or the peroneal vessels requires a reconstruction of the defect using the contralateral free VFG.

The femur is a bone surrounded by a thick layer of muscles and soft tissue, with a well-represented vascular supply coming from deep femoral artery branches. The anatomical structures potentially infiltrated by diaphyseal tumors in the femur include:

- Quadriceps muscle, in particular the vastus intermedius and vastus medialis/lateralis
- Deep femoral artery: its branches are usually adopted as recipient vessels for VFG
- Superficial femoral artery: its infiltration by the tumor contraindicates the reconstruction using a VFG

Assessment

Intercalary resection of the femur and tibia and reconstruction with VFG with or without massive allograft represents a high-demanding surgery that requires the availability of a microsurgical team in case of contralateral fibula harvesting and vessel anastomoses; for this reason, this reconstructive option should be reserved for patients with primary bone tumors with good prognosis.

Important structures to be critically evaluated before resection include:

- Tumor extension, through a contrast-enhanced MRI. At least 1 cm of safe residual bone in both epiphyses should remain after a resection with adequate margins.
- Subcutaneous and skin tissue over the anteromedial aspect of the leg. The need to excise a skin area could require a flap coverage.
- Superficial femoral artery. The tumor involvement of this artery contraindicates the reconstruction with a VFG.
- Fibula: it's mandatory, through a simple X-ray of both legs, to exclude fracture or deformity of the fibula harvested for the reconstruction.
- Deep and superficial femoral, anterior and posterior tibial, and peroneal vessels, through a preoperative CT angiography, in order to evaluate the presence of a tumor involvement of the vessels and to assess the vascular supply of the fibula. It's mandatory to evaluate both legs.

Adamantinoma of the Tibia Arisen on Osteofibrous Displasia of Long Bones

These figures show an adamantinoma of the left tibia arising from osteofibrous displasia (OFD) of long bones in a 36-year-old female. X-rays show an aggressive lesion of the tibial diaphysis with valgus and procurvate deformity of the bone. CT scan images show a subtotal involvement of the tibia by the tumor extension that spares the proximal and distal epiphyseal bone. MRI confirms the subtotal involvement of the tibia, without extraosseous mass except for the anteromedial aspect of the proximal third of the tibia, in which an extraosseous extension can be assessed. The fibula was not involved by the tumor, nor were the neurovascular structures of the leg (Fig. 3a–d).

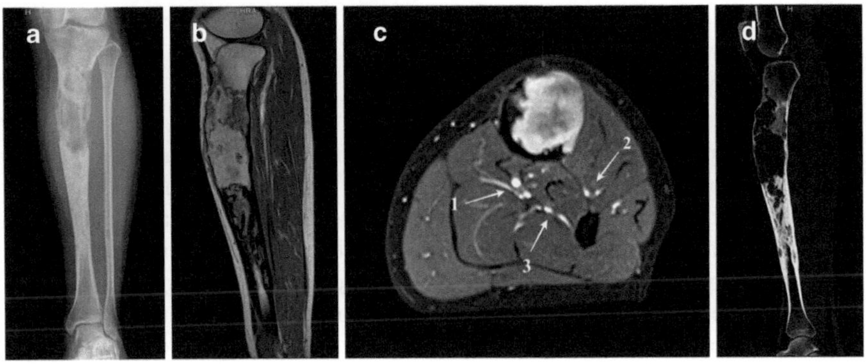

1. Posterior tibial vessels
2. Anterior tibial vessels
3. Peroneal vessels

Diaphyseal Osteoblastic Osteosarcoma of the Femur

Series of X-ray and MRI figures show an osteoblastic osteosarcoma of the right femur in a 16-year-old female. MRI shows the absence of distal epiphyseal tumor extension, with extraosseous mass on the posterior-medial side. The main neurovascular structures were not involved (Fig. 3e–g).

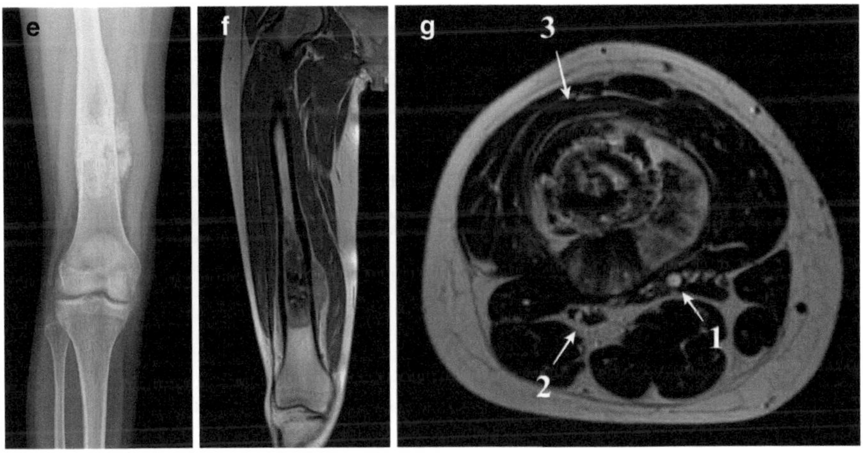

1. Superficial femoral vessels
2. Sciatic nerve
3. Vastus intermedius muscle

Surgical Steps

Intercalary Tibial Resection Surgical Steps

- Anteromedial or anterolateral approach to the tibial diaphysis, with medial or lateral parapatellar proximal extension according to tumor extension.
- Extensive mobilization of the fasciocutaneous flap exposing the anterior tibial vessels and deep peroneal nerve branch, after retracting the tibialis anterior and extensor hallucis longus muscles and tendons laterally. When infiltrated by the tumor, the anterior tibial vessels can be resected, leaving the proximal stump as recipient vessels for the vascular anastomoses of the VFG.
- Extensive mobilization of the medial fasciocutaneous flap, exposing the posterior tibial neurovascular structures, after pes anserinus tendon detachment and retracting medial gastrocnemius and soleus muscles posteriorly. In tumor without posterior extraosseous extension, the exposition of posterior tibial vessels and nerves is not always required.
- Section of the interosseous membrane
- Proximal and distal tibial osteotomy according to the tumor extension assessed on preoperative MRI.

Intercalary Femoral Resection Surgical Steps

- Lateral approach to the femoral diaphysis with, if required, a lateral parapatellar distal extension.
- Exposure of femoral diaphysis, after retracting the quadriceps muscle anteriorly. Usually, the vastus intermedius and part of vastus lateralis muscles are left as soft tissue cuff covering the tumor.
- Extensive mobilization of the sciatic nerve and the distal part of superficial femoral vessels, after the section of lateral intermuscular septum and retracting femoral biceps muscle posteriorly.
- Proximal and distal femoral osteotomy according to the tumor extension assessed on preoperative MRI.
- Once the osteotomies are performed, section the medial intermuscular septum and adductors muscles insertions and complete dissection of deep femoral vessels.

Options for Bone Reconstruction

After intercalary resection of the long bones, several reconstructive options have been reported:

- Intercalary prosthesis
- Massive allografts
- Bone transport
- Osteoinductive membrane technique
- Recycled autografts
- Vascularized fibula combined or not with a massive allograft

VFG combined with massive allograft represents our preferred reconstructive option after intercalary resection of the femur and tibia, as this method combines the immediate stability of the allograft with long-term biological potential of the VFG.

- The free VFG is firstly harvested from the contralateral leg through a posterolateral approach, exposing the peroneal vessels after retracting the soleal muscle posteriorly and after detaching the peroneus longus and flexor longus hallucis form the fibula. The fibula harvesting is done by a microsurgical team using separate instruments, who takes care to avoid contamination between the two surgical fields. It's mandatory to perform an accurate dissection to avoid common peroneal nerve injuries in the proximal third of the fibula and to preserve the peroneal vessels intact (Fig. 3h, i). Alternately, the ipsilateral fibula can be medialized as pedicle flap, without requiring a microsurgical anastomosis. The length of the fibula graft should be at least two centimeters longer than the bone resection in order to obtain at least 1 cm of overlap for each osteotomy.

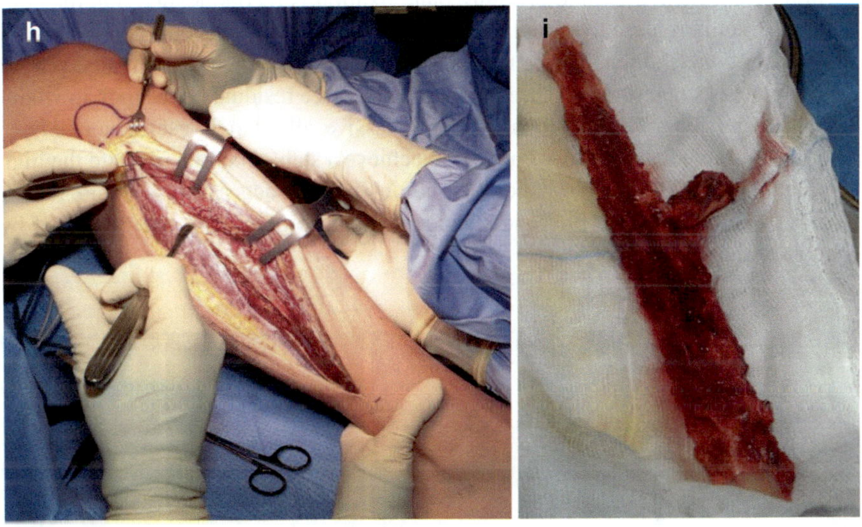

- The massive allograft is thawed and then shaped according to the length of the intercalary defect using custom made cutting guide, creating a slot inside the medullary canal in order to insert the vascularized fibula. It's mandatory to create a wide cortical window on the anterolateral or posterior part of the allograft, according to the site of recipient vessels, in order to avoid the compression of the vessels that supply the fibula graft (Fig. 3j, k).
- The VFG is inserted inside the medullary canal of host bone, surrounded by the massive allograft. It's important to shape the massive allograft to obtain the best match between the graft and host bone in order to facilitate the osteotomies' healing.

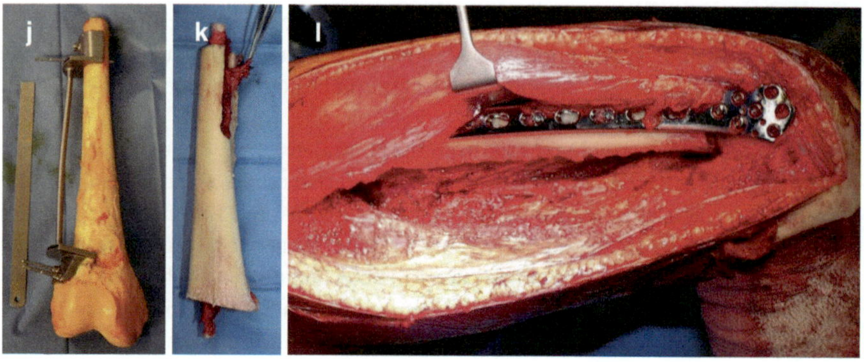

- The entire construct is finally fixed. If the proximal and distal residual bone is longer than 2 cm, a long bridging plate and screw fixation are advocated, to reduce the risk of graft fractures (Fig. 3l). In patients with long intercalary resection over 20 cm, a double bridging plate fixation is recommended. On the contrary, in children receiving intra-epiphyseal resection or in young patients with residual bone shorter than 2 cm a non-bridging fixation with cannulated screws and plate is suggested; in these patients with scarce residual bone stock in whom a bridging fixation is not possible, the massive allograft is useful not only to provide immediate stability but also to achieve a stable fixation, despite the high fracture risk. On the other hand, the bridging fixation acts as stress shield, reducing the fibula hypertrophy and remodeling that, on contrary, are enhanced by non-bridging fixation.

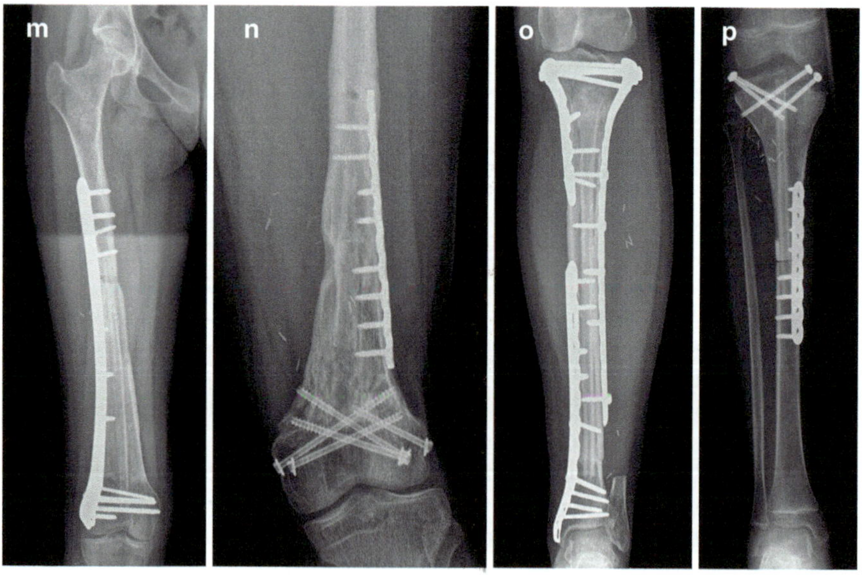

Figure showing different options using either bridging or non-bridging fixation of allograft fibula composite in intercalary diaphyseal reconstructions of the femur and tibia (Fig. 3m–p)

- In tibial intercalary resections in which the patellar tendon was detached, the tendon was then reattached to the graft tendon with a non-absorbable suture.
- After surgery, in tibial resection in whom the patellar tendon was reattached and in all pediatric patients, the operated leg was protected with a long leg cast for 4 weeks; controlled passive movements of the hip, knee, and ankle were then allowed. On the contrary, in young and adult patients the passive movements of the joints were allowed postoperatively. No weight-bearing was allowed until radiographic evidence of VFG union; then the patient could walk with partial weight-bearing. Full weight-bearing was started after evidence of complete allograft union. The donor leg was left free postoperatively, encouraging active and passive movements of the knee, ankle, and toes. Full weight-bearing on the donor side was allowed after 3 weeks from surgery.

3D Printed Cutting Guides in Multiplanar Joint-Sparing Resection and Allograft Reconstruction

Introduction

The surgical treatment of bone tumors occurring in the periarticular region can have a significant impact on the patient's quality of life. Indeed, in this setting, achieving a wide margin preserving the joint is challenging, and joint replacement with a megaprosthesis is often required. However, when feasible with safe surgical margins, a joint-sparing resection has to be preferred, particularly in young patients.

In multiplanar joint-sparing resections, the traditional free-hand approach exposes to the risk of contaminated margins as well as excessive ablation of healthy tissue. In this situation, the use of custom-made patient-specific cutting guides improves the accuracy of the osteotomies. The same technique can be adopted to adequately shape the allograft using allograft-specific custom-made cutting guides in order to achieve a precise matching of the defect.

Evaluation

The periarticular region presents a complex anatomy that must be carefully evaluated by the surgeon before planning and designing the cutting templates. Together with the articular surface of the joint, an adequate portion of subchondral bone must be preserved to prevent osteochondral necrosis and collapse. Preservation of ligamentous and tendinous insertions is crucial in order to maintain joint stability and muscular function, allowing an early and effective functional recovery. The aim is to maintain as much cortical bone integrity as possible to preserve mechanical strength, decreasing the risk of fractures.

Based on these issues, the number and orientation of the cutting planes and the morphology and position of the cutting templates are decided.

When planning a cutting guide, it is very important to consider the surgical approach and consequently the exposed surfaces of bone in order to design a device adequately matching the bone anatomy. Ligaments and tendinous insertions must be considered to plan a correct contact to the bone surface, avoiding the need for unnecessary detachment of important soft tissue structures.

The study of the anatomy is based on CT and MRI fusion, from which a three-dimensional model of the anatomical region with the tumor is obtained. The segmentation process of the tumoral tissue is achieved, providing an offset of the desired surgical margins, which could be larger or thinner, aiming to preserve crucial anatomical structures (articular joint surface, ligament, or tendinous insertions). On this model, through dedicated software, the cutting planes are decided and the cutting guides are planned and designed.

Through 3D printing, it is then possible to create also a three-dimensional template that will aid the surgeon in pre- and intra-operative visualization of the anatomy and cutting guide positioning.

The selection of the allograft to be used for reconstruction is made by comparing CT images of allografts from bone banks' databases with patient's CT. Once a matching bone segment is selected, an allograft-specific cutting template is designed to adequately shape the graft to match the bone defect for reconstruction.

Preoperative Planning and Design of Cutting Template

A case of juxta-articular peripheral chondrosarcoma of the lateral portion of the tibia. MRI and CT images show the extent of the tumor between the proximal epiphysis of the tibia and fibula, which required a hemicortical resection of the tibia with extra-articular resection of the tibio-fibular joint (Fig. 4a, b).

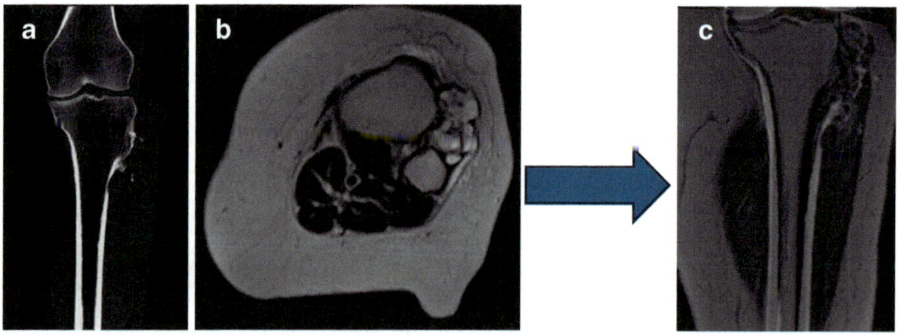

Fusion of CT and MRI images was performed, allowing imaging details of both soft tissues and bone (Fig. 4c).

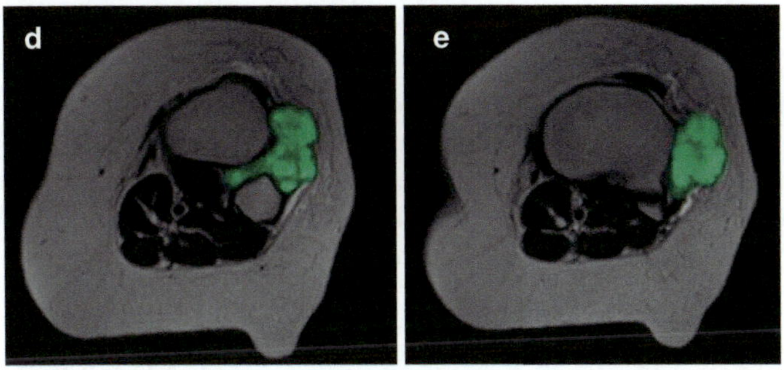

Slice-by-slice segmentation of the tumor from CT and MRI images (Fig. 4d, e).

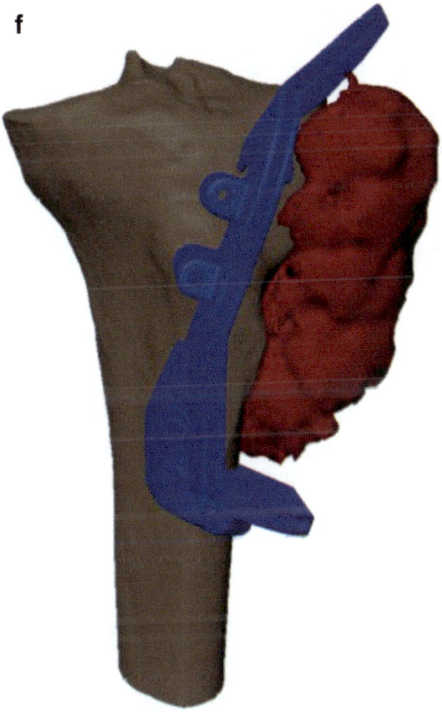

Creation of a three-dimensional rendering of the structures obtained from segmentation and the cutting template made by CAD software (Fig. 4f).

Surgical Steps

Tumor resection and allograft shaping. Both surgical steps were guided by a specific cutting template. Correct and accurate positioning of the cutting guide is crucial to respect the planning of site and orientation of cutting planes (Fig. 4g, h).

The hemicortical allograft was then fixed by a plate. The lateral collateral ligament, detached from the fibula, was anchored to the proximal epiphysis of the tibia (Fig. 4i).

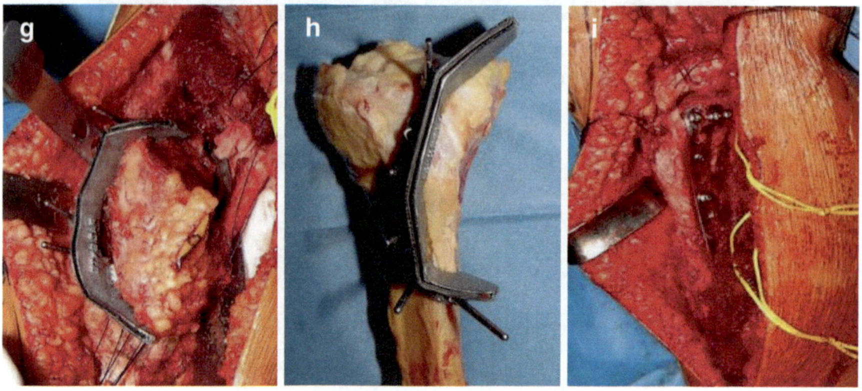

Follow-Up

Every patient is subjected to specific oncological follow-up protocols, according to the tumor histology and grade. Allograft reconstructions are followed with clinical examination and X-ray and CT sequential scans to assess proper osteotomy union. This is crucial to define the rehabilitation program, which has to be tailored to every single case.

CT scan at 1 year from surgery and X-rays at 3 years showing osseointegration between the allograft and the patient's bone (Fig. 4j, k).

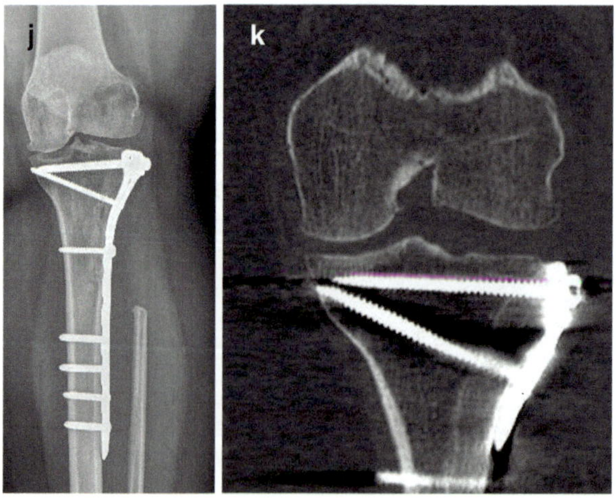

Hemicortical Resection of a Peripheral Chondrosarcoma of the Proximal Tibia

Peripheral chondrosarcoma of the proximal meta-epiphysis of the tibia in its posterior portion (Fig. 5a, b).

MRI shows the tumor extension close to the insertion of the posterior cruciate ligament.

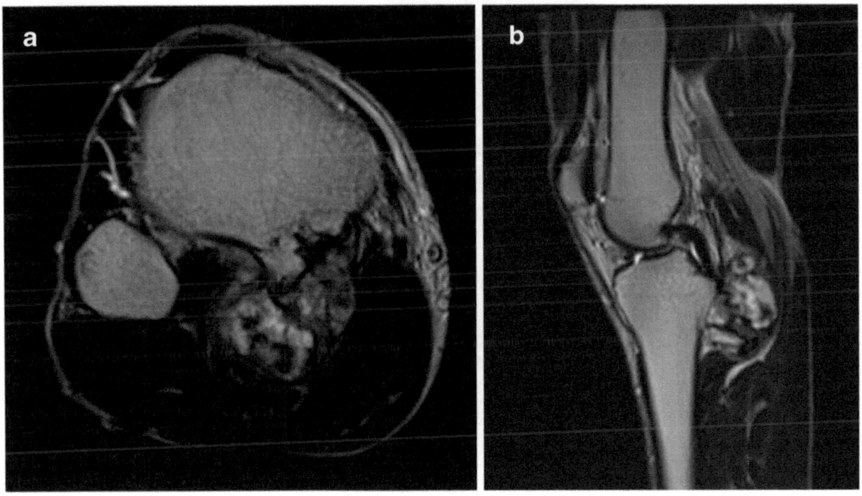

A three-dimensional model from the CT and MRI scans showing the close spatial relationship between the tumor and the posterior cruciate ligament insertion (Fig. 5c).

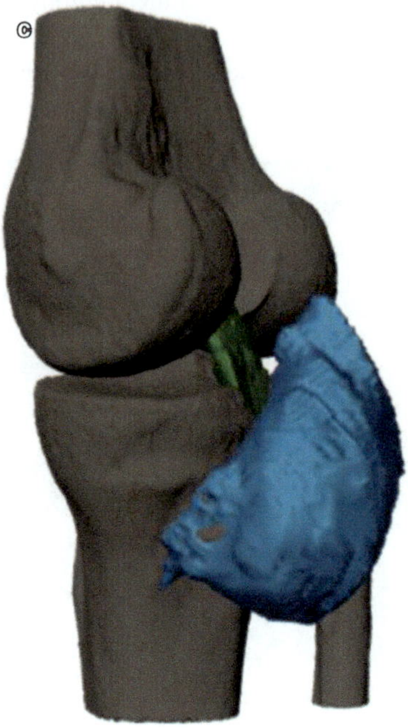

3D planning of the cutting guide based on MRI and CT images (Fig. 5d).

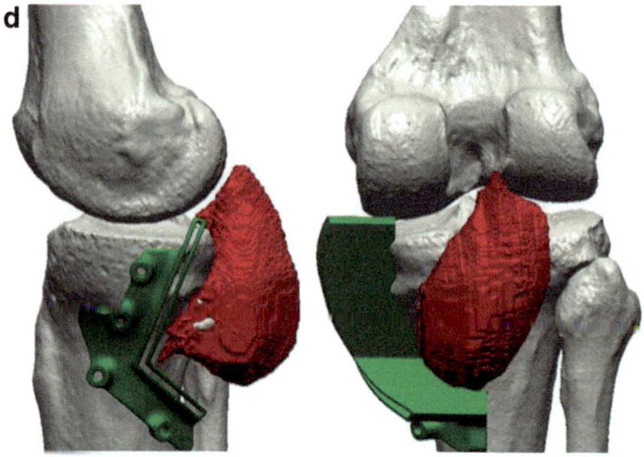

A posterior approach to the knee was used to perform the resection. Once the superficial fascia was incised, the popliteal vascular bundle, the tibial nerve, and the common peroneal nerve were isolated and retracted laterally. The tendinous insertion of the medial gastrocnemius was detached from the medial femoral condyle. The inferior geniculate vessels were ligated and cut. The popliteus muscle was left to cover the mass and the cartilaginous cap (Fig. 5e–g).

The cutting guide was carefully placed on the posteromedial margin of the tibia using a 3D model of the tibia with the tumor and cutting template as a reference. When the positioning was considered adequate, the cutting guide was fixed by K-wires to proceed with resection.

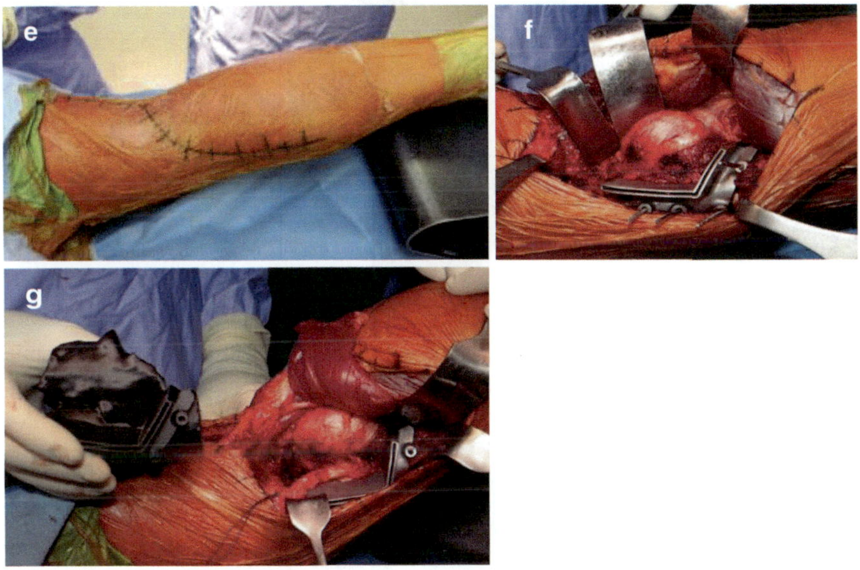

The allograft, previously selected by CT imaging matching, was shaped using an allograft-specific cutting guide to obtain a hemicortical allograft of the appropriate size to fill the bone defect resulting from the multiplanar osteotomy (Fig. 5h).

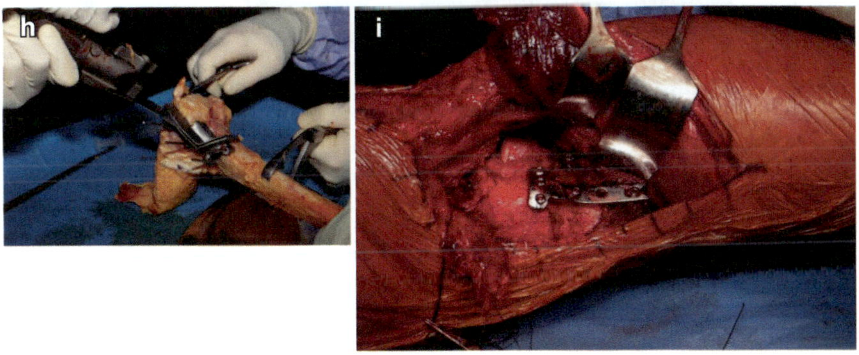

Fixation of the allograft was accomplished with a posterior plate. The suture of the native posterior capsule to the graft capsule was performed (Fig. 5i).

3D model of the reconstruction as planned. Allograft is displayed in blue (Fig. 5j).

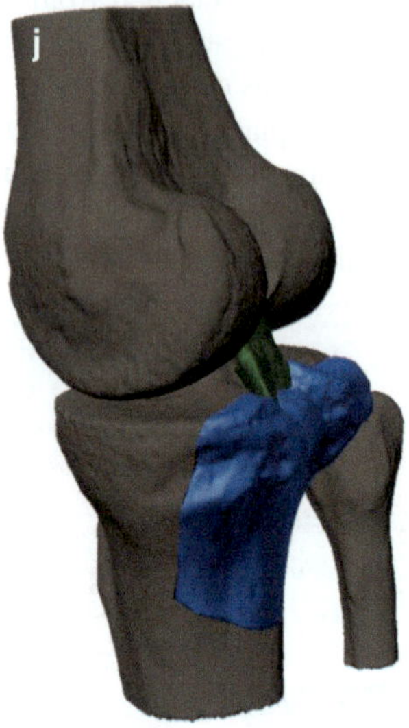

Once the resection is performed, we usually obtain a CT scan of the anatomic specimen. The CT image is compared digitally with the preoperative planning, checking the cutting precision obtained (Fig. 5k, l).

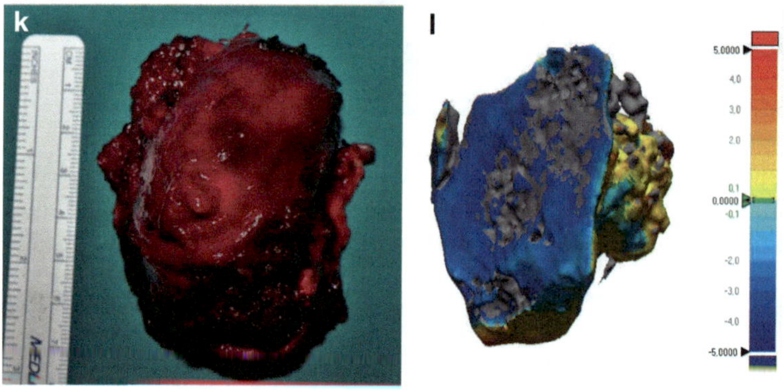

X-rays at 1 year from surgery show complete osseointegration between the hemicortical allograft and the host (Fig. 5m).

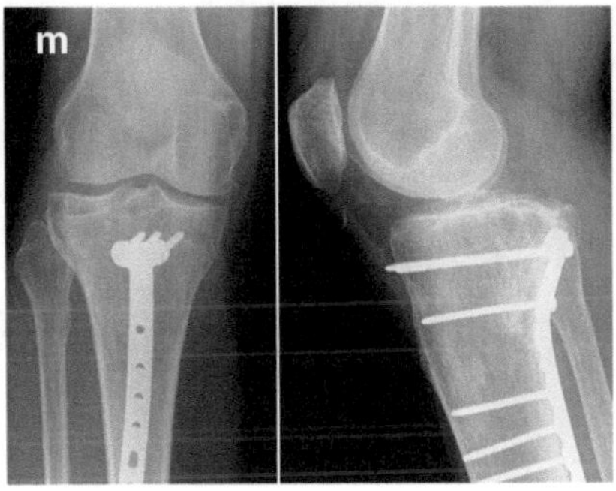

Hemicortical Resection of Osteosarcoma of the Distal Femur with Allograft Reconstruction

Osteosarcoma arising in the medial metaphysis of distal femur (Fig. 6a).

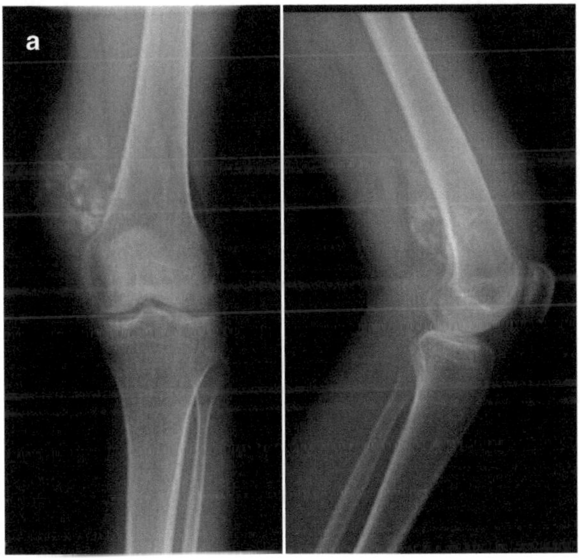

3D planning of the cutting guide based on MRI and CT images (Fig. 6b).

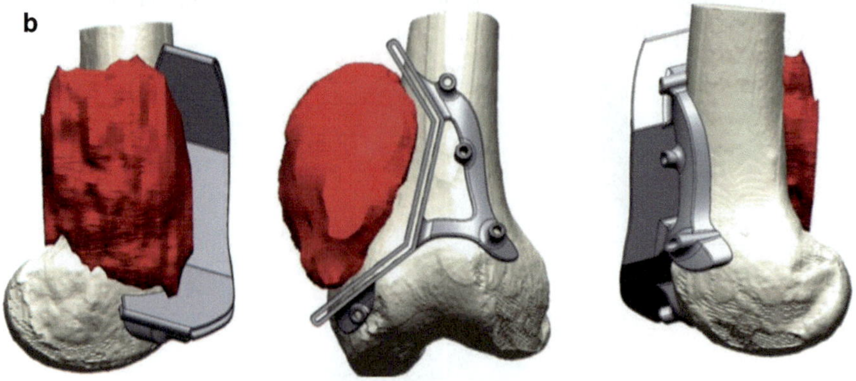

The resection was performed through a medial incision. The vastus medialis was retracted, leaving part of its medial fibers to cover the tumor. The medial intermuscular septum and great adductor tendon were sectioned (Fig. 6c).

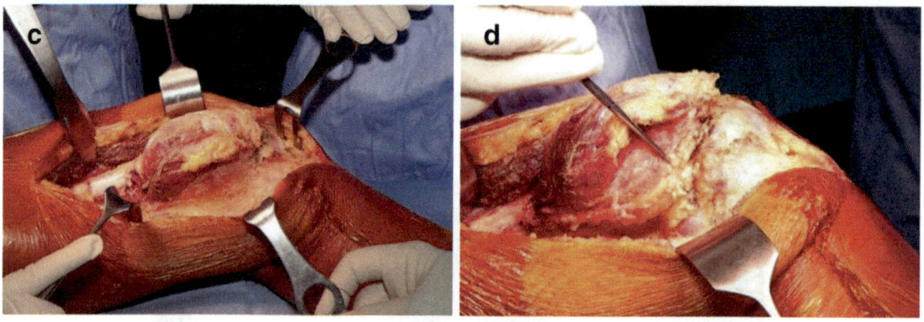

The femoral and popliteal vessels were isolated and retracted posteriorly. The anterior cortical surface of the femur, the articular surface, and the insertion of the medial collateral ligament were exposed (Fig. 6d).

Custom-made cutting guides were applied, and multiplanar joint-sparing medial hemicortical osteotomy of the distal femur was performed (Fig. 6e–g).

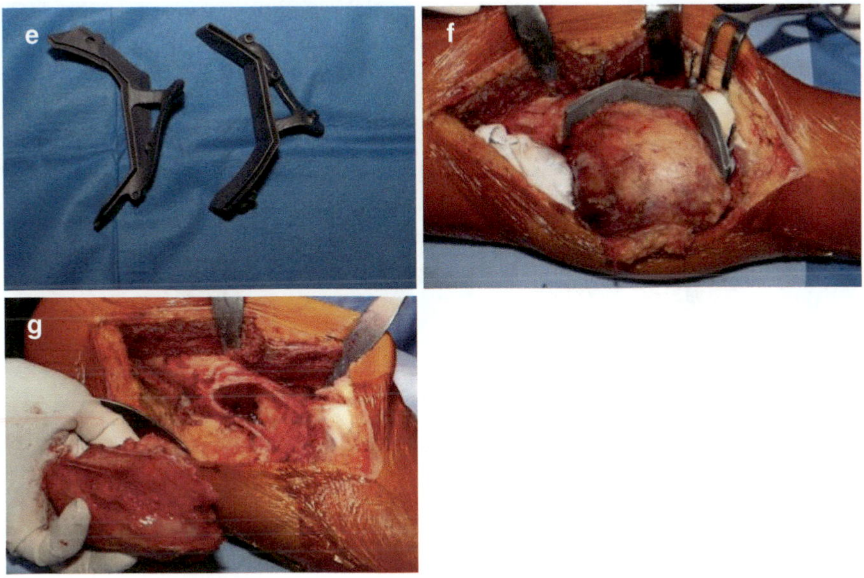

The anatomic specimen was sent for CT scan and histologic examination (Fig. 6h).

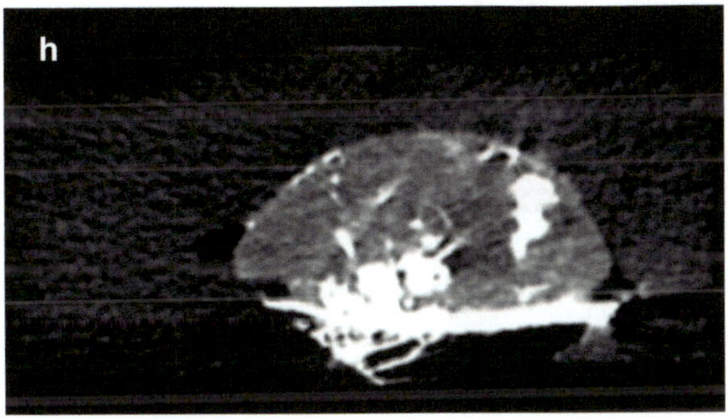

Using an allograft-specific cutting guide, the hemicortical graft was shaped and implanted to restore the bone defect (Fig. 6i–k).

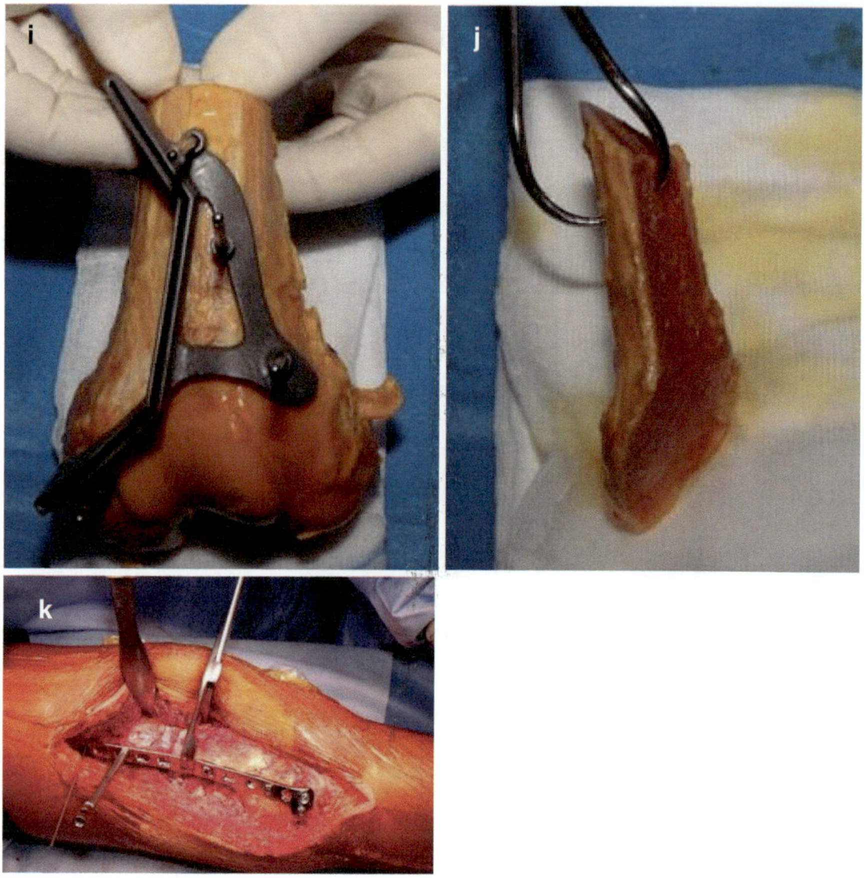

Postoperative X rays at 4 months (Fig. 6l).

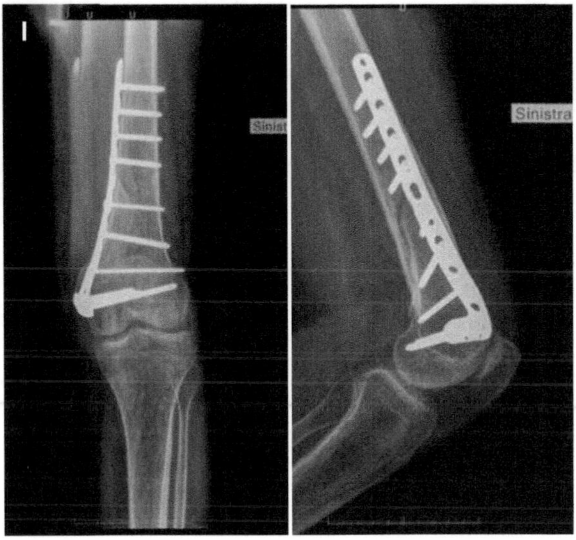

Resection of Chondrosarcoma of the Humerus Reconstructed with an Allograft and Vascularized Fibula

The patient presented with a pathologic fracture on cartilaginous lesion with an aggressive aspect at imaging. The thru-cut biopsy revealed a diagnosis of atypical cartilaginous tumor. Due to the aggressive aspect of imaging and pathologic fracture, an intercalary resection was planned through an accurate evaluation of MRI and CT scan (Fig. 7a–c).

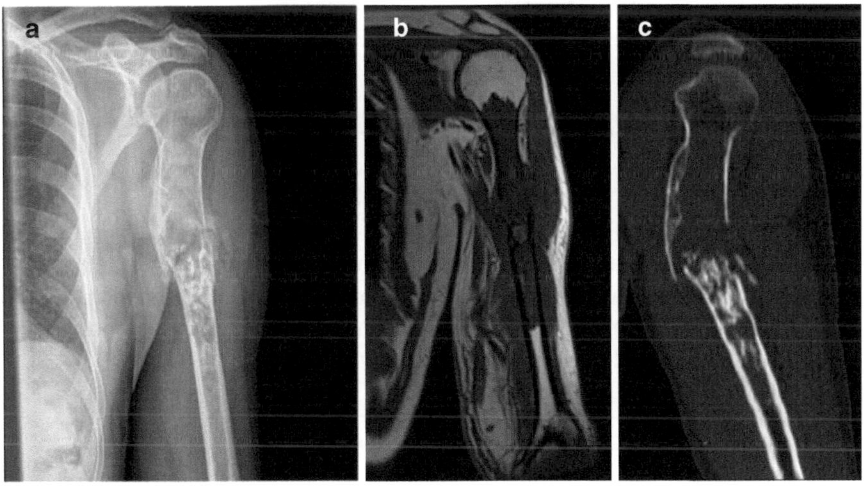

A multiplanar joint-sparing proximal osteotomy was planned. A matching allograft was selected from the Bone Bank. Custom-made cutting guides were designed for proximal humerus osteotomy in order to preserve the epiphysis and rotator cuff and subscapularis tendinous insertions (Fig. 7d).

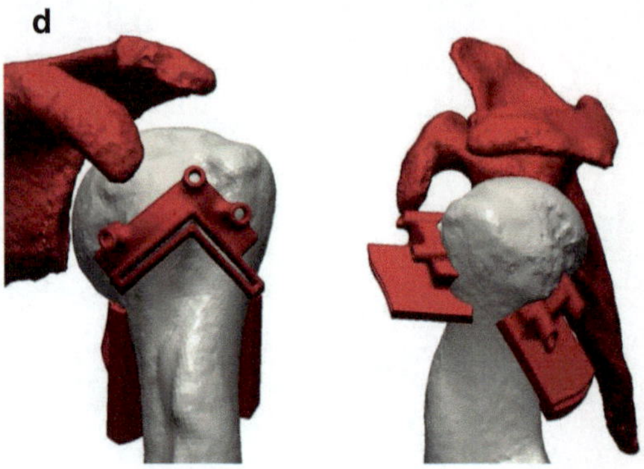

A 3 D model of the residual bone (in white) and allograft reconstruction (in blue) (Fig. 7e).

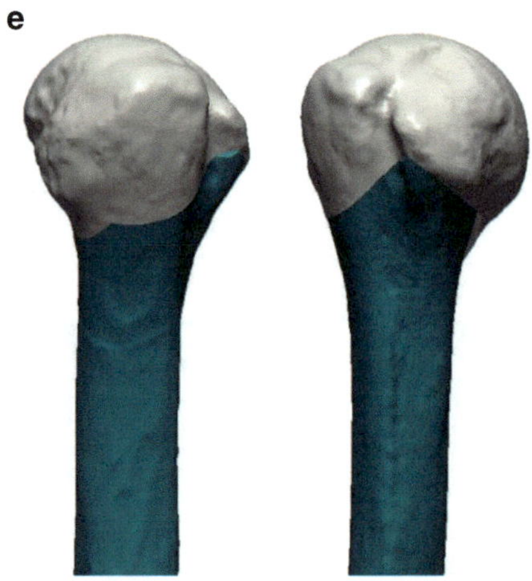

An extended anterolateral approach to the shoulder and arm was performed. The distal osteotomy was done freehand after measuring the distance from the tip of the greater tuberosity. Then, cutting guides were positioned anteriorly and posteriorly to perform the proximal joint-sparing osteotomy (Fig. 7f, g).

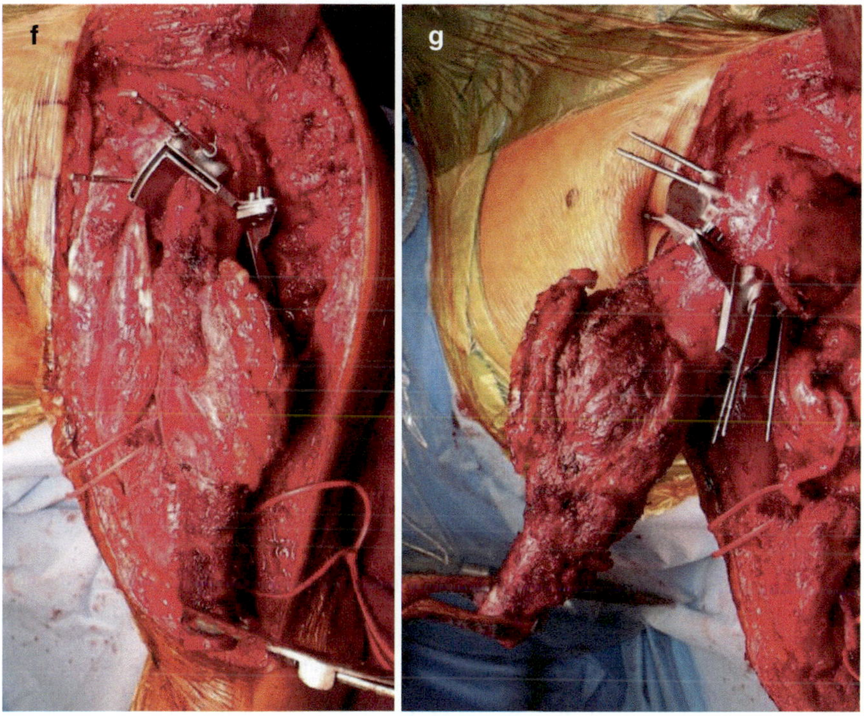

The allograft was then shaped using an allograft-specific cutting guide, and it was combined with a vascularized fibula in a concentric assembly (Fig. 7h, i).

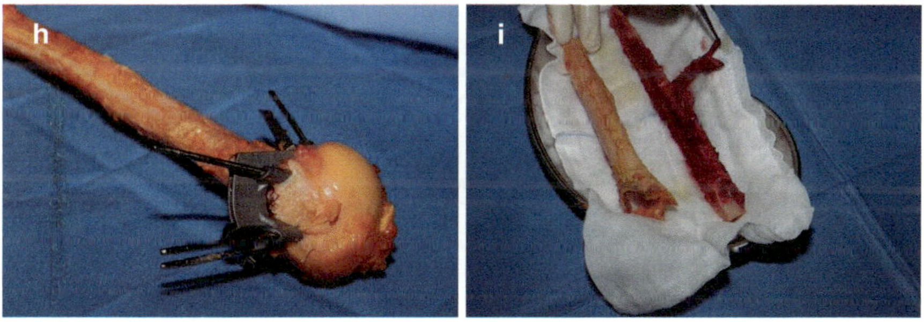

Radiographs at 1-year follow-up showed nonunion of the distal osteotomy (Fig. 7j). Non-union was treated with autograft from the iliac crest, resulting in subsequent complete healing. At the last follow-up, the patient had no functional limitations and an MSTS score of 30/30 (Fig. 7k).

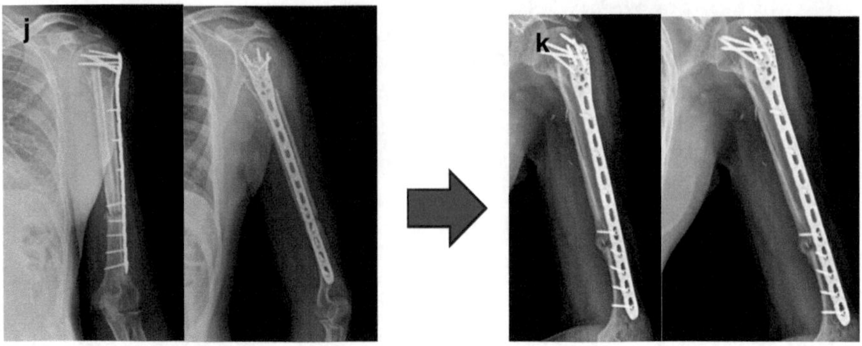

All pictures courtesy and © prof. DA Campanacci

Suggested Reading

1. Biau DJ, Dumaine V, Babinet A, Tomeno B, Anract P. Allograft-prosthesis composites after bone tumor resection at the proximal tibia. Clin Orthop Relat Res. 2007;456:211–7.
2. Campanacci DA, Totti F, Puccini S, Beltrami G, Scoccianti G, Delcroix L, Innocenti M, Capanna R. Intercalary reconstruction of femur after tumour resection: is a vascularized fibular autograft plus allograft a long-lasting solution? Bone Joint J. 2018;100-B(3):378–86. https://doi.org/10.1302/0301-620X.100B3.BJJ-2017-0283.
3. Campanacci DA, Scanferla R, Innocenti M, Muratori F, Puccini S, Scoccianti G, Beltrami G, Capanna R, Innocenti M. Are vascularized fibula autografts a long-lasting reconstruction after intercalary resection of the humerus for primary bone tumors? Clin Orthop Relat Res. 2023:1–13. https://doi.org/10.1097/CORR.0000000000002739.
4. Campanacci DA, Scanferla R, Marsico M, Scolari F, Scoccianti G, Beltrami G, Delcroix L, Innocenti M, Capanna R. Intercalary resection of the tibia for primary bone tumors: are vascularized fibula autografts with or without allografts a durable reconstruction? Clin Orthop Relat Res. 2024;482(6):960–75. https://doi.org/10.1097/CORR.0000000000003007.
5. Clatworthy MG, Gross AE. The allograft prosthetic composite: when and how. Orthopedics. 2001;24:897–8.
6. Donati D, Giacomini S, Gozzi E, Mercuri M. Proximal femur reconstruction by an allograft prosthesis composite. Clin Orthop Relat Res. 2002;394:192–200. https://doi.org/10.1097/00003086-200201000-00023.
7. Donati D, Colangeli M, Colangeli S, Di Bella C, Mercuri M. Allograft-prosthetic composite in the proximal tibia after bone tumor resection. Clin Orthopaed Relat Res. 2008;466(2):459–65. https://doi.org/10.1007/s11999-007-0055-9.
8. Gilbert NF, Yasko AW, Oates SD, Lewis VO, Cannon CP, Lin PP. Allograft-prosthetic composite reconstruction of the proximal part of the tibia. An analysis of the early results. J Bone Joint Surg Am. 2009 Jul;91(7):1646–56. https://doi.org/10.2106/JBJS.G.01542.
9. Gitelis S, Piasecki P. Allograft prosthetic composite arthroplasty for osteosarcoma and other aggressive bone tumors. Clin Orthop Retat Res. 1991;270(197):201.
10. Harris AI, Poddar S, Gitelis S, Sheinkop MB, Rosenberg AG. Arthroplasty with a composite of an allograft and a prosthesis for knees with severe deficiency of bone. J Bone Joint Surg Am. 1995;77:373–86.
11. Helguero CG, Kao I, Komatsu DE, Shaikh S, Hansen D, Franco J, Khan F. Improving the accuracy of wide resection of bone tumors and enhancing implant fit: a cadaveric study. J Orthop.

2015;12(Suppl 2):S188–94. https://doi.org/10.1016/j.jor.2015.10.010. PMID: 27047222; PMCID: PMC4796577.
12. Hirn M. Long intramedullary stems of prosthetic components reduce complications, when allograft-prosthesis composite is used in tumor reconstruction. J Surg Oncol. 2002;79:201–3. https://doi.org/10.1002/jso.10068.
13. Muratori F, Totti F, D'Arienzo A, Scorianz M, Scoccianti G, Beltrami G, Campo FR, Citarelli C, Capanna R, Campanacci DA. Biological intercalary reconstruction with bone grafts after joint-sparing resection of the lower limb: is this an effective and durable solution for joint preservation? Surg Technol Int. 2018;32:346–5. PMID: 29791703.
14. Muscolo DL, Farfalli GL, Aponte-Tinao LA, Ayerza MA. Proximal femur allograft-prosthesis with compression plates and a short stem. Clin Orthop Relat Res. 2010;468(1):224–30. https://doi.org/10.1007/s11999-009-0903-x. Epub 2009 Jun 2.
15. Scanferla R, Scolari F, Muratori F, Tamburini A, Delcroix L, Scoccianti G, Beltrami G, Innocenti M, Campanacci DA. Joint-sparing resection around the knee for osteosarcoma: long-term outcomes of biologic reconstruction with vascularized fibula graft combined with massive allograft. Cancers (Basel). 2024;16(9):1672. https://doi.org/10.3390/cancers16091672.
16. Scorianz M, Guariento L, Campanacci DA. The 3D printing production procedure. In: Zoccali C, Ruggieri P, Benazzo F, editors. 3D printing in bone surgery. Cham: Springer; 2022. https://doi.org/10.1007/978-3-030-91900-9_3.

Cryotherapy in Malignant Bone Tumor 'Tips and Trick Surgical Technique'

Shinji Miwa, Katsuhiro Hayashi, Yuta Taniguchi, and Hiroyuki Tsuchiya

Introduction

Patients with malignant bone tumors require surgical resection, chemotherapy, and radiation therapy. To cure the disease, surgical tumor resection with a sufficient surgical margin is necessary. After the tumor resection, the bone defects require reconstruction using tumor prosthesis or bone graft, including iliac or fibular bone graft, allograft, or devitalized tumor bone graft treated with irradiation, liquid nitrogen, or pasteurization. Although tumor prosthesis is widely used due to the simple procedure and early rehabilitation, the long-term outcomes and functional outcomes are unsatisfactory due to difficulty in reattachment of tendons and muscles to the tumor prosthesis. On the other hand, biological reconstruction can be expected to have long-term durability due to revitalization. Furthermore, good limb function can be achieved through adhesion of muscles and tendons. Among biological reconstructions, tumor-bearing autografts treated with liquid nitrogen have several advantages, including good osteoconduction, osteoinduction, simple procedure, perfect fit, low cost, and preservation of bone morphogenic proteins. In this section, several procedures of tumor-bearing autografts treated with liquid nitrogen are described.

Indication and Contraindication of Reconstruction Using Tumor-Bearing Frozen Autograft

To utilize the tumor-bearing bone for reconstruction of bone defects, the strength of the bone is important. Histologically, osteoblastic osteosarcomas are preferable for frozen autografts, and chondroblastic or fibroblastic osteosarcomas without severe

S. Miwa (✉) · K. Hayashi · Y. Taniguchi · H. Tsuchiya
Department of Orthopedic Surgery, Graduate School of Medical Sciences, Kanazawa University, Kanazawa, Japan

A. Puri, W. F. N. B. W. Ismail (eds.), *Atlas of Orthopedic Oncology Volume 1*,
https://doi.org/10.1007/978-981-95-8958-6_24

destruction of cortical bone are acceptable. In case of a mild osteolytic lesion, the tumor-bearing bone can be used for reconstruction after the treatment with liquid nitrogen if the osteolytic lesion can be augmented with bone cement or bone graft. In contrast, contraindications of tumor-bearing frozen autografts include pathological fractures and severe osteolytic lesions. In cases with pathological fractures and severe osteolytic lesions, other methods such as tumor prosthesis or distraction osteogenesis should be considered.

Freezing Procedure

Freezing Procedure and Perioperative Management

The freezing methods are classified into free freezing, pedicle freezing, and hemicortical freezing (Figs. 1, 2 and 3). The tumor-bearing bone is treated with liquid nitrogen as following steps: freezing of the tumor-bearing bone in liquid nitrogen (−196 °C) for 20 min, thawing at room temperature for 15 min, and thawing in distilled water for 10 min. During the treatment with liquid nitrogen, surgeons need to be careful to prevent fracture, dissemination of the tumor tissue, and surgical site infection. Volume of water in the bone marrow is increased by the freezing, and the increased volume of the water may cause fracture of the graft. Before the treatment with liquid nitrogen, intramedullary canals are curetted to reduce bone marrow containing blood to prevent the fracture during the procedure. To prevent dissemination

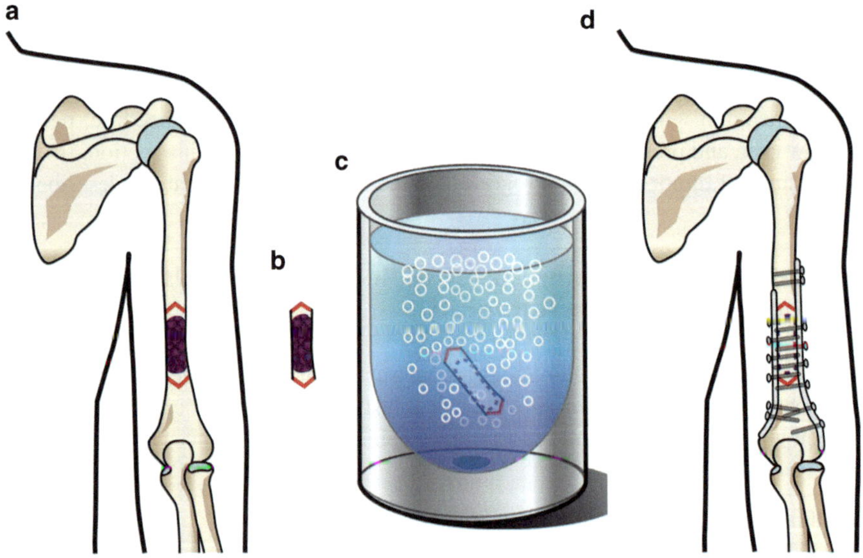

Fig. 1 Free freezing procedure (**a**) Two-site osteotomy (**b**) Tumor resection and curettage (**c**) Freezing in liquid nitrogen (**d**) Reconstruction

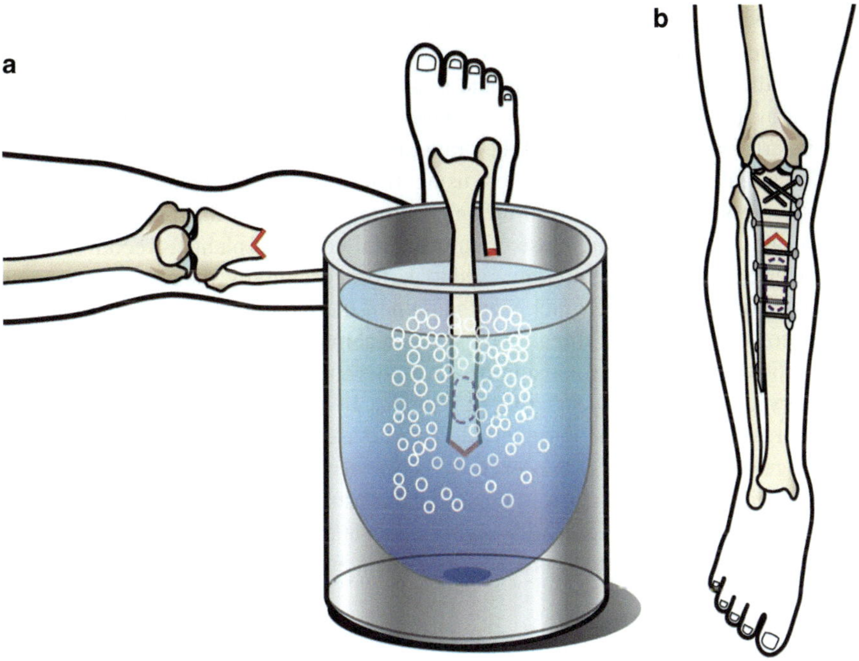

Fig. 2 Pedicle freezing procedure (**a**) Pedicle freezing in liquid nitrogen after one-site osteotomy and curettage of tumor (**b**) Reconstruction

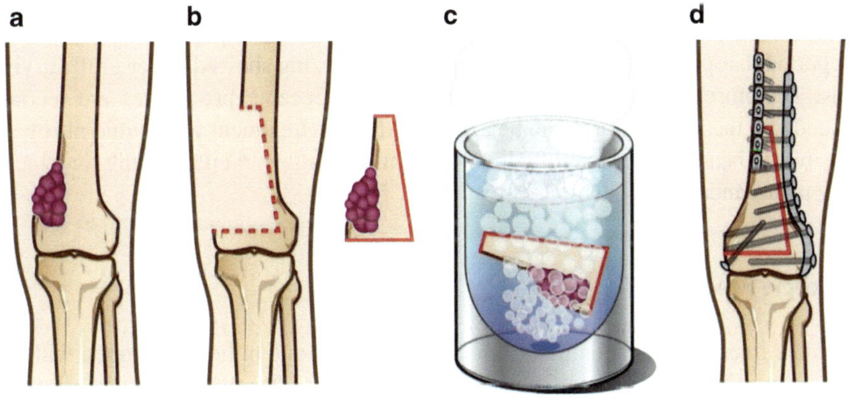

Fig. 3 Hemicortical freezing procedure (**a**) Eccentric tumor location in the long bone (**b**) Hemicortical resection of the tumor (**c**) Freezing in liquid nitrogen (**d**) Reconstruction

of tumor cells during osteotomy and curettage of the tumor lesion, these procedures are performed in a separated or distant area. After the freezing in liquid nitrogen, tumor-bearing frozen autograft is used for reconstruction. The frozen autograft is fixed by long locking plates, intramedullary nails, or long-stemmed prostheses. Soft tissues, including ligament and tendon, are sutured to the original site. After the surgery, curetted tumor tissue and extraskeletal mass are histologically evaluated to confirm the histological diagnosis and to assess therapeutic effect. Surgical drains are removed when the amount of drainage is ≤50 mL, and intravenous antibiotic administration is continued until the drain tube is removed.

Complications of reconstruction using frozen autograft include surgical site infection, non-union or delayed union, fracture, and osteoarthritis. To reduce the risk of surgical site infection, use of antibacterial-coated implants is recommended. Although a bone saw is commonly used to perform osteotomy, the use of a bone saw makes an osteotomy gap, which may cause non-union or delayed union. To reduce the osteotomy gap, use of thread-wire saw is recommended. In patients treated with osteoarticular reconstruction using frozen autograft, destructive change of the joint is observed within a few years after the surgery. In patients who require freezing of larger area than half of the joint part, composite use of prosthesis is recommended.

Range of movement (ROM) exercise is allowed immediately after the surgery. Partial weight-bearing is allowed 2 months after surgery, and full weight bearing is permitted based on the degree of bridging callus at the host-graft junction. The graft survival rates were reported to be 83% at 5 years and 70% at 10 years.

Free Freezing

Free freezing procedure comprises resection of the bone lesion by proximal and distal site osteotomies with an appropriate surgical margin, curettage of the bone, and freezing in liquid nitrogen (Fig. 1). Free freezing procedure is performed in case of bone tumors in the distal femur, distal humerus, and pelvis. We previously reported that pedicle freezing and hemicortical freezing showed better graft survivals. Therefore, pedicle freezing or hemicortical freezing procedures are recommended if these procedures can be applied. After the treatment with liquid nitrogen, the tumor-bearing bone is grafted in the original position and fixed using long locking plates and/or long-stemmed prosthesis.

Pedicle Freezing

Pedicle freezing is a technique to freeze the tumor bone in liquid nitrogen without excision of the tumor bone from the body (Fig. 2). After the separation of tumor bone with surgical margin from the surrounding normal tissues, the tumor-bearing bone is exposed by one-site osteotomy or dislocation of the joint. The surrounding soft tissue and normal bone are protected by surgical sheets to prevent freezing damage to normal tissue. Osteotomy, curettage, and reaming are performed to remove the bone marrow and tumor tissue to prevent fracture of the tumor-bearing bone due to watery volume expansion during the freezing. The tumor lesion with continuity with the affected limb is carefully rotated and frozen in liquid nitrogen container. The tumor-bearing bone is treated with liquid nitrogen for 20 min, thawed at room temperature for 15 min, and thawed in distilled water for 10 min. During the pedicle freezing of the tumor-bearing bone, normal tissue approximately 2 cm from the area treated with liquid nitrogen is frozen. The surgical margin of the tumor-bearing bone is positioned at the surface level of the liquid nitrogen. The pedicle freezing procedure is performed under tourniquet to prevent bleeding and dissemination of the tumor tissue. The frozen autograft is used for reconstruction using long locking plates and/or long-stemmed prosthesis.

Regarding indications, appropriate anatomical sites for the pedicle freezing method include the proximal femur, proximal humerus, proximal tibia, and shaft of the femur, humerus, and shaft of the tibia. In these sites, tumor bone can be rotated and treated with liquid nitrogen with continuity with the limb. In case of a bone tumor in the tibia, osteotomy of the distal fibula is needed to rotate the proximal tibia.

Hemicortical Freezing

Hemicortical freezing is a procedure to freeze hemicortical tumor lesions while preserving contralateral cortical bone in cases with eccentric tumor locations in the bone (Fig. 3). All-round detachment of surrounding soft tissue is needed to protect surrounding normal tissue, including nerves and vessels. After the protection of the surrounding normal tissues, hemicortical resection of the tumor-bearing bone with an appropriate surgical margin is performed. Tumor bone is curetted, and surrounding tissues are resected. The bone is treated with liquid nitrogen for 20 min, thawed at room temperature for 15 min, and thawed in the distilled water for 10 min. Then, the frozen autograft is positioned at the original site and fixed by long locking plates.

Indication of the procedure is localized lesion that occurs unilaterally and does not extend to the other side of the bone.

Freezing Procedure in Each Location

Proximal Humerus

In the case of bone tumors in the proximal humerus, pedicle freezing procedure can be applied (Fig. 4). Tumor resection is performed with appropriate surgical margin, including the biopsy tract. In cases where the tumor does not extend to the humeral head, an osteotomy is performed 2 cm from the proximal site of the tumor margin. V-shaped osteotomy using a thread-saw is recommended to reduce osteotomy gap and to increase the contact area and stability. In bone tumors that are close to the humeral head, proximal humerus with surgical margin and biopsy tract is exposed by cutting soft tissues around the proximal humerus. The extraskeletal masses and soft tissues are removed, leaving muscle insertions, ligaments, and joint capsules for reattachment. To prevent fracture of the graft due to increased water volume during freezing, intramedullary canal is curetted to remove the tumor tissue and bone marrow. After the freezing in liquid nitrogen, the frozen bone is grafted to the

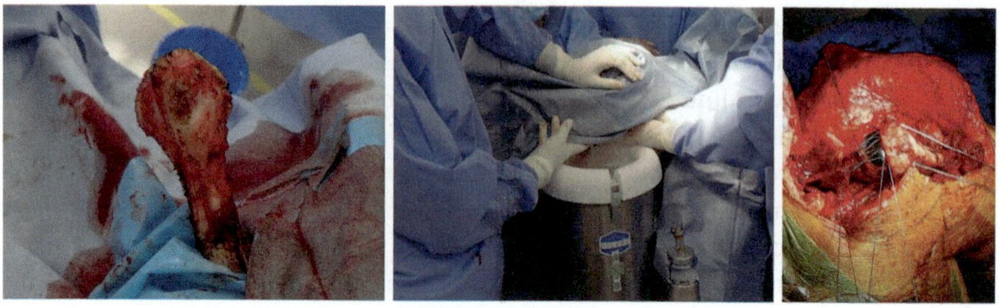

Fig. 4 Pedicle freezing procedure in the proximal humerus

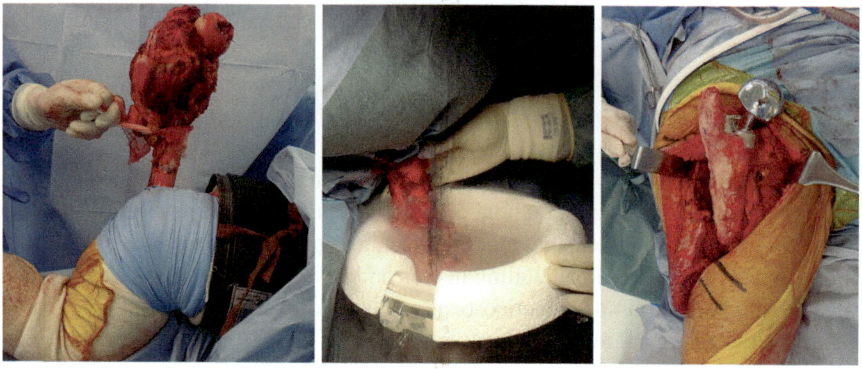

Fig. 5 Pedicle freezing procedure in the proximal femur

original site. Iliac bone graft or bone cement is used for mechanical support, if necessary. If possible, the tendons or ligaments are sutured to the original corresponding structures. During the pedicle freezing procedure, soft tissue is divided along the humerus beyond the surgical margin to rotate adequately. Surgical sheets are used to protect the surrounding normal tissue. Tumor-bearing bone connected to the humerus is carefully rotated and treated with liquid nitrogen while the surrounding normal tissue is protected with surgical sheets. The level 2 cm away from the tumor margin is positioned at the surface level of the liquid nitrogen. The frozen autograft is positioned at the original site and fixed by long locking plates and/or long-stemmed prosthesis.

Proximal Femur

In cases with bone tumors in the proximal femur, the pedicle freezing procedure can be applied (Fig. 5). The tumor-bearing bone with biopsy tract and extraskeletal mass is widely excised with an adequate surgical margin. The gluteus medius is peeled from the greater trochanter, and muscles and tendons are detached from the proximal femur to safely rotate the proximal femur and immerse it in liquid nitrogen. After separation of the freezing area by surgical sheets, intertrochanteric osteotomy is performed, and the greater trochanter is preserved. Tumor tissue and bone marrow are removed from intramedullary cavity to prevent frozen autograft fracture. To prevent dissemination of the tumor tissue, the surrounding normal tissues are protected by surgical sheets before curettage and drilling of the tumor-bearing bone. During the treatment with liquid nitrogen, 2 cm away from the margin of the tumor is positioned at the surface of the liquid nitrogen. To prevent bleeding and dissemination of the tumor tissue, a tourniquet is used during the pedicle freezing procedure. Long-stemmed prosthesis with bone cement is used for reconstruction. The gluteus medius is sutured to the greater trochanter of the femur. Postoperatively, joint motion range training is performed immediately from day 1. Full weight-bearing is performed at 6 weeks after the reconstruction.

Distal Femur

Free freezing is commonly used for bone tumors in the distal femur (Figs. 6 and 7). In case with eccentric tumor location in the bone, hemicortical freezing procedure can be a treatment option. Bone lesion is detached from the surrounding soft tissues with appropriate surgical margin. After retraction of major nerves and vessels, K-wire is inserted into the osteotomy line under fluoroscopy. Then, en-bloc tumor excision is performed with a microsurgical saw or thread wire saw. The surrounding soft tissue is removed, and tumor lesion is curetted. The tumor bone is treated with liquid nitrogen for 20 min, thawed at room temperature for 15 min, and thawed in distilled water for 15 min. The frozen bone is replaced and fixed with long locking plates and/or long-stemmed prostheses. If there remains large bone defect, iliac bone, allograft, or artificial bone graft is used.

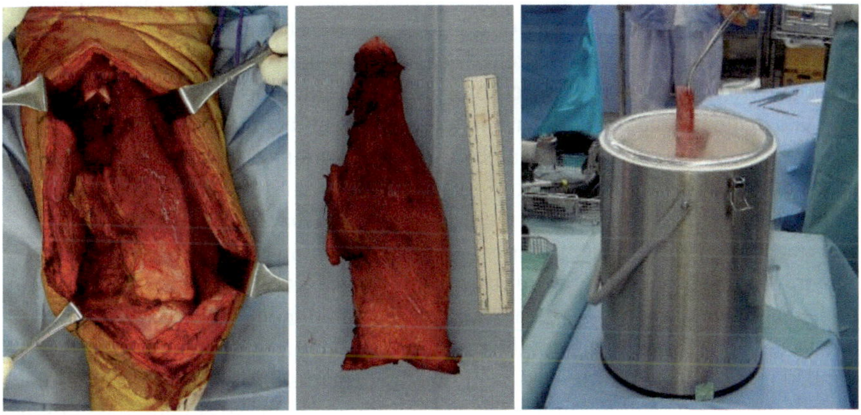

Fig. 6 Free freezing procedure in the distal femur

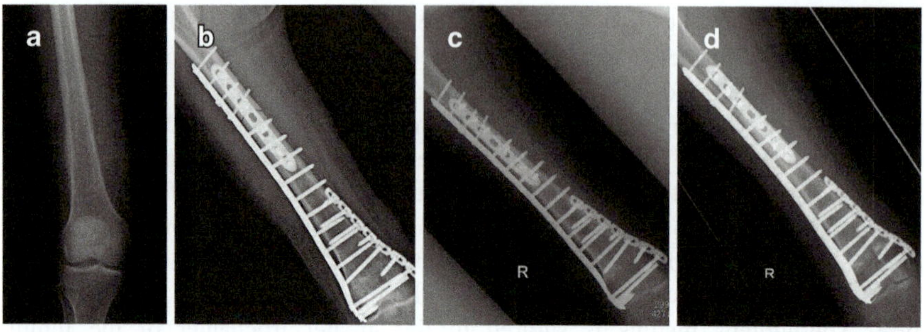

Fig. 7 Follow-up X-ray (**a**) Pre-operative X-ray (**b**) Post-operative X-ray (**c**) X-ray (1 year after operation) (**d**) X-ray (6 years after operation)

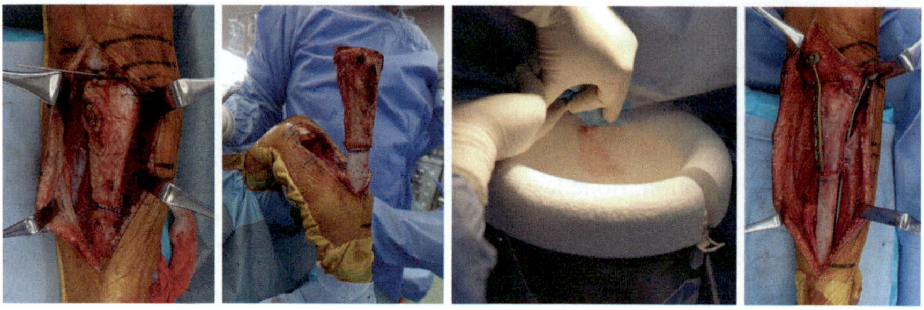

Fig. 8 Pedicle freezing procedure in the proximal tibia

Proximal Tibia

In case of bone tumors in the proximal tibia, pedicle freezing can be applied (Fig. 8). Bone tumor lesion with an appropriate surgical margin is separated from the surrounding soft tissue. After retraction of major nerves and vessels, K-wire is inserted into the osteotomy line under fluoroscopy. Then, en-bloc tumor excision is performed using microsurgical saw or thread wire saw. The surrounding soft tissue is removed, and tumor lesion is curetted. In case of lesions that are close to the cartilage, the proximal tibia is exposed by cutting anterior cruciate ligament, posterior cruciate ligament, medial collateral ligament, and lateral collateral ligament. If sufficient surgical margin can be obtained without resection of the cartilage, osteotomy at the proximal site of the bone lesion is performed. After separation and retraction of the surrounding normal tissue with a safe surgical margin, the K-wire is inserted into the cutting line under fluoroscopy, and osteotomy is performed along the K-wire. The normal bone and soft tissue are isolated using cotton for cast padding, an Esmarch bandage, and surgical sheets to prevent tumor contamination and damage to the normal tissue during the treatment with liquid nitrogen. A tourniquet is applied to the affected limb to prevent bleeding and distant dissemination of tumor cells. After curettage of the tumor lesion and removal of the surrounding soft tissue, the tumor-bearing bone is cautiously rotated down into the liquid nitrogen. The bone tumor with surgical margin is frozen in liquid nitrogen for 20 min, thawed at room temperature for 15 min, and thawed in distilled water for 15 min. The frozen autograft is reimplanted to the original site. Locking plates and/or long-stemmed prostheses are used for the reconstruction and fixation. Patellar tendon is sutured to the tibial tuberosity. In case of difficulty in primary wound closure, rotation flap and/or skin graft are performed.

Conclusions

Reconstruction using tumor-bearing autograft treated with liquid nitrogen can be applied for various types, locations, and conditions of bone tumors. Each method of freezing and reconstruction has several advantages and disadvantages. Surgeons are needed to understand characteristics of the freezing procedures and reconstruction methods and should determine appropriate surgical procedures in each case.

Suggested Reading

1. Chen WM, Wu PK, Chen CF, Chung LH, Liu CL, Chen TH. High-grade osteosarcoma treated with hemicortical resection and biological reconstruction. J Surg Oncol. 2012;105(8):825–9.
2. Fiore M, Sambri A, Zucchini R, Giannini C, Donati DM, De Paolis M. Silver-coated megaprosthesis in prevention and treatment of peri-prosthetic infections: a systematic review and meta-analysis about efficacy and toxicity in primary and revision surgery. Eur J Orthop Surg Traumatol. 2021;31(2):201–20.
3. Hayashi K, Yamamoto N, Takeuchi A, et al. Clinical course of grafted cartilage in osteoarticular frozen autografts for reconstruction after resection of malignant bone and soft-tissue tumor involving an epiphysis. J Bone Oncol. 2020;24:100310.
4. Higuchi T, Yamamoto N, Nishida H, et al. Knee joint preservation surgery in osteosarcoma using tumour-bearing bone treated with liquid nitrogen. Int Orthop. 2017;41(10):2189–97.
5. Kimura H, Yamamoto N, Shirai T, et al. Clinical outcome of reconstruction using frozen autograft for a humeral bone tumor. Anticancer Res. 2016;36(12):6631–5.
6. Miwa S, Yamamoto N, Hayashi K, et al. Graft survivals after reconstruction using tumor-bearing frozen bone in the extremities. Cancers (Basel). 2023;15(15)
7. Shirai T, Tsuchiya H, Terauchi R, et al. The outcomes of reconstruction using frozen autograft combined with iodine-coated implants for malignant bone tumors: compared with non-coated implants. Jpn J Clin Oncol. 2016;46(8):735–40.
8. Tomita K, Kawahara N. The threadwire saw: a new device for cutting bone. J Bone Joint Surg Am. 1996;78(12):1915–7.
9. Tsuchiya H, Wan SL, Sakayama K, Yamamoto N, Nishida H, Tomita K. Reconstruction using an autograft containing tumour treated by liquid nitrogen. J Bone Joint Surg Br. 2005;87(2):218–25.
10. Tsuchiya H, Abdel-Wanis ME, Tomita K. Biological reconstruction after excision of juxta-articular osteosarcoma around the knee: a new classification system. Anticancer Res. 2006;26(1B):447–53.
11. Tsuchiya H, Nishida H, Srisawat P, et al. Pedicle frozen autograft reconstruction in malignant bone tumors. J Orthop Sci. 2010;15(3):340–9.
12. Xu G, Miwa S, Yamamoto N, et al. Pedicle frozen autograft-prosthesis composite reconstructions for malignant bone tumors of the proximal femur. BMC Musculoskelet Disord. 2020;21(1):81.

GPSR Compliance

The European Union's (EU) General Product Safety Regulation (GPSR) is a set of rules that requires consumer products to be safe and our obligations to ensure this.

If you have any concerns about our products, you can contact us on ProductSafety@springernature.com

In case Publisher is established outside the EU, the EU authorized representative is:

Springer Nature Customer Service Center GmbH
Europaplatz 3
69115 Heidelberg, Germany

Batch number: 10732076

Printed by Printforce, the Netherlands